Reproductive Health and Fertility

Reproductive Health and Fertility

Editor: Ross Bell

FOSTER ACADEMICS

www.fosteracademics.com

www.fosteracademics.com

FOSTER ACADEMICS

Cataloging-in-Publication Data

Reproductive health and fertility / edited by Ross Bell.
p. cm.
Includes bibliographical references and index.
ISBN 978-1-63242-805-9
1. Reproductive health. 2. Sexual health. 3. Fertility, Human. 4. Human reproduction.
5. Human biology. 6. Reproduction. I. Bell, Ross.
RG133 .R47 2019
618.178--dc23

Foster Academics,
118-35 Queens Blvd., Suite 400,
Forest Hills, NY 11375, USA

ISBN 978-1-63242-805-9 (Hardback)

Printed and bound in China.

Contents

Preface

Reproductive health refers to the physical and psychological well-being of a person with respect to their sexuality. It is also concerned with the reproductive processes and functions at all stages of life. It facilitates a safer sexual life, which is both, satisfying as well as responsible. One's natural capability to reproduce offspring is known as fertility. Nutrition, instinct, timing, emotions, culture, consanguinity, endocrinology and sexual behavior are some of the common factors, which affect human fertility. Fertility declines with age in both males and females. The various advancements in reproductive health and fertility are glanced at and their applications as well as ramifications are looked at in detail. It brings forth some of the most innovative concepts and elucidates the unexplored aspects of reproductive health and fertility. The extensive content of this book provides the readers with a thorough understanding of the subject.

This book is a result of research of several months to collate the most relevant data in the field.

When I was approached with the idea of this book and the proposal to edit it, I was overwhelmed. It gave me an opportunity to reach out to all those who share a common interest with me in this field. I had 3 main parameters for editing this text:

1. Accuracy - The data and information provided in this book should be up-to-date and valuable to the readers.

2. Structure - The data must be presented in a structured format for easy understanding and better grasping of the readers

3. Universal Approach - This book not only targets students but also experts and innovators in the field, thus my aim was to present topics which are of use to all

Thus, it took me a couple of months to finish the editing of this book.

I would like to make a special mention of my publisher who considered me worthy of this opportunity and also supported me throughout the editing process. I would also like to thank the editing team at the back-end who extended their help whenever required.

Editor

Knowledge and practice of exclusive breastfeeding among mothers in the tamale metropolis of Ghana

Ruth Nimota Nukpezah[1*], Samuel Victor Nuvor[2] and Jerry Ninnoni[3]

Abstract

Background: The prevalence of exclusive breastfeeding (EBF) for the first six months of life has remained low worldwide and in Ghana, despite strong evidence in support of its practice. This study was aimed at assessing the knowledge and practice of exclusive breastfeeding among mothers in the Tamale metropolis of Ghana.

Methods: In a descriptive cross-sectional study, 393 mother-infant pairs attending child welfare clinics from three health facilities in the Tamale Metropolis were surveyed. A structured item questionnaire was used to collect data on the socio-demographic Characteristics of the participants, their knowledge regarding breastfeeding and level of practice of exclusive breastfeeding (EBF). The results were presented in frequency counts, percentages and inferences were made using a contingency table and chi-square values were computed to check for the relationship between participants demographic characteristics, the Knowledge and the practice of EBF and *P* value was set at 0.05.

Results: The Analysis of the data was done with SPSS version 20. The study surveyed a total of 393 mothers from Tamale metropolis, of whom 27.7% reported having exclusively breastfed their infant for the first 6 months of life. The socio-demographic of the participants showed that they all had some level of education. The study revealed that 39.4% initiated breastfeeding within one hour after birth. Majority of participants had heard of EBF 277 (70.5%), about 344 (87.5%) of participants believed that EBF should be practised for 5 months in their locality. Pearson Chi-square test of the association between sociodemographic characteristics associated and EBF showed a significant association between EBF and the sex of the child, $X^2 = 4.177$, $P = .041$. Whiles, EBF and the Knowledge on child spacing was $X^2 = 17.769$, $P < .001$ and EBF and knowledge on Breast cancer reduction was also significant $X^2 = 4.384$, $P = .036$.

Conclusions: Although all the participants had some level of education background, a majority did not have adequate knowledge on EBF and EBF practice was low in the study community. Thus, we suggest improved education at the child welfare clinics and the media should be used as a platform to educate women adequately about importance of EBF.

Keywords: Exclusive breastfeeding, Knowledge, Practice, Tamale, Ghana

Plain English

The factors contributing to the reduced rate of EBF practice in developing countries such as those in Africa has been shown to include: lack of knowledge about benefits of breastfeeding, lack of maternal decision-making power, work schedules, recommencing work after maternity leave, lack of support, traditional beliefs and practices. To address the issue, this study explored the knowledge and practice of Exclusive breastfeeding among mothers attending post-natal clinics in the Tamale metropolis. In a descriptive cross-sectional study, 393 mother-infant pairs attending child welfare clinics from three health facilities in the Tamale Metropolis were surveyed.

A structured item questionnaire was used to collect data on the socio-demographic characteristics of the participants, knowledge of mother regarding breastfeeding and level of practice of exclusive breastfeeding. Data analysis was carried out with the aid of IBM Statistical Package for the Social Sciences (SPSS) version 20 for

* Correspondence: nimotaruth@gmail.com
[1]Department of Nursing, University for development studies, Tamale, Ghana
Full list of author information is available at the end of the article

Windows and reported using, tables and prose. The study revealed that though the participants all had some level of education, a majority believed that EBF for a child should be less than 6 months after birth, hence, majority of the participants had inadequate knowledge on EBF. To add to this, the rate of EBF practice was found to be low in the study area.

Background

Breast milk has the essential nutrients that a newborn need to grow healthy and strong. Infants who are exclusively breastfed develop fewer infections; have less severe illnesses and mothers who practice EBF enjoy the benefit of extended lactation amenorrhea [1]. Adequate knowledge about exclusive breastfeeding is said to be the fundamental tool that can direct the course of EBF practice among mothers [2, 3]. Yet [4], indicated that most mothers have knowledge of EBF 97.6%, but only 64.6% have adequate knowledge and mother's higher knowledge about breastfeeding correlated with longer duration of practice. Meanwhile [5], in a study on knowledge of the importance of EBF for the first 6 months, also showed that the knowledge level of participants was (35.7%), this figure was seen to be relatively high. Yet, only about half of the participants (17.9%) practised EBF.

The risk of conditions such as, breast and ovarian cancer is lessened among mothers who adequately practice EBF [1]. World health organization indicated that EBF protective effect is not limited to the lactation period; it persists for years even after termination of breastfeeding. The benefits of EBF are bigger in settings of poverty, poor nutrition and poor hygiene, where baseline disease rates are higher. This is because giving babies other feds before six months is often associated with errors of contamination during the preparation and administration process. These errors can further lead to diarrheal diseases like cholera and dysentery which can culminate in childhood mortality [1, 5].

According to [6], with EBF coverage of 90%, about 13% of deaths of children less than 5 years could be averted in low and middle-income countries. This assertion is in line with other researchers who opined that initiation of breastfeeding within the first hour of birth may lead to the prevention of about 20% of neonatal deaths [7, 8] In low-income/middle-income countries. And optimal breastfeeding has the potential of preventing 12% of all under-5 deaths [9]. Children who are exclusively breast fed have been shown to be less susceptible to childhood diseases and are 14 times more likely to endure ill-health compared with those who are not breastfed [10].

Childhood mortality is high in low and middle-income countries where EBF prevalence is low. In Ghana for instance, the recorded rate of infant mortality is 53 per 1, 000 live births while mortality rate of children younger than 5 years is 31 per 1000 live births and these death ratios is partly due to inadequate EBF practice of mothers [11].

Other studies undertaken in Ghana also concluded that neonatal deaths could be prevented if all infants start breastfeeding within the first hour of birth [12].

Some of the interventions and policies introduced in Ghana to help encourage EBF practice are infant and young child feeding (IYCF) program, convention on the rights of the child and baby friendly Hospital initiative [6]. Despite the enactment of these policies, the rate of EBF in Ghana is still lower than the WHO's set goal of 90% for EBF. A report from Ghana multiple indicator cluster surveys showed that EBF in Ghana dropped drastically from 63.7% in 2008 to 46% in 2011 [12]. More specifically, the rate of EBF in Tamale was 63.3%. In effect, the rate of EBF is low globally (39%), with 36% occurring in low-income countries [1]. Several factors have been identified as impediments to proper nutrition and infant feeding habits. Substantial among them are, the perceptions surrounding infants feeding practices and inadequate information and support on good feeding practises, especially EBF for the first six months of life [13]. However, from the literature reviewed at the start of this study, there was no documented literature on the related factors associated with the knowledge and practice of EBF in the Tamale metropolis and no study had coved a vast majority of EBF among lactating mothers in the major Hospitals of the Region. This paper discusses the knowledge and practice of EBF among mothers visiting the child welfare clinics at Tamale West Hospital, Tamale Central Hospital and the Tamale Teaching Hospital in Ghana.

Research methods

Study setting

Tamale is the capital of Northern Region of Ghana and the metropolitan assembly is one of the 20 administrative districts in the Region. The Metropolitan is divided into three Sub-Metros; Tamale North Sub-Metropolitan, Tamale Central Sub-Metropolitan and Tamale South Sub-Metropolitan. Tamale Teaching Hospital (TTH), Tamale West Hospital (TWH) and Tamale Central Hospital (TCH) are the three main public facilities in the Region. Tamale Teaching Hospital is a tertiary referral Centre for the three northern regions. Tamale West Hospital and TCH are secondary level service point. These health facilities provide maternal and neonatal Care services that enriched the study objectives.

Population

The study populations were resident, lactating mothers of the Tamale Metropolitan area with a child of at least six months and at most two years at the time of the research. The participants attended child welfare clinic (CWC) in Tamale Teaching Hospital, Tamale West Hospital or Tamale Central Hospital. Using mothers who attend CWC at these facilities was useful to the study because these facilities are the main public facility in the region and has lots of client's patronage at the CWC. The annual estimate of the population of women who attends CWC at the selected Hospitals in 2015 was: TTH = 5986, TWH = 2999 and TCH = 2995. Total = 17,960.

Inclusion criteria

Lactating mothers who had children from ages 6 months - 2 years attending the Child Welfare Clinic (CWC) at Tamale Teaching Hospital, Tamale West Hospital and Tamale Central Hospital.

Exclusion criteria

The study excluded lactating mothers having children with Medical Conditions that prevented the practice of EBF such galactosemia and mothers who were unwilling and mothers with children less than 6 months.

Sampling procedure

Sample size determination

The desired sample was obtained using the Cochran's formula for calculating sample size $n = z^2pq/d^2$ [14].

Where: n = desired minimal sample population.

z = standard normal deviate which is 1.96 at 95% confidence level.

$p = 63.3\%$ (2011 estimated figure of exclusive breastfeeding rate in Tamale [12]).

d = degree of accuracy 5%.

q = 1-p.

Hence substituting the value into the formula: $n = z^2pq/d^2$.

$$n = \frac{(1.96)^2(0.633 \times 0.367)}{(0.05)^2}$$

$$n = 356.97 \approx 357$$

To address the possibility of non-response/incomplete questionnaires and attrition, 20% was added to the calculated sample size.

Hence, a total sample size of 428 working mothers with infant pairs was estimated for the study.

Sampling methods

Three types of sampling methods were used at different stages of the study. First and foremost, three Hospitals in Tamale Metropolis were purposively sampled. The Hospitals were: Tamale Teaching Hospital (TTH), Tamale West Hospital (TWH) and Tamale Central Hospital (TCH). These Hospitals were selected as these facilities are the major Hospital in the metropolis, the Hospitals serves as referral centers for clients from the surrounding district and the Hospitals had a child welfare clinic. Secondly, a quota sampling was used to calculate the sample size for each Facility [14]. Described quota sampling as a type of non-probability sampling where participants were selected non-randomly, based on their known proportion to the population.

The sample size for each facility was estimated proportional to their population size. We recruited an equal proportion of working mothers with infant's pair from Tamale West Hospital and Tamale Central Hospital, but the proportion was doubled in Tamale Teaching Hospital because of the population size was twice of the Tamale West Hospital and Tamale Central Hospital respectively. Thus, TTH = 5986, TWH = 2999, TCH = 2995, summing up to 17,960 population size. Using, *Sample fraction* $(f) = \frac{sample\ size\ (n)}{targeted\ population\ (N)}$ [14].

This extrapolates to sample size of Tamale Teaching Hospital 214, the sample size of Tamale West Hospital 107, and 107 for Tamale Central Hospital. This gives a total of 428 sample size.

Thirdly, at the facility level, simple random Probability sampling method was used to select the participants. [14] indicated that probability sampling allowed researchers to make a generalization to the population defined by the sampling frame, whereas nonprobability sampling does not make room for generalization to be made beyond the sample. This assertion informed the researcher's decision to use a simple random sampling technique to enlist the participants.

The participants were recruited by the researcher within eight (8) consecutive weeks in each of the health facilities. Simple random sampling (balloting) technique was utilized. On each clinic day, a list of mothers-infants pair who were registered for weighting and immunization was used as a sampling frame, they were assigned identification (ID) numbers. The numbers were listed in separate pieces of papers and placed into a bag. The papers were shuffled after which ballots were drawn from the bag without replacement. This exercise was repeated on each clinic day until the required sample of 428 (100%) participants was attained.

Pretesting

The pilot study was conducted among 10 mother-infants pair of similar age (6 to 24 months) in Savelugu Hospital which is a neighbouring community. Based on the responses that were received, appropriate modifications were made to the questionnaires to ensure accuracy, clarity and reproducibility. In addition, Correlation coefficient to check for the instrument's internal consistencies was also determined using SPSS Cronbach correlation formula· The tools were accepted with the coefficient of 0.877.

Data collection procedure

The research instrument used was a self-administered questionnaire. According to [14], questionnaire enhances greater privacy and reduces the incidence of bias responses which is often associated with other data of collection instrument such as interviews. The questionnaire consisted of two sections derived from the aim of the study: Knowledge and the practice of Exclusive breastfeeding.

Data were collected at the child welfare clinic of the selected hospitals and the mothers were given an average time of 15-min each to answer the questionnaires. About 428 questionnaires were given out. Only the 393 questionnaires which were completely answered were used for the final analysis. The data collection instrument (questionnaire) was in the English language. For participants who could not read well/understand some of the questions, the question items were read to them and appropriate options chosen by the clients was marked. The questionnaire comprised Yes/No questions on the level of practice of EBF and some categorical itemized questions about the participant's knowledge of EBF. The total number of questions were 25.

Data processing and analysis

Data analysis was carried out in June with the aid of IBM Statistical Package for the Social Sciences (SPSS) version 20 for Windows and reported using, tables and prose. The process for the data analysis included; data coding, sorting, cleaning, editing and checking for errors and biases by doing a thorough counting of the study question items and frequency of occurrences, the grouping of collected data, checking for minimum and maximum counts and analysing and discussing of data. The questionnaire was given to my supervisors to review and the analysis that was done after the study was also given to them to cross-check for approval. A descriptive table was drawn to show the socio-demographic, practice of EBF and Knowledge of participants about EBF. Further inferences were made using a contingency table and chi-square values was computed to check for the relationship between participants demographic characteristics, the Knowledge and the practice of EBF and P value was set at 0.05.

Results and discussion

The data were analysed using frequencies, percentages and prose. The analysis also included cross-tabulation and Pearson chi square test. Some responses were scored dichotomously as Yes = 1 and No = 0 and some questions were multi choice responses. Eight (8) knowledge questions and 8 demographic characteristics questions were presented respectively, whiles the practice Item questions were Nine (9). In carrying out this study, the researcher used a sample of 428 respondents and a total of 428 questionnaires was distributed to the lactating mothers. However, 393 questionnaires were returned fully answered with other questionnaires having 35 missing data. Therefore, the sample size for answering the research questions was 393 indicating 91.8% of total response rate.

Results

Results on socio-demographic characteristics of participants

The distribution of demographic data of respondents involved in the study. From Table 1, the majority, 204 (51.9%) of the respondents were JHS level and lower, SHS were 100 (25.4%), and lastly, those who had attained tertiary levels were 89 (22.6%). The study, therefore, revealed that majority of the respondents involved in the study were having some form of education. Other sociodemographic characteristics of respondents are summarized in Table 1.

Results on practice of EBF among participants

From Table 2, only 109 (27.7%) practiced EBF and 157 (39.9%) still breastfeed baby. In addition, 52 (13.2%) expressed breast milk when away from baby. In conclusion more than half of the participants claimed that their index child has being having episodes of childhood common ailment 260 (66.2%).

Table 3 also showed that the majority, 155 (39.4%) of the respondents-initiated breast feeding within one hour after birth. Again, 195 (49.6%) of the respondents indicated they gave prelateral feeds to their infants during the first six months, 124 (31.6%) indicated not applicable and 74 (18.8%) indicated they give mashed family foods to their infants during the first six months.

The participants gave a lot of reasons for introducing early feeds to their baby as summaries in the table. Regarding the age at which mothers started giving food to their babies, it was realized that majority had introduced feeds to their baby as early as first (1) and second (2) months respectively. At five months, 31 (7.8%) started taking feeds and at six month, 17 (4.3%) babies also started eating.

Results on the knowledge of EBF among participants

The result on knowledge as seen in Table 4, majority 277 (70.5%) of the participants had heard about EBF, surprisingly most people choose the electronic media 209 (53.2%) as compared to health professionals 135 (34.4%) as their major source of information. Concerning initiation, the majority concorded that EBP should be started immediately after birth 290 (73.8%). It was

Table 1 Socio-demographic data of the respondents

Variables	Frequency	Percent (%)
Education of mother		
JHS and lower	204	51.9
SSS	100	25.4
Tertiary	89	22.6
Total	393	100.0
Form of employment		
Unemployed	137	34.9
Worker	256	65.1
Total	393	100.0
Monthly Income (Ghana cedi)		
Low: ≤ 1000	135	34.4
Middle: 1000–2000	209	53.1
High: ≥ 2000	49	12.5
Total	393	100.0
Age of mother		
≤ 25 years	239	60.8
≥ 25 years	154	39.2
Total	393	100.0
Total number of children		
1	142	36.1
≥ 1	251	63.9
Total	393	100.0
Place of birth		
Non-Health Facility	143	36.4
Health facility	250	63.6
Total	393	100.0
Sex of child		
Female	277	57.8
Male	166	42.2
Total	393	100.0
Age of child		
6–24 Months	209	53.2
6 months	184	46.8
Total	393	100.0

Source: Field data, (2016)

also noted that majority believed that EBF should be practice for less than 5 months for a child. The table further summarised the rest of the discriptive findings on the knowledge of the participants on EBF.

Results on the factors associated with EBF

Tables 5 and 6 shows the summary of cross tabulation between EBF, demographic characteristics and some knowledge Characteristic respectively.

Table 2 Mode and period of breastfeeding infants by the lactating mothers

Statement	Yes		No	
	Freq	(%)	Freq	(%)
I gave breast milk only for six months	109	27.7	284	72.3
I still breastfeed baby	157	39.9	236	60e1
I expressed breast milk down for baby when away from baby	52	13.2	341	86.8
Episodes of childhood common ailment	260	66.2	133	33.8

Source: Field data, (2016)

Discussions of research findings

This research study surveyed a total of 393 mothers from Tamale metropolis, of whom 27.7% reported having exclusively breastfed their infant for the first 6 months of life. The socio-demographic of the participants showed that they all had some level of education. Secondly, most of the lactating women were workers and were middle-income earner who earned between 1000 and 2000 per month. A great majority were matured, they were above 25 years. Literature has shown that there is substantial evidence that breastfeeding women encounter demographic challenges that may affect the initiation and duration of BF. Women who graduated from high school were 70% more likely to breastfeed than those who did not; women who attended college were four times more likely to breastfeed than women who graduated from high school [13]. In a national study in rural Ghana, education, occupation, economic factors and marital status were the factors affecting EB [15]. In contrast, to this finding, an inverse relationship was observed in developing countries. This was possibly due to a perception that 'breastfeeding was old fashioned' or an indication of 'lesser social status'. There is an association between higher education and socioeconomic status, this increases the mother's ability to purchase infant formula. In addition to educational attainment, maternal age has been identified as among the factors most strongly influencing the initiation, duration and level of infant feeding [16].

It was observed in this study that mothers who were practising EBF were 27.7% which was far below the WHO recommendation of 90% [1]. Also, in a recent study at Tuna, a rural co-district capital of the Sawla-Tuna-Kabla district in the Northern Region of Ghana, a slightly lower rate of 42.0% EBF was realized [17]. These demonstrate a wide gap between the desired and the actual practice of EBF in the study area. The low practices of EBF in this area could be due to low knowledge of EBF, since the study revealed that most mothers did not get information regarding EBF from their health providers. Hence, majority of the mothers were not having knowledge on the need to initiate breastfeeding

Table 3 Time of Initiation of breastfeeding and food supplement by the lactating mothers

Response	How soon after delivery did you start breast feeding the baby?	
	Frequency (393)	Percent (%)
Initiation of BF within one hour after birth	155	39.4
Initiation of BF after first one hour after birth	238	60.6
Total	393	100.0
Response	Types of food/drink giving to infants during first six months	
Prelacteal feeds	195	49.6
Mashed family foods	74	18.8
Not applicable	124	31.6
Total	393	100.0
Response	Reasons for giving foods and drinks	
Hot weather makes babies cry; hence they need water	143	36.4
Breast milk production problem	37	9.4
Not able to combine work with breastfeeding	176	44.8
Not applicable	37	9.4
Total	393	100.0
Response	At what age did you start giving other food	
Six months and above	17	4.3
Five months	31	7.8
Four months	33	8.4
Three months	36	9.2
Two months	117	29.8
One month and less	159	40.5
Total	393	100.0

Source: Field data, (2016)

Table 4 Knowledge of participants about exclusive breasting practice

Variables		Frequency (393)	Percentages (100%)
Have you Heard of EBF	NO	116	29.5
	YES	277	70.5
Majour Source of Knowledge	Health professionals	135	34.4
	Electronic media	209	53.2
	Others	49	12.5
Knowledge on Time to initiate Breastfeeding	Anytime the mother is ready	103	26.2
	Immediately after birth	290	73.8
Duration of EBF	6 months–24 months	49	12.5
	≤5 months	344	87.5
Does EBF improve a child's immunity?	No	63	16.0
	Yes	330	84.0
Does EBF allows Child spacing?	No	349	88.8
	Yes	44	11.2
Does EBF reduce risk of breast and varian cancer	No	358	91.1
	Yes	35	8.9
Knowledge on how to express breastmilk down for baby	No	350	89.1
	Yes	43	10.9

Source: Field data, (2016)

Table 5 Cross tabulation of EBF and some Sociodemographic predictors of exclusive breastfeeding

Variables		Exclusive breast feeding		Total	Pearson Chi-square value	*P*-values
		No	Yes			
Education of mother	JHS and lower	151	53	204	3.708	.157
	SSS	65	35	100		
	Tertiary	68	21	89		
Total		284	109	393		
Employment Status	Unemployed	96	41	137	.504	.478
	Worker	188	68	256		
Total		284	109	393		
Sex of child	Female	173	54	227	4.177	.041
	Males	111	55	166		
Total		284	109	393		
Age of mother	25 years and below	180	59	239	2.828	.093
	25 years and more	104	50	154		
Total		284	109	393		
Income-Status	Ghc1000 and less (low income)	99	36	135	.554	.758
	Ghc1000–2000 (middle income)	148	61	209		
	Ghc2000 and more (high Income)	37	12	49		
Total		284	109	393		

Source: Field data, (2016)

within early. Majority of the lactating mother had some form of academic education, but this did not translate to their practice of EBF. As seen in the demographic characteristics. The low EBF could be due to lack of time to breastfeed the babies, or the social acceptance and recognition's given to breast baby feeds or the inadequate knowledge on EBF. Furthermore, the study was carried out on mothers at the antenatal clinics of the hospitals in the Tamale metropolis, a regional capital, and one would have expected them to acquire enough knowledge about EBF and practice EBF, but that was not the cause among the people of Tamale metropolis. In addition, it was also realized that inefficient baby-friendly initiative program might have also been practised at the hospital centers where the study was conducted. Mothers who delivered in baby friendly hospital units are more likely to be knowledgeable about EBF than mothers who did not attend these facilities [17]. A similar observation was also noted in Kware town of Sokoto State of Nigeria where only 31% of the mothers had adequate knowledge of exclusive breastfeeding [18]. Another related study in a similar socio-cultural background also revealed that only 31% of the mothers had adequate knowledge regarding EBF [19]. The knowledge about exclusive breast

Table 6 Cross tabulation EBF and some knowledge questions

Variables		Exclusive breast feeding		Total	Pearson Chi-square value	*P*-values
		No	Yes			
Does EBF Improves Immunity?	No	40	23	63	2.881	.090
	Yes	244	86	330		
Total		284	109	393		
Does EBF allow child spacing?	No	264	85	349	17.769	<.001
	Yes	20	24	44		
Total		284	109	393		
Does EBF reduce the risk of breast cancer?	No	264	94	358	4.384	.036
	Yes	20	15	35		
Total		284	109	393		

Source: Field data, (2016)

feeding (EBF) and the practice may depend upon the hospital facilities and their policies in caring for pregnant and lactating mothers after delivery. If there has been a policy to educate pregnant mothers on EBF before and after delivery at various hospitals it would have reflected in their care of the newborns. However, high EBF was noted in some other part of Nigeria where the practice of EBF rate was 75.6% among nursing mothers [20]. It was asserted that the high prevalence of EBF in those studies was because the mothers were mostly workers and took their children with them when they were working, and this makes easier the fostering of EBF practice among mothers. This assertion was also noted by Gladzah, with non-working mothers who were constantly available to breast feed their babies [21]. The Tamale metropolis is in the temperate zone, and because of the sunny and draughty nature of the weather, this might have compiled the mothers to state complementing breastmilk with other liquid diets for the child for six months of age.

Pearson Chi square test of the sociodemographic characteristics associated with EBF showed a significant association between EBF and the sex of the child, $X^2 = 4.177$, $P = .041$. Whiles, EBF and the Knowledge on child spacing was $X^2 = 17.769$, $P < .001$ and EBF and knowledge on Breast cancer reduction was $X^2 = 4.384$, $P = .036$.

This means that mothers who had adequate knowledge about EBF did practice exclusive breastfeeding. This current finding confirms the observation by Mercer on the maternal role attainment theory [22, 23], that stated that in the first stages of "commitment, attachment, and preparation" during pregnancy, the mother acquires the knowledge of breastfeeding and makes a psychological adjustment and prepares for the expectations of her new role. Thus, from the time of birth of infants when motherhood is implicit and understood in the contexts of her social structure, mother's knowledge of EBF influences the practice [21]. This clearly shows that mothers in this study had not fully achieved this phase of knowledge involved in maternal role identity and EBF decisions making. Similar to this finding [18], opined that knowledge on EBF significantly influenced exclusive breastfeeding among working mothers. In fact, the understanding of the importance of breastfeeding helped mothers adhere to EBF practice.

Limitations

This study was mainly a cross-sectional study design. Also, the study participants may present recall bias since infants up to 2 years were included. And lastly, from literature reviewed, perception of mothers was one of the factors that affected EBF, but this was not measured in the current study.

Conclusions

Though majority of the participants had some level of education in the Tamale Metropolis, they had inadequate knowledge about EBF and the rate of EBF was awfully low. Therefore, there was poor knowledge and practice with regards to EBF for the first six months among postpartum mothers in the Tamale Metropolis. These underscore the need to give individual counselling sections to the women at every available opportunity, telling them the importance of EBF to their babies and the women themselves to improve their knowledge about breastfeeding and ultimately their breastfeeding practices.

Abbreviations

CWC: Child welfare clinic; EBF: Exclusive breastfeeding; TCH: Tamale Central Hospital; TTH: Tamale Teaching Hospital; TWH: Tamale West Hospital

Acknowledgements

The authors acknowledge the mothers in the Tamale Metropolis who provided the information used for the study. The University of Cape Coast, Tamale Teaching and the other associated district hospitals also appreciated for the opportunity given to us to carry out this research.

Authors' contributions

This article is an extract from the findings of my Master of Nursing thesis. RNN designed the study, developed the questionnaire and wrote the paper. SVN and J N were my first and second supervisors respectively, they both helped in making sure that I chose the right research methods and they gave suggestions to the appropriate tools to use. All authors coordination and helped to draft the manuscript. All authors read and approved the manuscript.

Competing interests

The authors declare that they have no competing interests.

Author details

[1]Department of Nursing, University for development studies, Tamale, Ghana. [2]School of Medical Sciences, University of Cape Coast, Cape Coast, Ghana. [3]School of Nursing and Midwifery, University of Cape Coast, Cape Coast, Ghana.

References

1. World Health Organization. Infant and young child feeding: model chapter for textbooks for medical students and allied health professionals; 2009. http://www.ncbi.nlm.nih.gov/books/NBK148965/.
2. Ayawine A, Ayuurebobi K. Determinants of exclusive breastfeeding: a study of two sub-districts in the Atwima Nwabiagya District of Ghana. The Pan African Medical Journal. 2015;22. https://doi.org/10.11604/pamj.2015.22.248.6904

3. Kiragu R, Neupane JE, Kandel S. Knowledge, attitude and challenges of exclusive breastfeeding among primigravidas; 2014. https://www.theseus.fi/bitstream/handle/10024/71668/student_reginah.
4. Odu S, Deji SA, Amu E, Aduayi V. Knowledge, Attitude and Practice of Exclusive Breastfeeding Among Mothers Attending an Infant Welfare Clinic in Osogbo, Osun State, Nigeria. European Journal of Preventive Medicine. 2016;4(2):39–43. https://doi.org/10.11648/j.ejpm.20160402.13.
5. Motee A, Ramasawmy D, Pugo-Gunsam P, Jeewon R. An assessment of the breastfeeding practices and infant feeding pattern among mothers in Mauritius. J Nutri Metabol. 2013;2013:1–8. https://doi.org/10.1155/2013/243852.
6. Jones G, Steketee RW, Black RE, Bhutta ZA, Morris SS. How many child deaths can we prevent this year? Lancet. 2003;362(9377):65–71. https://doi.org/10.1016/S0140-6736(03)13811-1.
7. Neovita Study Group. Timing of initiation, patterns of breastfeeding, and infant survival: prospective analysis of pooled data from three randomised trials. Lancet Glob Health. 2016;4:e266. PubMed. https://doi.org/10.1016/S2214-109X(16)00040-1.
8. Debes AK, Kohli A, Walker N, et al. Time to initiation of breastfeeding and neonatal mortality and morbidity: a systematic review. BMC Public Health. 2013;13(Suppl 3):S19. https://doi.org/10.1186/1471-2458-13-S3-S19. [PMC free article] [PubMed]
9. Black RE, Victora CG, Walker SP, et al. Maternal and child undernutrition and overweight in low-income and middle-income countries. Lancet. 2012;382: 427–51. PubMed. https://doi.org/10.1016/S0140-6736(13)60937-X.
10. Black RE, Allen LH, Bhutta ZA, et al. Maternal and child undernutrition: global and regional exposures and health consequences. Lancet. 2008;371: 243–60. PubMed. https://doi.org/10.1016/S0140-6736(07)61690-0.
11. Tawiah-Agyemang C, Kirkwood BR, Edmond K, Bazzano A, Hill Z. Early initiation of breast-feeding in Ghana: barriers and facilitators. J Perinatol. 2008;28:S46–52. https://doi.org/10.1038/jp.2008.173.
12. Ghana Statistical Service (GSS). GHANA multiple Indicator cluster surveys with an enhanced malaria module and biomarker. Final report; 2011.
13. Fosu-Brefo R, Arthur E. Effect of timely initiation of breastfeeding on child health in Ghana. Heal Econ Rev. 2015;5(1). https://doi.org/10.1186/s13561-015-0044-8.
14. Cochran WG. Sampling Techniques (3rd ed.). New York: John Wiley. 1977. https://archive.org/details/Cochran1977SamplingTechniques_201703.
15. Polit DF, Beck CT. Resource manual for nursing research: generating and assessing evidence for nursing practice. 9th ed. Philadelphia: Wolters Kluwer Health/lippincott Williams & Wilkins; 2012.
16. Emmanuel A. Breastfeeding intentions and practices of women in Plateau state, Nigeria: a cross-sectional study of women attending antenatal clinics in selected hospitals. University of Cape Town: Doctoral dissertation; 2014. http://hdl.handle.net/11427/13138.
17. Pérez-Escamilla R. Breastfeeding and the nutritional transition in the Latin American and Caribbean region: a success story? Cadernos de saude publica. 2003;19(1):S119–27. https://doi.org/10.1590/S0102-311X2003000700013.
18. Mogre V, Dery M, Gaa PK. Knowledge, attitudes and determinants of exclusive breastfeeding practice among Ghanaian rural lactating mothers. Int Breastfeed J. 2016;11(1). https://doi.org/10.1186/s13006-016-0071-z.
19. Leshi O, Samuel FO, Ajakaye OM. Breastfeeding knowledge, attitude and intention among female young adults in Ibadan, Nigeria. Open Journal of Nursing. 2016;6(1):11–23. https://doi.org/10.4236/ojn.2016.61002.
20. Oche M, Umar A, Ahmed H. Knowledge and practice of exclusive breastfeeding in Kware, Nigeria. Afr Health Sci. 2011;11(3):518–52.
21. Iliyasu Z, Kabir M, Abubakar IS, Galadanci NA. Current knowledge and practice of exclusive breastfeeding among mothers in Gwale local government area of Kano state. Nigerian Medical Practitioner. 2005;48(2):50–5. https://doi.org/10.4314/nmp.v48i2.28764.
22. Gladzah ND. Challenges of exclusive breastfeeding among female health Workers in two Hospitals in Accra: University of Ghana; 2013. Retrieved from http://ugspace.ug.edu.gh/handle/123456789/5863.
23. Mercer RT. Becoming a mother versus maternal role attainment. J Nurs Scholarsh. 2004;36(3):226–32. https://doi.org/10.1111/j.1547-5069.2004.04042.x.

2

Validation of the person-centered maternity care scale in India

Patience A. Afulani[1*], Nadia Diamond-Smith[1], Beth Phillips[1], Shreya Singhal[2] and May Sudhinaraset[3]

Abstract

Background: Person-centered care during childbirth is recognized as a critical component of quality of maternity care. But there are few validated tools to measure person-centered maternity care (PCMC). This paper aims to fill this measurement gap. We present the results of the psychometric analysis of the PCMC tool that was previously validated in Kenya using data from India. We aim to assess the validity and reliability of the PCMC scale in India, and to compare the results to those found in the Kenya validation.

Methods: We use data from a cross-sectional survey conducted from August to October 2017 with recently delivered women at 40 government facilities in Uttar Pradesh, India ($N = 2018$). The PCMC measure used is a previously validated scale with subscales for dignity and respect, communication and autonomy, and supportive care. We performed psychometric analyses, including iterative exploratory and confirmatory factor analysis, to assess construct and criterion validity and reliability.

Results: The results provide support for a 27-item PCMC scale in India with a possible score range from 0 to 81, compared to the 30-item PCMC scale in Kenya with a 0 to 90 possible score range. The overall PCMC scale has good reliability (Cronbach alpha = 0.85). Similar to Kenya, we are able to group the items in to three conceptual domains representing subscales for "Dignity and Respect," "Communication and Autonomy," and "Supportive Care." The sub-scales also have relatively good reliability (Cronbach alphas range from 0.67 to 0.73). In addition, increasing scores on the scale is associated with future intentions to deliver in the same facility, suggesting good criterion validity.

Conclusions: This research extends the PCMC literature by presenting results of validating the PCMC scale in a new context. The psychometric analysis using data from Uttar Pradesh, India corroborates the Kenya analysis showing the scale had good content, construct, and criterion validity, as well as high reliability. The overlap in items suggests that this scale can be used across different contexts to compare women's experiences of care, and to inform and evaluate quality improvement efforts to promote comprehensive PCMC.

Keywords: Person-centered care, Maternity care, Measurement, Validation, Developing settings, India

Plain English summary

Disrespect, abuse, and mistreatment during childbirth are commonly reported in both the global scientific community and popular media. Yet till recently, there has been no standardized way to measure women's experiences of respectful and responsive care, which we refer to as person-centered maternity care (PCMC). In our previous work in Kenya we developed and tested a scale for measuring PCMC, and we wanted to learn how that scale worked in a different setting. We therefore administered the PCMC scale to over 2000 women in India who had recently delivered a baby at a government health facility. To determine if the scale was credible in India, we ran statistical tests to see how the questions in the scale hung or grouped together. The results showed that the PCMC scale worked best in the India sample as 27 questions that gave a holistic measure of women's experiences during childbirth. Similar to what we found in Kenya, the PCMC scale covered dignity and respect, communication and autonomy, and supportive care. Women with higher PCMC scores were more likely to

* Correspondence: Patience.Afulani@ucsf.edu
[1]School of Medicine, Institute for Global Health Sciences, University of California, San Francisco, USA
Full list of author information is available at the end of the article

plan to deliver at the same facility again—implying high credibility. These findings suggest the PCMC scale can be used across many different contexts to compare women's experiences of maternity care. A standard measurement tool combined with clear policy guidelines can help to improve accountability of facilities, support staff in understanding how to provide person-centered care, and ensure women's voices, preferences, and values are front and center in the care they receive.

Background

Person-centered care during childbirth is recognized as a valued dimension of quality of maternal and newborn care [1]. Poor person-centered care during childbirth has, however, increasingly been documented around the globe [2–5]. This recognition has prompted recent recommendations by the World Health Organization (WHO) on intrapartum care for a positive childbirth experience [6]. Person-centered maternity care (PCMC) refers to "maternity care that is respectful of and responsive to individual women and their families' preferences, needs, and values" [7, 8]. The WHO recommendations highlight respectful maternity care, effective communication, and companionship during labor and childbirth as key dimensions of PCMC that should be provided to every women throughout labor and birth [6]. These recommendations are based on a human rights-based approach, as well as on evidence of the potential impacts of these interventions to reducing maternal morbidity and mortality [6].

Although we conceptualize PCMC as a broader construct which includes respectful maternity care, they highly overlap given the broad domains of respectful maternity care that have been proposed [9]. A recent review that synthesized data from sixty-seven studies from 32 countries identified twelve domains of respectful maternity care: being free from harm and mistreatment; maintaining privacy and confidentiality; preserving women's dignity; prospective provision of information and seeking of informed consent; ensuring continuous access to family and community support; enhancing quality of physical environment and resources; providing equitable maternity care; engaging with effective communication; respecting women's choices that strengthen their capabilities to give birth; availability of competent and motivated human resources; provision of efficient and effective care; and continuity of care [10]. These domains greatly overlap with previously identified domains of PCMC, which include dignity, autonomy, privacy/confidentiality, communication, social support, trust, supportive care, and the health facility environment [8, 11].

PCMC is important for increasing demand for facility deliveries, as well as for improving maternal and neonatal health outcomes for facility-based deliveries [12–14]. Facility-based deliveries have increased dramatically in India in the last decade. In 2015–16, about 79% of women in India reported that they delivered in a health facility compared to 39% in 2005–6, representing a two-fold increase [15]. Rates are slightly lower in Uttar Pradesh (the setting for our study), where about 68% of women in 2015–16 reported their last delivery was in a facility (up from 21% in 2005–6) [16]. This dramatic increase in facility deliveries is partly fueled by a cash incentive program, called Janani Suraksha Yojana (JSY), offered to women for delivering in a public facility. However, other factors, such as the relationship with community health workers have also played an important role in decision-making around place of birth [17, 18]. Despite the large increase in facility deliveries, India has not seen the expected reductions in maternal and neonatal mortality. Research exploring the impact of JSY on maternal and neonatal mortality generally has pointed to JSY having no impact on these adverse outcomes [19, 20]. It has been hypothesized that poor quality of care, due in part to overburdened health personnel because of the large increase in the number of deliveries, is contributing to the lack of change in maternal and neonatal health outcomes [20]. Past research in Uttar Pradesh specifically have found poor quality of care for delivery and newborn services, and a high prevalence of unqualified providers [21].

In India, alongside evidence of poor maternal and newborn clinical care is increasing evidence of poor PCMC [22–24]. Research in Uttar Pradesh, the most populous state in India, has documented that between 20 to 57% of women who recently delivered in health facilities reported some form of mistreatment during childbirth [23, 24]. In one study, the most commonly reported forms of poor person-centered care included verbal abuse, requests for bribes, not being allowed a companion, and discrimination [23]. Observational data of deliveries at facilities in Uttar Pradesh confirmed women's reports of mistreatment [25]. Other studies have documented factors associated with mistreatment, including women's empowerment, presence of support person, and type of providers [24, 26, 27]. Women were more likely to experience mistreatment if they were less empowered [27], had no companions [26], and received care from nurses compared to physicians or midwives [24]. Research in Uttar Pradesh also found that women who reported mistreatment at the time of delivery were more likely to have a complicated delivery or postpartum complications [24]. All of these studies have used different types of tools focused on measuring mistreatment or disrespect and abuse.

Increased awareness of the problem of poor PCMC has highlighted the need for validated measures for it

[2, 28, 29]. Afulani et al. (2017) recently validated the first scale to measure person-centered maternity care in Kenya. This validated scale includes 30 items (indicators or questions) with three sub-scales measuring dignity and respect, communication and autonomy, and supportive care. The scale was validated in two populations in Kenya, one rural and one urban. Validation in one country is important for moving this measurement agenda forward; however, the question remains as to how the measurement of a concept as complex and potentially culturally nuanced as person centered care can be translated from one country to another. To our knowledge, there has been no tool validated to holistically measure person-centered maternity care in India. Thus, as part of facility-based quality improvement project being implemented in Kenya and India, we sought to develop a person-centered maternity care scale that was potentially applicable to multiple settings including Kenya and India. The goal of this paper is to present the results of the psychometric analysis of the same tool validated by Afulani et al. 2017 in Kenya in an Indian population.

Methods

The development of this scale followed standard procedures for scale development and included the following: (1) Literature review to define the construct of person-centered maternity care and identify domains; (2) Item generation based on existing tools with additional questions; (3) Expert reviews in with experts in Kenya, India (Uttar Pradesh), and the US to assess content validity—whether the items represent all possible indicators relevant to the construct [30]; (4) Cognitive interviews with potential respondents in Kenya and in two public health facilities Uttar Pradesh, India to assess how participants internalize the questions and if the questions were being interpreted as intended. It was also used to evaluate problems with the wording of questions and whether questions are context appropriate and salient [31–33]; (5) Pretesting to finalize the scale items and full survey tool; and (6) Structured interviews in surveys with recently delivered women. Iterative revision of items followed each step. Similarly, the items were first translated into Hindi for the cognitive interviews with iterative translations following each revision. Details of the activities carried out in each of these steps up to finalizing the items for the survey are described in Afulani et al. 2017, where the process towards developing the final items and psychometric analysis based on survey data from Kenya are presented [8].

All study activities in India took place in Uttar Pradesh, a state in northern India. Uttar Pradesh is the most populous state in India (current population of 204.2 million), with 75 districts spread across four culturally and geographically distinct zones. The vast majority of Uttar Pradesh residents are considered rural (77%, Census 2011), though nearly all Uttar Pradesh residents live within 50 km of urban or peri-urban areas. A near final version of the PCMC tool was translated and administered to 867 women at nine government facilities in two districts of Uttar Pradesh, as part of the baseline surveys for a quality improvement intervention. However, minor edits were made to the items after this initial survey to obtain the final set of 38 items that were administered in Kenya and used for the analysis that yielded the 30 item PCMC scale. The 30 items from the Kenya validation, in addition to two other items—whether the woman was asked for bribes and whether she was asked to buy items from outside the facility—which we believed were important to the Indian context from our preliminary work in India, were then translated to Hindi and back translated to ensure accuracy. This set of 32 items was added to the study questionnaire for a cross-sectional study on quality of maternity care in Uttar Pradesh, and pre-tested with 10 recently delivered women at Lucknow District Women's Hospital in June 2017.

The final questionnaire was then administered to 2018 women in 40 high volume public health facilities in 20 districts of Uttar Pradesh. This data is used for the psychometric analysis presented in this paper. The survey was conducted from August through October 2017. Respondents were women aged 18 to 46 years who delivered in the 48 h preceding the survey at any of the 40 participating health facilities. Eligible women were identified by facility staff and subsequently invited by study staff to participate in the survey. Recruitment and consenting took place at the post-natal ward, and respondents were given the option of continuing with the interview in a private space at the facility or at their bed. Most interviews (2015 out of 2018) occurred on the post-natal ward at the patient's bed. All interviews were conducted in Hindi. All participants provided written informed consent after receiving information about the research. Interviews were conducted using the CommCare platform on tablets, with data uploaded to the server at the end of each day. About fifty women were interviewed per facility depending on facility delivery load (per the study design). Ethical approval for this study was provided by the ethics review boards of University of California, San Francisco and the Community Empowerment Lab in India.

Psychometric analyses

The psychometric analysis followed the same process as in the Kenya PCMC validation [8].We first examined the distributions of all the items. In instances where questions had responses in the "not applicable" category, we converted the "not applicable" category into the highest category to obtain a uniform scale for the psychometric analysis. This approach is conservative as it assumes the highest quality rating for each "not applicable" response. Only one item (explaining medications) had to be recoded in this format. We also reverse coded negative items in order for responses to reflect a scale of 0 as the lowest level to 3 as the highest level.

We used iterative exploratory and confirmatory factor analysis to assess construct validity—the degree to which the items represent the underlying conceptual structure. Kaiser-Meyer-Olkin (KMO) value of 0.5 or above was used as the criterion for sampling adequacy [34]. The Eigenvalues (the amount of information captured by a factor) and scree plots (plots of Eigenvalues) were used to determine the number of factors to extract. We used both Kaiser's rule of retaining only factors with eigenvalues exceeding unity and the "break" in the scree plot to decide on how many factors to retain [30, 35, 36]. We then conducted subsequent factor analysis and examined the item loadings to determine which items to retain or delete. Since most of the items had been vetted in the Kenya validation and the goal was not item reduction at this stage, we used a relaxed cut-off of 0.1 to retain items in this analysis [37]. We used oblique rotation, which, allows for correlation between the rotated factors and aligns the factor axes as closely as possible to the groups of the original variables [31, 34, 35]. We compared the factor structure to that obtained in the Kenya validation and tested our final factor structure with confirmatory factor analysis.

We assessed criterion validity—whether the measure is related to other measures or outcomes in theoretically predictable ways—by regressing the final scale on whether not the woman responded she would deliver in the same facility if she were to have another baby [30, 38]. We assessed the internal consistency reliability using Cronbach's alpha, with Cronbach's alpha of 0.7 or higher generally considered sufficient evidence of reliability [35]. We used STATA version 14 to perform the statistical analyses.

Results

We performed the psychometric analysis using data from the full sample ($N = 2018$). Table 1 shows the demographic characteristics of respondents. The average age of the women was about 25 years (range of 18 to 46) with an average parity of 2 (range of 1 to 8 children). Almost all (99%) of the women were married, and 34% had less than primary education. Nearly 85% of the sample resided in the rural portions of the districts.

Table 2 shows the original domains, the questions for each domain, and comments on decisions taken related to that item. The distributions for the items are shown in Appendix. The Kaiser-Meyer-Olkin (KMO) measure of sampling adequacy for all items are greater than 0.5, with an overall KMO of 0.91, indicating that overall the variables are satisfactory for factor analysis. The initial exploratory factor analysis with all 32 items yielded four factors (Fig. 1) accounting for 87% of the total variance, although the scree plot showed only one dominant factor. Also, the third and fourth factors in the un-rotated solution did not have any items loading positively on them suggesting a two-factor solution. When the oblique rotation was applied, only the items on labor and delivery support loaded on the fourth factor. When reduced to three factors (i.e. applying the Kenya three-factor structure), only labor and delivery support still loaded on the third factor. For the two-factor solution, 16 items loaded on the first factor and 11 on the second factor. These 27 items also loaded on the single factor. Four items that had factor loadings of less than 0.1 on the retained factors at each stage were dropped. These items

Table 1 Distribution of selected demographic variables ($N = 2018$)

Variables	No.	%	
Age: Mean (SD)	2018	25	(4)
Parity: Mean (SD)	2018	2.2	(1.3)
Marital status			
Married	2013	99.8	
Widowed	2	0.1	
Divorced/Separated	3	0.2	
Education			
No school/Primary	941	46.6	
Post-primary/vocational/Secondary	828	41	
College or above	249	12.3	
Employed			
No	1905	94.4	
Yes	113	5.6	
Pregnancy complications			
No	425	21.1	
Yes	1593	78.9	
Religion			
Christian	1	0.1	
Muslim/other	342	17	
Hindu	1675	83	
Caste			
Scheduled caste/scheduled tribe	574	28.4	
General	332	16.5	
Other backwards caste	1112	55.1	
Total	2018	100	

Table 2 Items for person-centered maternity care scale

Original Domain	Question	Referred to in text as	Comment
Dignity/Respect	1. How did you feel about the amount of time you waited? Would you say it was very short, just a little long, somewhat long, or very long?	Time to care	Retained but loads at less than 0.3
Dignity/Respect	2. During your time in the health facility did the doctors, nurses, or other health care providers introduce themselves to you when they first came to see you?	Introduce self	Retained but loads at less than 0.3
Dignity/Respect	3. Did the doctors, nurses, or other health care providers call you by your name?	Called by name	Retained
Dignity/Respect	4. Did the doctors, nurses, or other staff at the facility treat you with respect?	Treated with respect	Retained
Dignity/Respect	5. Did the doctors, nurses, and other staff at the facility treat you in a friendly manner?	Friendly	Retained
Dignity/Respect	6. Did you feel the doctors, nurses, or other health providers shouted at you, scolded, insulted, threatened, or talked to you rudely?	Verbal abuse	Retained
Dignity/Respect	7. Did you feel like you were treated roughly like pushed, beaten, slapped, pinched, physically restrained, or gagged?	Physical abuse	Retained but loads at less than 0.3
Privacy/Confidentiality	8. During examinations in the labor room, were you covered up with a cloth or blanket or screened with a curtain so that you did not feel exposed?	Visual privacy	Retained
Privacy/Confidentiality	9. Do you feel like your health information was or will be kept confidential at this facility?	Record confidentiality	Retained
Autonomy	10. Did you feel like the doctors, nurses or other staff at the facility involved you in decisions about your care?	Involvement in care	Retained
Autonomy	11. Did the doctors, nurses or other staff at the facility ask your permission/consent before doing procedures and examinations on you?	Consent to procedures/exams	Retained
Autonomy	12. During the delivery, do you feel like you were able to be in the position of your choice?	Delivery position choice	Retained
Communication	13. Did the doctors, nurses or other staff at the facility speak to you in a language you could understand?	Language	Retained but loads at less than 0.3
Communication	14. Did the doctors and nurses explain to you why they were doing examinations or procedures on you?	Explain exams/ procedures	Retained
Communication	15. Did the doctors and nurses explain to you why they were giving you any medicine?	Explain medicines	Retained
Communication	16. Did you feel you could ask the doctors, nurses or other staff at the facility any questions you had?	Able to ask questions	Retained but loads at less than 0.3
Social Support	17. Were you allowed to have someone you wanted (outside of staff at the facility, such as family or friends) to stay with you during labor?	Labor support	Retained
Social Support	18. Were you allowed to have someone you wanted to stay with you during delivery?	Delivery support	Retained
Supportive Care	19. Did the doctors and nurses at the facility talk to you about how you were feeling?	Talk about feeling	Retained
Supportive Care	20. Did the doctors, nurses or other staff at the facility support your anxieties and fears?	Support anxiety	Deleted based on wording of question
Supportive Care	21. Do you feel the doctors or nurses did everything they could to help control your pain?	Control pain	Retained
Supportive Care	22. When you needed help, did you feel the doctors, nurses or other staff at the facility paid attention?	Attention when need help	Retained
Trust	23. Did you feel the doctors, nurses or other staff at the facility took the best care of you?	Took best care	Retained
Trust	24. Did you feel you could completely trust the doctors, nurses or other staff at the facility with regards to your care?	Trust	Retained
Facility environment	25. Do you think there was enough health staff in the	Enough staff	Retained

Table 2 Items for person-centered maternity care scale *(Continued)*

Original Domain	Question	Referred to in text as	Comment
	facility to care for you?		
Facility environment	26. Thinking about the labor and postnatal wards, did you feel the health facility was crowded?	Crowded	Deleted: low loading
Facility environment	27. Thinking about the wards, washrooms and the general environment of the health facility, will you say the facility was very clean, clean, dirty, or very dirty?	Clean	Retained but loads at less than 0.3
Facility environment	28. Was there clean drinking water available in the facility?[a]	Water	Deleted: low loading
Facility environment	29. Was there electricity in the facility?	Electricity	Deleted: low loading
Facility environment	30. In general, did you feel safe in the health facility?	Safe	Retained but loads at less than 0.3
Predictability & transparency of payments	31. Did the doctors, nurses or other staff at the facility ask you or your family for money other than the official cost?[b]	Bribe	Retained but loads at less than 0.3
Predictability & transparency of payments	32. Were you or your family asked to buy anything from outside the health facility for your care?[b]	buy supplies	Deleted: low loading

Notes: All items retained loaded at > 0.1 on the final main scale
[a]Question asked as was there water in Kenya version (drinking water added by India survey team)
[b]All items in scale validated from Kenya data except these two questions

are: "Was there clean drinking water available in the facility?", "Thinking about the labor and postnatal wards, did you feel the health facility was crowded?" and "Were you or your family asked to buy anything from outside the health facility for your care?". We also dropped the item on "Did the doctors, nurses or other staff at the facility support your anxieties and fears" because the question was identified as ambiguous based on feedback on the original scale.

Factor analysis of the remaining 27 items still yielded four factors with one dominant factor (Fig. 2), with item distributions on the factors as in the full set. However, all the items had loadings of > 0.1 (with most greater than 0.3) on the retained factors, including when the factors were constrained to a single factor (Table 3). This suggests high construct validity for a single dominant 27 item PCMC scale based on the India data. However, because the domains of PCMC are overlapping, the items loading on the two factors (which was the best multiple factor solution for the India data) did not represent clear conceptual domains. For instance, the first factor includes items from the domains dignity and respect and supportive care. It however also includes the items on "being spoken to in a language they understand" and "being able to ask questions," which conceptually should have loaded on the second factor, which has more items on communication and autonomy (but also includes the items on privacy and confidentiality). We therefore

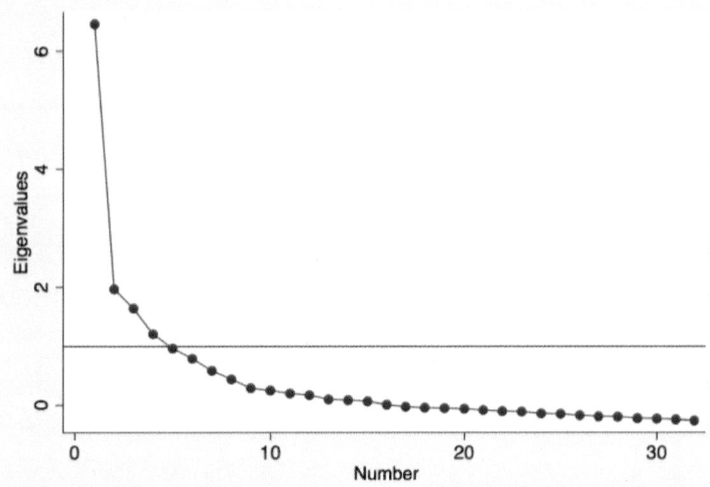

Fig. 1 Scree plot for 32 items after exploratory factor analysis

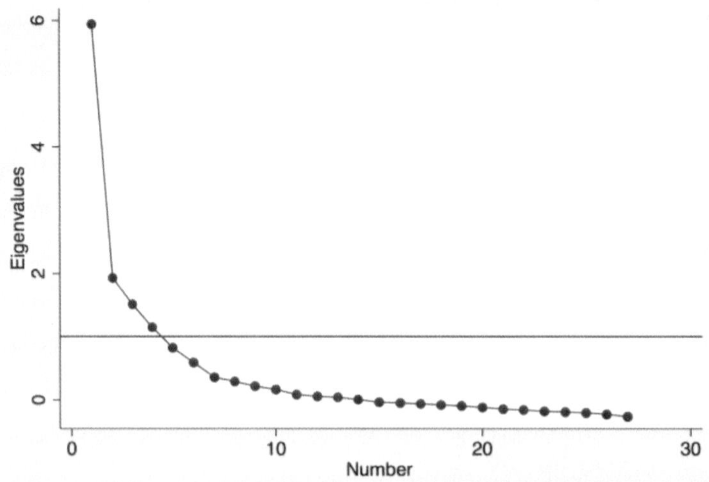

Fig. 2 Scree plot for 27 items after exploratory factor analysis

regrouped the retained items into three conceptual domains as in the Kenya analysis, to provide the sub-scales for Dignity and respect, Communication and autonomy, and Supportive care. These are theoretically derived categories rather than data driven. However, when factor analysis is run on each set, the items load well on the factor representing each domain, except for the question on "being able to ask questions" which loads negatively on the communication and autonomy domain and positively on the dignity and respect domain, although conceptually it should group under communication and autonomy (Table 4).

The overall PCMC scale has a Cronbach's alpha of 0.85, suggesting good reliability. The sub-scales also have relatively good reliability (alphas from 0.67 to 0.73 in Table 5). The average PCMC score for the sample based on the sum of the 27 items is 50 (where 0 is the minimum possible score and 81 is the maximum possible score (range for the sample is 16 to 79). In addition, increasing scores on the scale is associated with future intentions to deliver in the same facility (Table 6), suggesting good criterion validity.

Discussion

Person-centered care is a recognized dimension of quality of care; however, until recently, there has not been a validated scale for person-centered care for maternity services in low resource settings [8]. This paper extends the PCMC literature by presenting the results of validating the PCMC scale in a new context –India. The analysis provides support for a 27-item multidimensional PCMC scale in Uttar Pradesh, India, in comparison to the 30-item scale derived from the Kenya validation of the same scale. The possible range of scores for the 27-item scale is therefore from 0 to 81 (compared to 0 to 90 for the 30-item Kenya scale). Similar to Kenya, the items can be grouped into three conceptual domains representing subscales for "Dignity and Respect," "Community and Autonomy," and "Supportive Care." These subscales are in general supported by the empirical analysis. The scale has good reliability (Cronbach alpha = 0.85). The subscales also have good reliability (Cronbach alpha ranging from 0.67–0.73), suggesting that future studies may use these individual subscales or the full scale when examining women's experiences in labor and delivery. The preliminary work towards the development of this scale ensured it had good content validity. The psychometric analysis using data from Uttar Pradesh, India corroborates the Kenya analysis showing the scale had good construct and criterion validity, as well as high reliability.

Validating the PCMC scale in a different context is necessary to highlight potential cultural and social differences in the conceptualization of person-centered care. We, however, do not find very significant differences. One potential reason is that the foundational work that led to the development of the final set of items included expert and cognitive interviews from India. Twenty-six items are common across the India and Kenya PCMC scales and could facilitate comparison across the two countries. While the validation of the PCMC tool with data from India demonstrates a similar set of items to that from the Kenya validation, there were a few notable exceptions. First, the item on "provider support anxieties" has been dropped from the current version of the scale because the question was identified as ambiguous

Table 3 Rotated factor loadings of items on dominant factor for main scale ($N = 2018$)

Variable	Factor loadings
Time to care	0.26
Introduce self	0.12
Called by name	0.42
Treated with respect	0.77
Friendly	0.79
Visual privacy	0.48
Record confidentiality	0.34
Involvement in care	0.63
Consent to procedures/exams	0.42
Delivery position choice	0.38
Language	0.17
Explain exams/procedures	0.48
Explain medicines	0.57
Talk about feeling	0.51
Able to ask questions	0.21
Labor support	0.37
Delivery support	0.35
Attention when need help	0.63
Control pain	0.68
Verbal abuse	0.47
Physical abuse	0.20
Enough staff	0.55
Took best care	0.71
Trust	0.45
Bribe	0.16
Clean	0.12
Safe	0.20

Table 4 Rotated factor loadings of items on dominant factor for sub-scales ($N = 2018$)

Subscale	Variable	Factor loadings
Dignity and respect		
	Treated with respect	0.92
	Friendly	0.92
	Verbal abuse	0.51
	Physical abuse	0.25
	Visual privacy	0.43
	Record confidentiality	0.30
Communication and autonomy		
	Introduce self	0.18
	Called by name	0.25
	Involvement in care	0.68
	Consent to procedures	0.70
	Delivery position choice	0.35
	Language	0.17
	Explain exams/ procedures	0.80
	Explain medicines	0.75
	Able to ask questions	−0.05
Supportive care		
	Time to care	0.25
	Labor support	0.54
	Delivery support	0.52
	Talk about feeling	0.42
	Attention when need help	0.67
	Took best care	0.76
	Control pain	0.68
	Trust	0.49
	Safe	0.26
	Enough staff	0.64
	Clean	0.05
	bribe	0.19

based on feedback from in-country partners and reviewers of the original scale. Thus, this difference is not based on the empirical analysis, as it could have been retained based on its loading.

Second, the three items related to health facility environment—water, electricity, and crowding—that were included in the Kenya "Supportive care" sub-scale do not hang well with the rest of the items in India validation; therefore, they have been removed from this version of the scale. It is unclear why these items load much poorer in India than in Kenya. One reason is the difference in distribution in this sample, which affects the factor loading. Another potential reason is that this sample is from high-volume delivery facilities, and perceptions of person-centered care may be more closely related to the interpersonal relationships than to the broader health facility environment in this context. It should be noted that in the Kenya validation, "crowding" loaded well in urban samples, but not in rural samples. The majority of women in this sample were from rural areas of Uttar Pradesh. Therefore, the importance of health facility environment factors in influencing person-centered care may be more related to urban/rural context as opposed to Kenya vs. India. Also, the rewording of the question on availability of "water" to "drinking water" in India may have affected its relationship to the other items in the scale.

Since publishing the 30-item scale in Kenya, we have had discussions with various experts on whether to include the health facility environment items as part of the scale. While we have felt that the health facility environment is an important aspect of person-centered care, supported by a recent qualitative evidence synthesis on

Table 5 Reliability and distribution of Full PCMC scale and sub-scales ($N = 2018$)

	Alpha	Mean	SD	Min	Max	Possible range
Full PCMC Scale (27 items)	0.85	50.3	10.9	16	79	0–81
Sub-scales						
Dignity and respect (6 items)	0.70	14.1	3.48	2	18	0–18
Communication and autonomy (9 items)	0.67	9.6	4.3	0	25	0–27
Supportive Care (12 items)	0.73	26.7	5.19	6	36	0–36

respectful maternity care [10], others have argued the health facility environment influences PCMC but is not necessarily part of it. The poor loading of these health facility environment related items might support this counter argument. Regardless, it is interesting to note the nuances of what is important to person-centered care across different contexts and cultures.

Third, the item on "being asked for bribes," which was dropped from the Kenya scale has been retained in the India scale. The role of bribes is central to the mistreatment literature in India, as past studies have identified that poor and disadvantaged women, in particular, are asked to pay bribes in order to receive care [23, 39]. In cognitive interviews for the present study, women and providers in Kenya were both much less likely to report facility staff asking for bribes. However, in line with extant literature, bribes were much more common in cognitive interviews in India. It is therefore not surprising that this indicator would be retained in the India PCMC scale. The question used in the scale to get at bribes is "Did the doctors, nurses or other staff at the facility ask you or your family for money other than the official cost?". But the complexity of the issue of bribes in this context is highlighted in other qualitative work by our team. These findings show women sometimes give providers tips, without being asked, when they feel providers are delaying care for them because they want bribes, even when this might not be the case; or when they are happy with the outcome of their pregnancies. In such cases they may be unhappy if the provider refuses to take the money. This suggests more than one question will be needed to unpack what is considered a bribe and what is not.

The differences across India and Kenya highlight the need for careful consideration of which items are most

Table 6 Bivariate linear regression of person-centered maternity care score on future intentions to deliver in the same facility ($N = 2018$)

	Coef.	*p*-value	[95% Conf.	Interval]
Will deliver in same facility again in future				
No (ref)				
Yes	16.99	< 0.00	14.30	19.68
Cons	33.87	< 0.00	31.22	36.51

relevant across contexts as well as attention to the wording of items for different contexts. Validation in other settings is needed, and application of the full set of items in other parts of India followed by psychometric analysis will help to develop a tool that can be applied to all of India. But, given that not every study has the capacity to go through the process of validating a tool to use in the study, we believe the PCMC scale can be reasonably used across settings. It appears the 30-item version works well in settings like Kenya and the 27-item version works well in settings like Uttar Pradesh, India. Researchers and practitioners could therefore choose the version of the scale they believe will work best in their setting. However, given none of the samples used in the validation was nationally representative, it might be best to administer the full set of items if the length is not a concern. Analysis could then be conducted to assess whether the full set or only a subset will work best as a scale.

As in any study, there are a number of limitations. First, it should be noted that the sample is not generalizable to all of India—or even all of Uttar Pradesh. Women were recruited from public facilities that are all high volume (> 200 deliveries/month). Although we recruited women from a variety of facility levels, including primary health care centers and community health care centers, in addition to district hospitals, the sample excludes women who attend private and lower volume facilities and those who do not make it to a facility. The sample is however representative of women in Uttar Pradesh who gave birth in public health facilities, which represents 44% of all births and 66% facility-based births in Uttar Pradesh [16]. According to the recent National Family Health Survey (NFHS) survey (2015–16), among women who gave birth in the last 5 years in public facilities, about 86% resided in rural areas; 16% were Muslim and 84% were Hindus. Also, 99% were married, with an average age of 25 years and an average parity of 2 children; 56% had less than a secondary education and almost all (99.7%) belonged to the most vulnerable castes (Other backward caste (OBC) and Scheduled caste/Scheduled tribe (SCST)) [16]. This is similar to the characteristics of our sample which included 85% rural residents, 17% Muslim and 83% Hindi, with 99% married, average age of 25 years and parity of

2; and 47% with less than secondary education and majority (83.5%) from the most vulnerable castes. The characteristics of our sample are also somewhat similar to the general population of Uttar Pradesh, which is 73% rural, 18% Muslim and 81% Hindu, and 78% belong to the most vulnerable castes [16]. These similarities suggest that the PCMC scale may be applied to Uttar Pradesh, but it is possible that the factor structure may differ across different sub-populations within India, as was found in Kenya [8]. Nonetheless, given that data from two settings in Kenya and India all show one dominant factor, we believe the single multidimensional scale is likely stable across settings.

In addition, the data are self-reported, thus subject to recall bias and social desirability bias. Women may not clearly remember their experiences during their labor, and their recall may also be clouded by the outcome of their deliveries (although women who had an infant death were excluded). Recall is however likely not be a major issue with this sample given interviews occurred within 48 h of delivery. Social desirability bias on the other hand is a bigger issue as the interviews occurred in the post-natal ward. Prior research suggests women are more likely to report more positively on their experiences when interviewed close to the time of delivery and within the health facility [8, 28, 29]. Studies in India have also shown that women tend to report more positively in interviews when compared to direct observations due to normalization of certain mistreatment [25]. Thus, the levels of PCMC found in this study likely overestimates the quality of actual levels of PCMC in the study facilities. Finally, the 27-item scale may be considered too long for facilities wishing to include the tool as part of quality improvement initiatives. We used a relaxed cut-off to retain items in this analysis because the goal was not item reduction, but to assess construct validity of comprehensive scale with high content validity. This conservative approach is acceptable in early stages of scale development [30]. Future studies may, however, wish to use a more data-driven approach in order to focus the scale on a smaller set of indicators.

Despite these limitations, this study contributes in a number of ways to existing literature on person-centered care and quality of care for maternity services. In particular, this study validated an existing PCMC scale in a new context and found significant overlap in indicators across India and Kenya, two very different contexts. The overlap should not be very surprising in the light of a recent qualitative evidence synthesis on respectful maternity care, which concluded that globally, women's perspectives of what constitutes respectful maternity care are quite consistent [10]. The overlap in items suggests that this scale can be used across many different contexts to compare women's experiences of care.

It is important to note that the items in this scale capture all but one of the 12 domains of respectful maternity care from the recent review [10]. That the PCMC tool captures all of these domains, except continuity of care, is not surprising given the initial work towards its development involved a review of the literature including that on mistreatment/disrespect and abuse/respectful maternity care. Thus, the person-centered maternity care scale is an effective tool for holistically measuring respectful maternity care and might be among the best tools currently available for this purpose. An additional question on continuity of care may however be needed to complete it. Future studies looking at person-centered care measures across the continuum of reproductive care, including family planning will also help improve continuity of care.

Finally, a recent review of quantitative studies on disrespect and abuse highlighted how differences in study tools as well as other methodological differences affect comparison of different studies, hence the need for more consistent methodologies if we are to be able to compare studies across settings (while taking into account key contextual differences) [39]. We believe the PCMC tool having so far been validated in three settings in two countries addresses one of the key steps towards responding to this call.

Conclusions

This study presents the results of validating the PCMC scale in Uttar Pradesh, India. The PCMC scale provides a valuable tool for the growing number of quality improvement initiatives in India, and beyond. The scale may also be used to support policy and programmatic efforts to improve the quality of maternity care. Five years ago, the Government of India developed broad quality assurance guidelines for quality of care, and several years later issued a maternal and neonatal health care manual to guide providers about importance of patient-centered care during labor and delivery [40, 41]. However, it is unclear how to measure and evaluate women's experiences of care across different facilities in India. This scale will help to bridge this gap. In addition, this scale will be valuable for assessing implementation of the WHO recommendations on intrapartum care for a positive childbirth experience [6]. Providing clear guidelines and standard measurement tools will help improve accountability of facilities, support providers/staff in understanding how to provide person-centered care, and ensure women's voices, preferences, and values are front and center in the care they receive.

Abbreviations

CA: Communication and Autonomy; DR: Dignity and Respect; HFE: Health Facility Environment; KMO: Kaiser-Meyer-Olkin; PCMC: Person-centered maternity care; SC: Supportive Care; WHO: World Health Organization

Acknowledgements

We would like to thank all the people who contributed to the development of the tool first validated in Kenya. We are also grateful to all the members of the SPARQ and CEL teams. Finally, we would like to express our gratitude to all our data collectors and study participants in India.

Funding

This work was funded the Bill and Melinda Gates Foundation [OPP1127467]. During the period of this work, PA was supported by the University of California, San Francisco PTBi transdisciplinary post-doctoral fellowship, which is in turn funded by the Bill and Melinda Gates Foundation [OPP1107312]; and Marc and Lynne Benioff. The funders had no role in the study design, data collection and analysis, decision to publish, or preparation of the manuscript.

Authors' contributions

PA led the development of the tool, conceived the manuscript, conducted the analysis, and led the writing. ND and MS supported the development of the tool and the writing of the manuscript. BP and SS supported the data collection and writing of the manuscript. All authors read and approved the final manuscript.

Competing interests

The authors declare that they have no competing interests.

Author details

[1]School of Medicine, Institute for Global Health Sciences, University of California, San Francisco, USA. [2]Community Empowerment Lab, Lucknow, India. [3]Jonathan and Karin Fielding School of Public Health, University of California, Los Angeles, USA.

References

1. Tunçalp Ö, Were W, MacLennan C, Oladapo O, Gülmezoglu A, Bahl R, et al. Quality of care for pregnant women and newborns—the WHO vision. BJOG Int J Obstet Gynaecol. 2015;122:1045–9.
2. Bohren MA, Vogel JP, Hunter EC, Lutsiv O, Makh SK, Souza JP, et al. The mistreatment of women during childbirth in health facilities globally: a mixed-methods systematic review. PLoS Med. 2015;12:e1001847.
3. Warren CE, Njue R, Ndwiga C, Abuya T. Manifestations and drivers of mistreatment of women during childbirth in Kenya: implications for measurement and developing interventions. BMC Pregnancy Childbirth. 2017;17:102.
4. Afulani PA, Kirumbi L, Lyndon A. What makes or mars the facility-based childbirth experience: thematic analysis of women's childbirth experiences in western Kenya. Reprod Health. 2017:14. [cited 2018 Jan 7] Available from: https://www.ncbi.nlm.nih.gov/pmc/articles/PMC5747138/
5. Montesinos-Segura R, Urrunaga-Pastor D, Mendoza-Chuctaya G, Taype-Rondan A, Helguero-Santin LM, Martinez-Ninanqui FW, et al. Disrespect and abuse during childbirth in fourteen hospitals in nine cities of Peru. Int J Gynaecol Obstet Off Organ Int Fed Gynaecol Obstet. 2018;140:184–90.
6. World Health Organization. WHO recommendations: intrapartum care for a positive childbirth experience. WHO. 2018; [cited 2018 Feb 28]. Available from: http://www.who.int/reproductivehealth/publications/intrapartum-care-guidelines/en/
7. Institute of Medicine (US) Committee on Quality of Health Care in America. Crossing the Quality Chasm: A New Health System for the 21st Century. Washington (DC): National Academies Press (US); 2001. http://www.ncbi.nlm.nih.gov/books/NBK222274/. Accessed 22 Dec 2017.
8. Afulani PA, Diamond-Smith N, Golub G, Sudhinaraset M. Development of a tool to measure person-centered maternity care in developing settings: validation in a rural and urban Kenyan population. Reprod Health. 2017;14:118.
9. White Ribbon Alliance. Respectful Maternity Care. White Ribb Alliance. 2015; [cited 2017 Mar 28]. Available from: http://whiteribbonalliance.org/campaigns2/respectful-maternity-care/
10. Shakibazadeh E, Namadian M, Bohren MA, Vogel JP, Rashidian A, Pileggi VN, et al. Respectful care during childbirth in health facilities globally: a qualitative evidence synthesis. BJOG Int J Obstet Gynaecol. 2018;125(8):932–42.
11. Sudhinaraset M, Afulani P, Diamond-Smith N, Bhattacharyya S, Donnay F, Montagu D. Advancing a conceptual model to improve maternal health quality: the person-centered care framework for reproductive health equity. Gates Open Res. 2017;1:1.
12. Koblinsky M, Moyer CA, Calvert C, Campbell J, Campbell OMR, Feigl AB, et al. Quality maternity care for every woman, everywhere: a call to action. Lancet. 2016; [cited 2016 Sep 24]; Available from: http://linkinghub.elsevier.com/retrieve/pii/S0140673616313332
13. Miller S, Abalos E, Chamillard M, Ciapponi A, Colaci D, Comandé D, et al. Beyond too little, too late and too much, too soon: a pathway towards evidence-based, respectful maternity care worldwide. Lancet. 2016; [cited 2016 Sep 24]; Available from: http://linkinghub.elsevier.com/retrieve/pii/S0140673616314726
14. Shaw D, Guise J-M, Shah N, Gemzell-Danielsson K, Joseph K, Levy B, et al. Drivers of maternity care in high-income countries: can health systems support woman-centred care? Lancet. 2016; [cited 2016 Sep 24]; Available from: http://linkinghub.elsevier.com/retrieve/pii/S0140673616315276
15. National Family Health Survey - 4 201 5–16 India Fact sheet. [cited 2018 Mar 2]. Available from: http://rchiips.org/NFHS/pdf/NFHS4/India.pdf
16. National Family Health Survey - 4 201 5–16 Uttar Pradesh Fact sheet [Internet]. [cited 2018 Mar 2]. Available from: http://rchiips.org/NFHS/pdf/NFHS4/UP_FactSheet.pdf
17. Sabde Y, Chaturvedi S, Randive B, Sidney K, Salazar M, Costa AD, et al. Bypassing health facilities for childbirth in the context of the JSY cash transfer program to promote institutional birth: a cross-sectional study from Madhya Pradesh, India. PLoS One. 2018;13:e0189364.
18. Vellakkal S, Reddy H, Gupta A, Chandran A, Fledderjohann J, Stuckler D. A qualitative study of factors impacting accessing of institutional delivery care in the context of India's cash incentive program. Soc Sci Med. 2017;178:55–65.
19. Coffey D. Costs and consequences of a cash transfer for hospital births in a rural district of Uttar Pradesh, India. Soc Sci Med. 2014;114:89–96.
20. Randive B, Diwan V, Costa AD. India's conditional cash transfer Programme (the JSY) to promote institutional birth: is there an association between institutional birth proportion and maternal mortality? PLoS One. 2013;8:e67452.
21. Sharma G, Powell-Jackson T, Haldar K, Bradley J, Filippi V. Quality of routine essential care during childbirth: clinical observations of uncomplicated births in Uttar Pradesh, India. Bull World Health Organ. 2017;95:419–29.
22. Chattopadhyay S, Mishra A, Jacob S. 'Safe', yet violent? Women's experiences with obstetric violence during hospital births in rural Northeast India. Cult Health Sex 2017;0:1–15.
23. Sudhinaraset M, Treleaven E, Melo J, Singh K, Diamond-Smith N. Women's status and experiences of mistreatment during childbirth in Uttar Pradesh: a mixed methods study using cultural health capital theory. BMC Pregnancy Childbirth. 2016;16:332.
24. Raj A, Dey A, Boyce S, Seth A, Bora S, Chandurkar D, et al. Associations between mistreatment by a provider during childbirth and maternal health complications in Uttar Pradesh, India. Matern Child Health J. 2017:1–13.
25. Dey A, Shakya HB, Chandurkar D, Kumar S, Das AK, Anthony J, et al. Discordance in self-report and observation data on mistreatment of women by providers during childbirth in Uttar Pradesh, India. Reprod Health. 2017; 14 [cited 2018 Jan 8]. Available from: https://www.ncbi.nlm.nih.gov/pmc/articles/PMC5688759/
26. Diamond-Smith N, Sudhinaraset M, Melo J, Murthy N. The relationship between women's experiences of mistreatment at facilities during childbirth, types of support received and person providing the support in Lucknow, India. Midwifery. 2016;40:114 23.

27. Diamond-Smith N, Treleaven E, Murthy N, Sudhinaraset M. Women's empowerment and experiences of mistreatment during childbirth in facilities in Lucknow, India: results from a cross-sectional study. BMC Pregnancy Childbirth. 2017;17:335.
28. Sando D, Abuya T, Asefa A, Banks KP, Freedman LP, Kujawski S, et al. Methods used in prevalence studies of disrespect and abuse during facility based childbirth: lessons learned. Reprod Health. 2017;14:127.
29. Savage V, Castro A. Measuring mistreatment of women during childbirth: a review of terminology and methodological approaches. Reprod Health. 2017;14:138.
30. DeVellis RF. Scale development: theory and applications. 4th ed. Los Angeles: SAGE Publications, Inc; 2016.
31. Collins D. Pretesting survey instruments: an overview of cognitive methods. Qual Life Res Int J Qual Life Asp Treat Care Rehab. 2003;12:229–38.
32. Jobe JB, Mingay DJ. Cognitive research improves questionnaires. Am J Public Health. 1989;79:1053–5.
33. Nápoles-Springer AM, Santoyo-Olsson J, O'Brien H, Stewart AL. Using cognitive interviews to develop surveys in diverse populations. Med Care. 2006;44:S21–30.
34. Katchova A. Principal Component Analysis. Econom Acad. [cited 2017 Mar 14]. Available from: https://sites.google.com/site/econometricsacademy/econometrics-models/principal-component-analysis
35. Hinkin T, Tracey J, Enz C. Scale Construction: Developing Reliable and Valid Measurement Instruments. Artic Chapters. 1997; Available from: http://scholarship.sha.cornell.edu/articles/613
36. Afifi AA, Clark V, May S. Computer-aided Multivariate Analysis. 4th ed: CRC Press; 2004.
37. Spector PE. Summated rating scale construction: an introduction. 1st ed. Newbury Park: SAGE Publications, Inc; 1991.
38. Crosby RA, DiClemente RJ, Salazar LF. Research methods in health promotion. San Francisco: Jossey-Bass; 2006.
39. Sudhinaraset M, Beyeler N, Barge S, Diamond-Smith N. Decision-making for delivery location and quality of care among slum-dwellers: a qualitative study in Uttar Pradesh, India. BMC Pregnancy Childbirth. 2016;16:148.
40. Ministry of Health and Family Welfare, Government of India. Operational Guidelines on Quality Assurance in Public Health Facilities. 2013 [cited 2018 Mar 9]. Available from: http://www.rrcnes.gov.in/quality%20Assurance/Operational%20Guidelines%20on%20Quality%20Assurance%20%28Print%29.pdf.
41. Jhpiego. DAKSHATA Empowering Providers for Improved MNH Care during Institutional Deliveries A strategic initiative to strengthen quality of intra - and immediate postpartum care. 2015 [cited 2018 Mar 9]. Available from: http://www.nhmmp.gov.in/WebContent/MH/Schemes/Dakshata/Activity%20Report%20Final%20(Sep-15).pdf.

Long-acting reversible contraceptive use in the post-abortion period among women seeking abortion in mainland China: intentions and barriers

Zhongchen Luo[1], Lingling Gao[2*], Ronald Anguzu[3] and Juanjuan Zhao[2]

Abstract

Background: This study aimed to describe the intentions of and barriers to the use of long-acting reversible contraceptives (LARCs) in the post-abortion period among women seeking abortion in mainland China.

Methods: A cross-sectional study was conducted from July 2015 to December 2015 using a waiting room questionnaire. A total of 381 women seeking abortions were recruited at a public hospital abortion clinic. The outcome variable was an 'intention-to-use' LARCs in the immediate post-abortion period. Chi-square tests were used to assess associations between categorical variables. Statistically significant variables ($p \leq 0.05$) were then further analyzed by logistic regression.

Results: Among 381 respondents, 42.5% intended to use LARCs in the immediate post-abortion period; 35.2% intended to use intra-uterine devices (IUDs); and 13.9% intended to use implants. Previous use of LARC was a predictor for an intention to use LARCs (odds ratio [OR] = 2.41; 95% confidence interval [CI]: 1.06–5.47). Participants with one or no child had reduced odds for an intention to use LARC (OR = 0.32, 95% CI: 0.15–0.47 and OR = 0.29, 95% CI: 0.13–0.68, respectively). Women with a higher sex frequency (at least once per week) showed increased odds for LARC use (OR = 3.34; 95% CI: 1.03–10.78) and married women were more likely to use LARC than single women (OR = 1.57; 95% CI:1.00–2.47). Women who planned to have another baby within two years were more likely not to use LARCs in the immediate post-abortion period (OR = 0.97; 95% CI: 0.43–2.12). Barriers to the use of LARCs were anxiety relating to impaired future fertility (56.2%), LARCs being harmful to health (45.2%), irregular bleeding (44.3%), risk of IUD failure (41.6%) and lack of awareness with respect to LARCs (36.1%).

Conclusions: Intention to use LARCs was predicted by marital status, frequency of sexual activity, number of children, planned timing of next pregnancy, and previous LARC use. Impaired future fertility, being harmful to health, irregular bleeding, risk of complications, and lack of awareness with regards to LARCs were the main barriers in their potential use.

Keywords: Long acting reversible contraception, Intrauterine devices, Implants, Induced abortion, Intention, Barriers

* Correspondence: gaoll@mail.sysu.edu.cn
[2]School of Nursing, Sun Yat-sen University, 74#, Zhongshan Road II, Guangzhou 510089, China
Full list of author information is available at the end of the article

Plain English summary

Long-acting reversible contraceptives (LARCs) are the most cost-effective contraceptives for the prevention of unintended pregnancies, and the use of these medications during the post-abortion period reduces the rate of repeat abortions. However, the willingness of women to use LARCs during the post-abortion period remains uncertain; intentions and potential barriers to their use therefore require further investigation. This study explores the intentions and barriers to the use of LARC in the post-abortion period among pregnant women seeking abortion in mainland China.

Information was collected using a field questionnaire survey by convenience sampling methods. The survey contained 18 questions including socio-demographic information, sexual and reproductive health history, awareness, experience, intention, and barriers to use for each type of LARC in the immediate post-abortion period.

Of the 381 women seeking abortion with unintended pregnancy, approximately 42.5% were interested in using LARCs during the post-abortion period. 35.2% intended to use intra-uterine device (IUDs), while nearly 13.9% of the women intended to use the implant method during the post-abortion period, which suggested that this cohort of women preferred IUDs over implants. Intention to use LARCs was predicted by marital status, frequency of sexual activity, number of children, planned timing of the next pregnancy, and previous LARC use. Impaired future fertility, being harmful to health, irregular bleeding, risk of complications, and lack of awareness were the main barriers to the use of LARC. In order to increase access to LARCs in order to reduce unintended pregnancies in women, education and communication should focus on alleviating barriers to the use of LARCs.

Background

Unintended pregnancy is an important public health challenge cross the world, as well as in mainland China. Unintended pregnancy has negative effects on the health of the mother and baby, leading to a sizeable, and potentially avoidable, cost burden [1]. According to the Chinese 'health and family planning statistics annual publication' (2014), unintended pregnancy results in 6.62 million abortions in mainland China [2]. Moreover, the rate of repeat induced abortions due to unintended pregnancies is also high in mainland China, with nearly half of the women seeking abortion having had at least one previous induced abortion [3]. Unintended pregnancy usually occurs due to contraceptive issues including emergency contraception failure (33.1%), incorrect use of contraception or a lack of condoms (28.6%) and use of the rhythm method (21.9%). Short-term family planning methods are less effective, and have a higher risk of contraceptive failure [4].

Long-acting reversible contraceptives (LARCs) are a type of contraceptive that is easily reversed and do not rely on the user to maintain efficacy for at least three years. Typical examples include intra-uterine devices (IUDs) and implants [5]. These are user-independent and exhibit higher compliance than short-acting methods [6]. Almost all women of reproductive-age who use LARCs can return to a fertile state, as the effects are reversible [5]. The mean time until return to fertility following the use of implants or IUDs is within days of cessation; faster than all progestogen-only oral contraceptives [5]. Trussell and Hassan et al. conducted a study to estimate the relative costs of short-acting reversible methods and LARC methods, and reported that LARCs were more cost-effective than short-acting reversible methods such as oral contraceptives, the ring, the patch, or injections over a three-year period [7]. The American College of Obstetricians recommends LARCs as an effective method with which to reduce the risk of unintended pregnancy and abortion [8].

Previous evidence has also shown that the use of LARCs during the post-abortion period reduces repeat abortion rates [9, 10]. However, LARC methods have been under-utilized during the immediate post-abortion period in mainland China [11, 12]. To provide a wider choice of more effective methods, and to encourage the continuation of this method, it is important to understand the intentions and barriers to LARC use in women seeking abortion, so that effective counseling practices and promotional policies can be implemented. However, little is known about the intentions and barriers to LARC use in Chinese women seeking abortion. Thus, the present study explored the intentions for LARC use and the factors associated with contraceptive choices among women with unintended pregnancy and seeking abortion in mainland China. Barriers to LARC use in the immediate post-abortion period were also identified.

Methods

Study design and setting

A cross-sectional study was carried out between July and December 2015 in Guangzhou, a sub-provincial city located in Southeastern China. Guangzhou is the capital of the Guangdong Province, and has a population of approximately 16 million [13]. In Guangzhou, the sex ratio is 109.5 male for every 100 female; 68.6% of women in this region are of reproductive age (15–50 years old) [14]. The total number of health care institutions in Guangzhou is approximately 3749, including 165 hospitals and 16 maternity and child-care centers,. These institutions provide very similar family planning services [15] which are guided by the Post-abortion Care Consortium in May 2002 [16]. One hospital was randomly selected for the present study on the basis that it would provide a sufficient sample size.

The study hospital was A-level, has over 3000 beds and provides leading services for post-abortion care in mainland China. The eligible criteria for inclusion in the study were women seeking artificial abortion due to an unintended pregnancy and not having a diagnosed cognitive impairment. Participants received no incentives for participation in this study. Sample size was calculated using the modified Kish-Leslie formula [17].; this calculation told us that we required a sample of 363 women, based on 95% confidence intervals, 5% precision and the 38.2% prevalence of induced abortion in Guangzhou [18].

Data collection

Ethical approval was obtained from the study hospital. A trained research assistant (RA), who was a masters student majoring in Nursing, was responsible for collecting data. All eligible subjects who were waiting for their appointments at the abortion clinic of the study hospital were invited to participate in the study. The RA explained details of the purpose and procedure of the study to the women. All women who provided informed written consent were asked to fill in questionnaires in an interview room. The RA remained in the vicinity to answer questions and personally collect the returned questionnaires. A total of 399 women were approached, of whom 381 completed the questionnaires.

Measures

The immediate post-abortion period was defined as the period of time after undergoing medical or surgical abortion, but before resuming intercourse. LARC referred to the use of either implants or IUD contraceptives.

An 18-item questionnaire was used to collect data. Firstly, the definition of *"intention to use a LARC"* was described as *"intending to use either IUDs or implants in the immediate post-abortion period"*. Subsequently, women were asked whether they intended to use a LARC (Yes or No). Typical questions were *"Would you like to use an intra-uterine device for contraception in the immediate post-abortion period?"* and *"Would you like to use an implant for contraception in the immediate post-abortion period?"*. In addition, one question investigated personal barriers to the use of LARC. Women were asked to select as many factors as possible from a list of 20 that they perceived as barriers to their use of a LARC. In addition, 5 questions were included which pertained to socio-demographic characteristics including age, marital status, educational level, monthly income and occupation. Six questions referred to sexual and reproductive health history, and subjects were asked questions relating to intercourse frequency, contraceptive use, previous abortions, time from the latest abortion until present, number of children, and expected timing of the next pregnancy. Four questions also referred to awareness and experience regarding the use of any type of LARC.

The 18-item survey questionnaire was based on a comprehensive review of the literature relating to LARCs [19–25]. After the questionnaire was developed, it was reviewed for content validity by four obstetricians and five midwives. These experts provided written feedback on the clarity and relevance of the questionnaire but were not requested to provide a quantitative rating for each item. No item was revised. Before the investigation, the questionnaire was piloted with 10 women seeking abortion in this hospital. All women could understand and complete the questionnaire easily, so no changes were required. The 4-week test–retest correlation for the questionnaire was 0.93.

Statistical analyses

The Statistical Package for Social Sciences (SPSS) v20.0 was used for all data entry and analyses. Descriptive statistics summarized the socio-demographic characteristics of the participants, as well as sexual and reproductive health histories, awareness, experience and intention to use LARCs. Differences in the rate of the women's intention to use LARCs among groups with different socio-demographic and reproductive characteristics were computed using the chi-square test. Variables identified as being significant ($p < 0.05$) in these initial tests were then entered into a logistic regression model to determine predictors of the women's intention to use a LARC in the post-abortion period.

Results

Socio-demographic characteristics

Table 1 presents the demographic information of our participants. Almost all women (95.5%) were of Han ancestry with a mean age of 26.9 ± 5.7 years. More than half of the participants (55.6%) had at least a junior college education. The majority (85.0%) were employed and approximately half (50.4%) were single, had personal monthly incomes over 4000 RMB (60.9%), and had intercourse at least once a week (61.9%). Nearly half of the participants (45.1%) had a previous induced abortion, about one-third (28.3%) had a one-year interval from the latest abortion until present, 44.6% had at least one child, and 47.5% of the participants did not want any further children, at least for the next two years.

Awareness, experience and intention to use a LARC

The majority of participants (93.4%) had previous contraceptive experiences. Although the majority of women (88.7%) were aware of LARCs, few (8.4%) had

Table 1 Socio-demographic and reproductive characteristics of participants ($n = 381$)

Variable	Frequency f (%)
Age (years)[a]	
16–19	20 (5.2)
20–29	254 (66.7)
30–44	107 (28.1)
Marital status	
Married	189 (49.6)
Single	192 (50.4)
Level of education	
Junior high school or below	79 (20.7)
Middle special / senior high school	90 (23.6)
Junior college	111 (29.1)
College graduate or higher	101 (26.5)
Monthly income	
<4000 ¥	149 (39.1)
4000–7999 ¥	196 (51.4)
≥ 8000 ¥	36 (9.5)
Occupation	
Unemployed	57 (15.0)
Employed	324 (85.0)
Reproductive characteristics	
Frequency of intercourse	
At least one time per week	236 (61.9)
< 4 times per month	125 (32.8)
< 1 time per month	20 (5.2)
Have used contraception	
No	25 (6.6)
Yes	227 (93.4)
Have previously had an abortion	
No	207 (54.8)
Yes	172(45.7)
Interval between last two abortions ($n = 172$, months)	
< 6 months	23 (13.4)
6–11 months	26 (15.1)
≥ 12 months	123 (71.5)
Number of children	
0	211 (55.4)
1	111 (29.1)
≥ 2	59 (15.5)
Expected timing of next pregnancy (years)	
< 2 years	160 (42.0)
≥ 2 years	118 (31.0)
Do not want more children	63 (16.5)
Unknown	40 (10.5)

[a]Mean (SD) = 26.87 (5.70) years

previous experience using a LARC (7.8% had used IUDs and 1.1% had used implants). Less than half of the women (42.5%) intended to use a LARC during the post-abortion period, with 35.2 and 13.9% intending to use IUDs and implants, respectively (Table 2).

Predicting the intention of Chinese women to use a LARC

Women were more likely to intend to use a LARC during the post-abortion period if they were married, had a greater frequency of sexual activity, had more than one child, had not planned pregnancy within 2 years or had previously used a LARC ($\chi^2 = 11.89$, $p < 0.01$; $\chi^2 = 6.63$, $p = 0.04$; $\chi^2 = 20.87$, $p < 0.01$; $\chi^2 = 11.83$, $p < 0.01$; $\chi^2 = 7.63$, $p < 0.01$) (Table 3).

Variables that had significant correlation with a woman's intention to use a LARC were retained in a subsequent logistic regression model. A best-fit regression model indicated that marital status, intercourse frequency, number of live children, planned timing of next pregnancy and previous LARC use were all significant predictors of a woman's intention to use a LARC during the post-abortion period (Table 4).

Barriers to the use of LARCs during the immediate post-abortion period

Participants without intention to use a LARC during the post-abortion period ($n = 219$) were asked to report their perceived barriers to the use of LARCs. The barriers among this group varied. The most frequently mentioned

Table 2 Relationship with the use of LARCs during the immediate post-abortion period among Chinese women with unintended pregnancy seeking abortions ($n = 381$)

Item	Frequency f (%)
Are aware of LARC	
No	43 (11.3)
Yes	338 (88.7)
IUDs	338 (88.7)
Implants	50 (13.9)
Implants and IUDs	50 (13.9)
Previous LARC use	
No	349 (91.6)
Yes	32 (8.4)
IUDs	28 (7.8)
Implants	4 (1.1)
Intended to use LARC in immediate post-abortion period	
No	219 (57.5)
Yes	162 (42.5)
IUDs	134 (35.2)
Implants	53 (13.9)
Implants or IUDs	25 (6.6)

Table 3 Associations between demographic/reproductive factors and an intention to use LARCs within women with unintended pregnancy during the post-abortion period ($n = 381$)

	Intended to use LARC ($n = 162$) *f (%)*	No intended to use LARC ($n = 219$) *f (%)*	χ^2	*P*
Age (years)			4.02	0.13
16–19	7 (4.3)	13 (5.9)		
20–29	101 (62.3)	153 (69.9)		
30–44	54 (33.3)	53 (24.2)		
Marital status			11.89	**0.01****
Married	97 (59.9)	92 (42.0)		
Single	65 (40.1)	127 (58.0)		
Level of education			3.40	0.26
Junior high school or below	41 (25.3)	38 (17.4)		
Middle special/senior high school	38 (23.5)	52 (23.7)		
Junior college	42 (25.9)	69 (31.5)		
College graduate or higher	41 (25.3)	60 (27.4)		
Personal monthly income (RMB)			0.12	0.94
< 4000	65 (40.1)	84 (38.4)		
4000–7999	82 (50.6)	114 (52.1)		
≥ 8000	15 (9.3)	21 (9.6)		
Occupation			1.20	0.27
Unemployed	28 (17.3)	29 (13.2)		
Employed	134 (82.7)	190 (86.8)		
Reproductive characteristics				
Frequency of sexual activity			6.63	**0.04***
At least once a week	110 (67.9)	126 (57.5)		
< 4 times per month	48 (29.6)	77 (35.2)		
< 1 time per month	4 (2.5)	16 (7.3)		
Has used a contraceptive			2.31	0.13
No	7 (1.3)	18 (8.2)		
Yes	155 (95.7)	201 (91.8)		
Has had an abortion			2.68	0.10
No	81 (50.0)	128 (58.4)		
Yes	81 (50.0)	91 (41.6)		
Interval between last two abortions (n = 172, months)			0.89	0.64
< 6 months	12 (12.9)	11 (13.9)		
6–11 months	12 (12.9)	14 (17.7)		
≥ 12 months	69 (74.2)	54 (68.4)		
Number of children			20.87	**0.01****
0	78 (48.1)	133 (60.7)		
1	43 (26.5)	68 (31.1)		
≥ 2	41 (25.3)	18 (8.2)		
Expected timing of next pregnancy (years)			11.83	**0.01****
< 2 years	54 (33.3)	106 (48.4)		
≥ 2 years	56 (34.6)	62 (28.3)		
Does not want more children	36 (22.2)	27 (12.3)		

Table 3 Associations between demographic/reproductive factors and an intention to use LARCs within women with unintended pregnancy during the post-abortion period ($n = 381$) *(Continued)*

	Intended to use LARC ($n = 162$) *f (%)*	No intended to use LARC ($n = 219$) *f (%)*	χ^2	*P*
Unknown	16 (9.9)	24 (11.0)		
Aware of LARC			0.01	0.93
Yes	144 (88.9)	194 (88.6)		
No	18 (11.1)	25 (11.4)		
Previous LARC use			7.63	**0.01****
Yes	21 (13.0)	11 (5.0)		
No	141 (87.0)	208 (95.0)		

**statistically significant by χ^2 or t tests with $p < 0.05$*
*** statistically significant by χ^2 or t test with $p < 0.01$*

barrier was "worry about future fertility" (56.2%). Additionally, participants reported the following: "fear of harm to health" (45.2%), "concern about irregular bleeding or spotting" (44.6%), "anxiety about IUD-related reproductive tract infections, movement, or loss of the device" (44.3%), "lack of awareness about LARC", "fear of pain" (33.3%), and "the process to insert or remove IUDs is tedious" (23.7%; Table 5).

Table 4 Factors associated with an intention to use LARCs among women with unintended pregnancies seeking abortions ($n = 381$)

Socio-demographic characteristics	Intended to use LARC *OR (95% CI)*	*P*
Marital status		
Married	1.57 (1.00–2.47)	0.05
Single	1	
Frequency of sexual activity		
At least once per week	3.34 (1.03–10.78)	**0.04***
< 4 times per month	2.34 (0.71–7.71)	0.16
< 1 time per month	1	
Number of children		
0	0.29 (0.13–0.68)	**0.01****
1	0.32 (0.15–0.47)	**0.01****
≥ 2	1	
Expected timing of next pregnancy (years)		
< 2 years	0.97 (0.43–2.12)	0.94
≥ 2 years	1.79 (0.80–4.01)	0.15
Does not want more children	1.18 (0.48–2.88)	1.18
Unknown	1	
Previous LARC use		
Yes	2.41 (1.06–5.47)	**0.04***
No	1	

*statistically significant AOR with $p < 0.05$
**statistically significant AOR with $p < 0.01$

Discussion

This study identified that only around two-fifths of Chinese women seeking abortion were interested in using a LARC. One-third intended to use IUDs, while only one in seven intended to use the implant method during the post-abortion period. These findings were consistent with a previous study conducted in China [26], which suggested that consultation may enhance access to LARCs. Wei and Liu [26] found that only 11.1 and 1.8% of women seeking abortion chose IUDs and contraceptive implants during the immediate post-abortion period prior to consultation with health professionals. After consultation, the intended use of IUDs and implants increased to 19.7 and 2.7%, respectively.

The findings of the present study also indicated that women seeking abortion preferred IUDs to contraceptive implants. The one-child policy was introduced to control population in mainland China in 1979 [27]; however, since 2016, women in mainland China have been allowed to give birth to two children. During the period in which the one-Child policy was enforced, immediate post-placental insertion of an IUD was practiced as part of the standard care package received by all women following the birth of their first child [28]. This may have led to a high general level of acceptance of IUDs in China, while implants were relatively less known or under-used [26, 29].

Frequency of intercourse, marital status, number of living children, previous LARC use and excepted timing of next pregnancy were all shown to be significant predictors of a woman's intention to use a LARC. In contemporary mainland China, having sex before marriage is widely accepted among unmarried Chinese women, and this cohort showed a high intercourse frequency, as well as a high rate of induced abortion [30]. Research has also shown that the rate of IUD use among unmarried women is low (6304, 7.42%) [31] and that the majority of these women use short-acting contraceptives after abortion instead of LARCs [12]. However, post-placental

Table 5 Potential barriers among women who do not intend to use LARC during the post-abortion period ($n = 219$)

Women's perceptions	f(%)	Rank by frequency
Worry about future fertility	123 (56.2)	1
Fear of harm to health	99 (45.2)	2
Worried about irregular bleeding or spotting	97 (44.3)	3
Fear of complications such as pregnancy with IUDs, reproductive tract infections, movement, or loss from uterus	91 (41.6)	4
Lack of awareness about LARC	79 (36.1)	5
Fear of pain	73 (33.3)	6
Process to insert or remove IUDs is tedious[a]	52 (23.7)	8
Fear of the surgical process of insertion or removal	51 (23.3)	7
Might cause abnormal menstruation	48 (21.9)	8
Performance without hormones	45 (20.5)	9
Friends or relatives have had bad experiences with LARC	26 (11.9)	10
Worried about weight gain	17 (7.8)	11
Too expensive	10 (4.6)	12
Have not been in a long-term relationship	9 (4.1)	13
Partner opposed to it	9 (4.1)	13
Prevented by religion from using the method	5 (2.3)	14
Have another satisfying method of contraception	3 (1.4)	15
Ineligible for the method because of being single	3 (1.4)	15
Unsure of future family plan	2 (0.9)	16

[a]For instance, if a Procreation Certificate is needed, then one must go to a health care provider to have the device inserted or removed

insertion of an IUD is usually recommended to married women by health professionals [32]. The use of LARCs during the immediate post-abortion period is not the standard form of care. This indicates that LARCs might be under-utilized among unmarried women who have a high frequency of intercourse, and it is therefore important to address the barriers to LARC usage among unmarried women with high intercourse frequency and to promote its use among this group in order to reduce the risk of unintended pregnancy and repeated induced abortion.

Furthermore, the present study found that women with no or only one child, or planned to have a child within two years were found to have less intent to use a LARC. A previous study by Fleming and Sokoloff also showed that women with more than one child were more likely to be interested in using IUDs than nulliparous women [22]. A study conducted by Anguzu and Tweheyo similarly indicated that women who had living children were 1.5-times more likely to use a LARC compared to nulliparous women [20].

Previous LARC use was associated with whether participants were interested in LARC use in the post-abortion period. Evidence indicated that LARC users had a high degree of satisfaction with respect to this type of contraceptive [33]. Women who had previously used LARCs were 1.49-times more likely to intend to use a LARC [34].

Finally, this study indicated that barriers to the use of LARCs during the immediate post-abortion period included "worry about future fertility", "fear of harm to health", "may cause irregular bleeding", "fear of complications", and "lack of awareness about the methods". A previous study indicated that because women believed that LARC use would negatively impact upon their future fertility, they did not choose a LARC [35]. We similarly found that worry about future fertility was the main reason that women seeking abortion did not intend to use a LARC in the immediate post-abortion period. It is obvious that worries about the risk and side effects of LARCs was one of the main reasons preventing women from using LARCs. A study that surveyed women aged 16 to 25 years showed that factors influencing contraceptive technology choices included "familiarity with the methods", "whether or not the method contained hormones", "likely effect on periods", and "other side effects" [36]. A population of women who desired sterilization also had concerns about the side effects of LARCs [21].

Another barrier was a lack of awareness with regards to these methods. An internet-based study of 1982 female undergraduates at a large mid-western university in the United States found that lack of education about LARCs was the primary reason participants rejected this method [37]. Whitaker et al. [23] found that women aged 14–24 were likely to have positive attitudes around

IUD methods after undergoing a three-minute educational intervention, suggesting that such interventions may improve positive attitudes towards LARC use among women seeking abortions [9]. There remain many myths regarding the use of LARCs, particularly regarding its potential effect on future fertility, which may prevent women of reproductive age using it to avoid unwanted pregnancy [38]. In order to help women to make informed decisions, health care professionals should pay significant attention to providing women with information relating to LARCs, especially with regards to alleviating the barriers.

Our study has some limitations which should be taken into consideration. Firstly, this investigation was conducted in only one hospital and most participants were employed women of Han ancestry. These findings may not therefore be representative of other settings or apply to those who are not of Han ancestry or are unemployed. In addition, this study relied upon a questionnaire that relied upon self-reporting by the respondents. Thus, there was the potential for recall bias in these data. Finally, adding qualitative study questions could provide additional insights into these findings in future research.

Conclusions

This study has significant clinical utility for health care professionals working with Chinese women seeking abortion. To identify women seeking abortion who intend not to use LARCs, health care professionals should asses their marital status, frequency of sexual activity, number of children, planned timing of the next pregnancy, and previous LARC use.

Impaired future fertility, being harmful to health, irregular bleeding risk of IUD failure and lack of awareness with regards to LARCs were the main barriers to LARC use. It is important to promote the use of LARCs among unmarried Chinese women; particularly during the post-abortion period to reduce the risk of unintended pregnancy and repeated induced abortion. Health care professionals could develop strategies to enhance women's intentions to use LARCs, such as providing information to alleviate the barriers to LARC use.

Acknowledgments
The authors thank the Department of Post-Abortion Care (PAC) outpatient services of the Third Affiliated Hospital of Sun Yat-sen University for assistance with participant recruitment.

Funding
This study did not receive any specific grant from funding agencies in the public, commercial, or not-for-profit sectors.

Authors' contributions
LZ conceptualized and designed the article, implemented result analysis and explanation, and was a major contributor in writing the manuscript. GL was responsible for quality control and reviewing the articles, critically revised all manuscript drafts, and generally managed the article. RA critically revised all manuscript drafts. ZJ analyzed and interpreted patient data. All authors read and approved the final manuscript.

Competing interests
The authors declare that they have no competing interests.

Author details
[1]Nursing Department, Guizhou Provincial People's Hospital, Guiyang, China. [2]School of Nursing, Sun Yat-sen University, 74#, Zhongshan Road II, Guangzhou 510089, China. [3]School of Public Health, Makerere University, Kampala city, Uganda.

References

1. Trussell J, Henry N, Hassan F, Prezioso A, Law A, Filonenko A. Burden of unintended pregnancy in the United States: potential savings with increased use of long-acting reversible contraception. Contraception. 2012; https://doi.org/10.1016/j.contraception.2012.07.016.
2. National Health And Family Commission. China health and family planning statistical yearbook, vol. 2015. BeiJing: China Union Medical University Press; 2015. p. 225–6.
3. Guo P, Liu Y, Tang F, Yang Y, Li P, Wang W. Analysis of current status of artificial abortion of 2956 cases and the evaluation of the effect of post-abortion care in female reproductive health. Chin Gen Prac. 2016; https://doi.org/10.3969/j.issn.1007-9572.2016.24.023. [In Chinese]
4. Wang Y, Yang Q. Changes in the high-risk factors of induced abortion in 2003 and 2013. J Chin Med Univ. 2015; https://doi.org/10.3969/j.issn.0258-4646.2015.11.018. [In Chinese]
5. Kolman KB, Hadley SK, Jordahliafrato MA. Long-acting reversible contraception: who, what, when, and how. J Fam Pract. 2015;64:479–84.
6. Lotke PS. Increasing use of long-acting reversible contraception to decrease unplanned pregnancy. Obstet Gynecol Clin N Am. 2015; https://doi.org/10.1016/j.ogc.2015.07.008.
7. Trussell J, Hassan F, Lowin J, Law A, Filonenko A. Achieving cost-neutrality with long-acting reversible contraceptive methods. Contraception. 2015; https://doi.org/10.1016/j.contraception.2014.08.011.
8. ACOG Practice Bulletin No. 121. Long-acting reversible contraception: implants and intrauterine devices. Obstet Gynecol. 2011; https://doi.org/10.1097/AOG.0b013e318227f05e.
9. Rose SB, Lawton BA. Impact of long-acting reversible contraception on return for repeat abortion. Am J Obstet Gynecol. 2012; https://doi.org/10.1016/j.ajog.2011.06.102.
10. Kilander H, Alehagen S, Svedlund L, Westlund K, Thor J, Brynhildsen J. Likelihood of repeat abortion in a Swedish cohort according to the choice of post-abortion contraception: a longitudinal study. Acta Obstet Gynecol Scand. 2016; https://doi.org/10.1111/aogs.12874.
11. Zhong Y, Huang Z. Analysis and following-up study of 1450 cases of women who received post-abortion care. Reprod Contracept. 2014; https://doi.org/10.7669/j.issn.0253-357X.2014.04.0334. [In Chinese].
12. Wu X. Current situation analysis of contraception after abortion due to unintended pregnancy in unmarried women in Enping City[J]. China Modern Med. 2017;7:158–60. [In Chinese]
13. Guangzhou Bureau Of Statistics: The population scale and population distribution of Guangzhou in 2015. 2016. http://www.gzstats.gov.cn/tjgb/qtgb/201611/t20161108_24979.html. Accessed 12 Sept 2017.

14. Guangzhou Bureau Of Statistics: Census assembly, the sixth census in Guangzhou. 2013. http://www.gzstats.gov.cn/pchb/dlcrkpc/. Accessed 12 Sept 2017.
15. Guangzhou Bureau Of Statistics: 2016 Guangzhou Statistical Yearbook,Number of Health Institutions. 2016. http://data.gzstats.gov.cn/gzStat1/chaxun/njsj.jsp/. Accessed 12 September 2017.
16. Corbett MR, Turner KL. Essential elements of postabortion care: origins, evolution and future directions. Int Fam Plan Perspect. 2003; https://doi.org/10.1363/ifpp.29.106.03.
17. Kish L. Sampling organizations and groups of sizes. Am Sociol Rev. 1965;30:564–72.
18. Song X, Ma Y, Zuo L, Xu Y, Ling L. Status and influencing factors of induced abortion among childbearing women with different household registration in Guangzhou. Chin J Fam. 2013; https://doi.org/10.3969/j.issn.1004-8189.2013.11. [In Chinese]
19. Potter J, Rubin SE, Sherman P. Fear of intrauterine contraception among adolescents in new York City. Contraception. 2014; https://doi.org/10.1016/j.contraception.2014.01.011.
20. Anguzu R, Tweheyo R, Sekandi JN, Zalwango V, Muhumuza C, Tusiime S, et al. Knowledge and attitudes towards use of long acting reversible contraceptives among women of reproductive age in Lubaga division, Kampala district, Uganda. BMC Res Notes. 2014; https://doi.org/10.1186/1756-0500-7-153.
21. White K, Hopkins K, Potter JE, Grossman D. Knowledge and attitudes about long-acting reversible contraception among Latina women who desire sterilization. Womens Health Issues. 2013; https://doi.org/10.1016/j.whi.2013.05.001.
22. Fleming KL, Sokoloff A, Raine TR. Attitudes and beliefs about the intrauterine device among teenagers and young women. Contraception. 2010; https://doi.org/10.1016/j.contraception.2010.02.020.
23. Whitaker AK, Johnson LM, Harwood B, Chiappetta L, Creinin MD, Gold MA. Adolescent and young adult women's knowledge of and attitudes toward the intrauterine device. Contraception. 2009; https://doi.org/10.1016/j.contraception.2008.04.119.
24. Mekonnen G, Enquselassie F, Tesfaye G, et al. Prevalence and factors affecting use of long acting and permanent contraceptive methods in Jinka town, Southern Ethiopia: a cross sectional study[J]. Pan Afr Med J. 2014; https://doi.org/10.11604/pamj.2014.18.98.3421.
25. Burns B, Grindlay K, Dennis A. Women's awareness of, interest in, and experiences with long-acting reversible and permanent contraception[J]. Women's Health Issues. 2015; https://doi.org/10.1016/j.whi.2014.12.006.
26. Wei Z, Liu H. Influence of informed choice on induced abortion. Reprod Contracept. 2009;29:264–8. [In Chinese]
27. Yang X, Gao LL, Ip WY, Sally Chan WC. Predictors of breastfeeding self-efficacy in the immediate postpartum period: a cross-sectional study[J]. Midwifery. 2016; https://doi.org/10.1016/j.midw.2016.07.011.
28. Xu JX, Connell C, Chi IC. Immediate postpartum intrauterine device insertion-a report on the Chinese experience[J]. Adv Contracept. 1992;8(4):281–90.
29. Pan Y, Che Y, Zhu H, Shen J, Lu Z, Lu M. Intrauterine device utilization of married women of childbearing age in shanghai during 2004-2012. Reprod Contracept. 2015; https://doi.org/10.7669/j.issn.0253-357X.2015.04.0259. [In Chinese]
30. Xiao Y, Mao Z, Liu L, Yang Y, Zhu H. Analysis on reason of induced abortion of 569 unmarried female. Matern Child Health Care China. 2007; https://doi.org/10.3969/j.issn.1001-4411.2007.28.034. [In Chinese]
31. Zhao H. Current Status of Family Planning/Reproductive Health and Evaluation of Quality of Care among Internal Migrants in Three Chinese Large Cities. Shanghai: Fudan University; 2011. [Dissertation in Chinese]
32. Liu Y. Situation and trend of contraceptive use among reproductive aged women in China[J]. Chin J Fam Plann. 2014; https://doi.org/10.3969/j.issn.1004-8189.2004.05.001.
33. Diedrich JT, Desai S, Zhao Q, Secura G, Madden T, Peipert JF. Association of short-term bleeding and cramping patterns with long-acting reversible contraceptive method satisfaction. Am J Obstet Gynecol. 2015; https://doi.org/10.1016/j.ajog.2014.07.025.
34. Dassah ET, Odoi AT, Owusuasubonteng G. Prevalence and factors predictive of long-acting reversible contraceptive use in a tertiary hospital in urban Ghana. Eur J Contracept Reprod Health Care. 2013; https://doi.org/10.3109/13625187.2013.790951.
35. Bracken J, Graham CA. Young women's attitudes towards, and experiences of, long-acting reversible contraceptives. Eur J Contracept Reprod Health Care. 2014; https://doi.org/10.3109/13625187.2014.917623.
36. Rose SB, Cooper AJ, Baker NK, Lawton B. Attitudes toward long-acting reversible contraception among young women seeking abortion. J Women's Health. 2011; https://doi.org/10.1089/jwh.2010.2658.
37. Hall KS, Ela E, Zochowski MK, Caldwell A, Moniz M, McAndrew L, et al. 'I don't know enough to feel comfortable using them': Women's knowledge of and perceived barriers to long-acting reversible contraceptives on a college campus. Contraception. 2016; https://doi.org/10.1016/j.contraception.2016.02.007.
38. Russo JA, Miller E, Gold MA. Myths and misconceptions about long-acting reversible contraception (LARC). J Adolesc Health. 2013; https://doi.org/10.1016/j.jadohealth.2013.02.003.

4

Long term trends in behaviour to protect against adverse reproductive and sexual health outcomes among young single African women

Mohamed M. Ali[1*] and John Cleland[2]

Abstract

Background: HIV and unintended pregnancy are major interrelated concerns in sub-Saharan Africa. Focussing on single women aged 15-24 years we assess trends in key behaviours that affect both outcomes.

Methods: We performed a secondary analysis of public-access data sets from 112 surveys from 36 countries in the region, conducted between 1991 and 2015. We examined trends over 20 years in primary abstinence (virginity), secondary abstinence (no sex in past 3 months) among sexually experienced women, current use of modern contraception and condom use at most recent coitus among sexually active women.

Results: Little change occurred in primary or secondary abstinence. Over the 20 year period, contraceptive use in the region rose from 14.7 to 33.4%, with significant increases observed in 18 of 30 countries with multiple surveys. Since 2001–2005, the proportion of contraceptive users reporting condoms as their method fell from 61.1 to 51.3%, while use of oral contraceptives or injectables rose from 19.9 to 24.0%. Between 1996 and 2000 and 2006–2010, condom use at last coitus rose from 21.3 to 40.5% but then plateaued. A strong correlation between condom use and national HIV prevalence was found. About half of condom users at last sex had earlier in interviews reported this method for pregnancy-prevention.

Conclusions: Though condoms tend to be overlooked by both HIV and family planning agencies, their contribution to the health of single women remains central. Current efforts to promote non-barrier contraceptive methods may inadvertently increase HIV risk. Condom promotion for pregnancy-prevention should be re-invigorated by social marketing campaigns and other means.

Plain English summary

Using data from 112 surveys conducted in 36 countries, we examine trends over the past 20 years in behaviours that protect against pregnancy and sexually transmitted infections. We focus on single women aged 15 to 24 years living in sub-Saharan Africa. About half of these young women reported no experience of sexual intercourse (ie virginity). Sexual encounters are infrequent for many: among non-virgins, only about half had sex in the 3 months before they were interviewed. Abstinence is clearly a major form of protection but has changed little over the 20 year period, suggesting that campaigns to promote it as a primary defence against HIV were largely ineffective. Trends in current use of contraception and condom use at most recent sex are encouraging. In 2011–5, one-third of women with sexual activity in the past 3 months said that they were using a contraceptive method and 42% reported using a condom at last sex. The proportion of contraceptive users relying on condoms has recently dipped from 61 to 51% while those relying on pills or injectables grew to 24%. We conclude that condoms remain the optimal method of contraception for young women for whom sex is infrequent and loving in localities the risk of infection is high. We call for a re-invigoration of condom social marketing. While non-barrier contraceptive methods are appropriate

* Correspondence: alim@who.int
[1]UNDP-UNFPA-UNICEF-WHO-World Bank Special Programme of Research, Development and Research Training in Human Reproduction (HRP), World Health Organization, 20 Avenue Appia, 1211 Geneva, Switzerland

for single women in more committed and intimate relationships, promotion should be cautious because their high contraceptive effectiveness has to be balanced against their lack of protection against infection.

Background

The health of young people, aged 15-24 years, has become a global priority, as demonstrated by the UN's Global Strategy for Women's, Children's and Adolescent's Health [1], reports from the UN Population Fund [2], the creation of a Lancet Commission in 2012, and innumerable other international declarations. Prominent among concerns are reproductive and sexual health, particularly in sub-Saharan Africa (henceforth Africa). Because of the combination of high birth rates and declining mortality, the youth population in this region is particularly large, accounting for 38% of the total. Rates of teenage childbearing and HIV/STI infections are much higher than in all other regions. Maternal mortality ratios in young women and abortion rates in unmarried women are estimated to be higher in Africa than elsewhere and, because of restrictive laws, many abortions are unsafe [3, 4].

A very large literature has accumulated on the reproductive and sexual health, and associated behaviour, of young women in Africa. Age at first marriage, or cohabitation, has increased [5, 6]. Age at first birth has also risen, due in large measure to improvements in girls' schooling [7]. The level of premarital sex has risen despite a trend towards delayed sexual debut [7, 8]. In some countries premarital childbearing has increased while in others it has declined or remained unchanged [5]. Contraceptive use among sexually active unmarried teenagers has increased though contraceptive failure and discontinuation are more common in this group than among older women [9]. Unmet need for contraception--non-use in those wanting to avoid pregnancy-- in African adolescents remains high [10].

Trends in HIV incidence are encouraging with a 42% decline of new infections among youth in Africa between 2001 and 2013 [11]. However, young women remain at much higher risk than young men and account for 25% of all new infections in adults. Several favourable trends have contributed to this decline and relevant information is available from the electronic data base of the Demographic and Health Survey (DHS) program [12]. Reported condom use at most recent coitus among those with a recent non-cohabiting partner, or with multiple partners, has increased in many countries though the level remains unsatisfactory. The percentage of sexually active young women who received an HIV test in the past 12 months and were told the results has increased greatly in East and Southern Africa. In 14 priority countries, 11.6 million men have been circumcised [11]. DHS data confirm the upward trend in circumcision [12].

In this paper we assess behavioural change by never married African women aged 15-24 years. Specifically, we analyse trends in abstinence, current contraceptive use and condom use at most recent sex drawing on all DHSs conducted since 1991. The inclusion of information on multiple partners would have provided a more comprehensive assessment of behavioural change but we decided against it because of convincing evidence that this information is particularly unreliable [13]. Our paper complements the extensive existing literature in several ways. First, we present a clear chronological record of change, starting with data from 1991 to 1995 and ending with the most recent quinquennium, 2011–2015. Second, we pay equal attention to pregnancy- and HIV-prevention in contrast to most publications that focus on only one of these intertwined behaviours. Third we examine changes in type of contraceptive method used and in double method protection. Fourth, we estimate the effect of structural shifts in the study population over the 20 year period, namely age, education and rural-urban residence, on reported behavioural change.

Methods

The main methods used in this paper were described in an earlier publication [14]. In brief, we downloaded the individual data files from all DHSs conducted in Africa from 1991 to 2015 that are publically available on 31 December 2016. A total of 112 surveys from 36 countries were used. The analysis population comprised single (i.e. never married) women aged 15-24 years. We focussed on 4 self-reported behavioural outcomes: primary abstinence (or virginity); secondary or temporary abstinence in sexually experienced women (defined as no intercourse in the 3 months preceding the survey); current use of modern contraceptive methods among women who had been sexually active in the 3 months preceding the survey; and condom use at most recent coitus among the sexually active. We chose a 3 month boundary for secondary abstinence rather than the more commonly used 12 month definition because of doubts about the meaning of reported "current" condom use by women who have been sexually inactive for several months. Estimates of these four outcomes were calculated for denominators with 100 or more women. Sample sizes and denominators for all 112 surveys are shown in Additional file 1.

To assess trends we grouped all surveys by date of fieldwork as follows: 199 1-95, 1996–2000, 2001–05, 2006–10, and 2011–2015. The number of surveys in each 5 year period ranged from 15 in the first period to 28 in the last. Estimates from individual surveys in each period are summarised by box plots, showing medians and inter-quartile ranges (IQRs). Exact 95% CIs for the median values were calculated from the binomial distribution. We were unable to estimate condom use last coitus for the period 1991–1995, owing to insufficient number of surveys with the relevant information.

We also present country-specific results in Additional files 1, 2, 3, 4, 5, 6, 7, 8 and 9. For the 30 countries with multiple surveys, we calculated the median date of fieldwork for first and most recent survey and estimated the annual rate of change in the prevalence of each of the 4 outcomes. We assessed the significance of within-country changes using logistic regression by including a binary indicator for survey round with robust standard errors. In addition to the crude percentages, standardized percentages were also computed, using the composition of the earliest survey for each country with respect to age (in 3 year bands), place of residence, education (primary school or less versus secondary or higher) as the standard population.

To assess whether trends had been distorted by variations in the countries represented in each time period, we re-did the analyses for the 16 countries with 4 or more DHSs. The comparison, shown in Additional file 2, showed a close similarity between all-survey and multiple surveys results. The survey-normalized weights were applied to take account of variations in probabilities of selection corrected for non-response. All analyses were carried out in Stata 14.2.

Results

Abstinence

Trends in primary abstinence (virginity) were modest and irregular, ranging from 62.3% (95%CI: 57. 9-68.7) in 200 1-5 to 54.8% (95%CI: 49. 1-67.9) in 201 1-5 with no statistically significant changes (Fig. 1 and Table 1). The inter-quartile ranges (IQRs) were wide in all periods except 200 1-2005, indicating large and persistent variability between countries. Of the 30 countries with two or more surveys, significant ($p < 0.01$) increases are apparent in six, notably Madagascar and Malawi, and significant decreases in four, notably Guinea, Lesotho and Rwanda (Additional file 3).

Trends in secondary abstinence were also irregular and non-significant, ranging from 48.4% (95%CI: 42.1–62.8) to 48.4% (95%CI: 42.1–62.8) in different periods (Fig. 2 and Table 1). Statistically significant changes were apparent in only 6 countries (Additional file 3). Levels of secondary abstinence are high and, in conjunction with with primary abstinence suggest that, on average, only about 25% of young women were exposed to potential risk in the past 3 months.

Contraception

The median level of current use of a modern method of contraception among women who had sex in the past 3 months rose sharply and significantly from 14.7% (95%CI: 5.1–26.5) in the early 1990s to 33.4% (95%CI: 28. 5-46.6) in the most recent period. However, the big increase occurred between the early 1990s and the early 2000s and change since then have been modest have been modest (Fig. 3 and Table 1). A clear correlation with education only emerged in the past decade, rising to 0.64 ($p < .0001$) in the most recent quinquennium (Additional file 4). Inter-country variability changed little as indicated by the IQRs. Statistically significant increases are observed in 18 countries, and the mean annual increase exceeded 2% in Cameroon, Congo

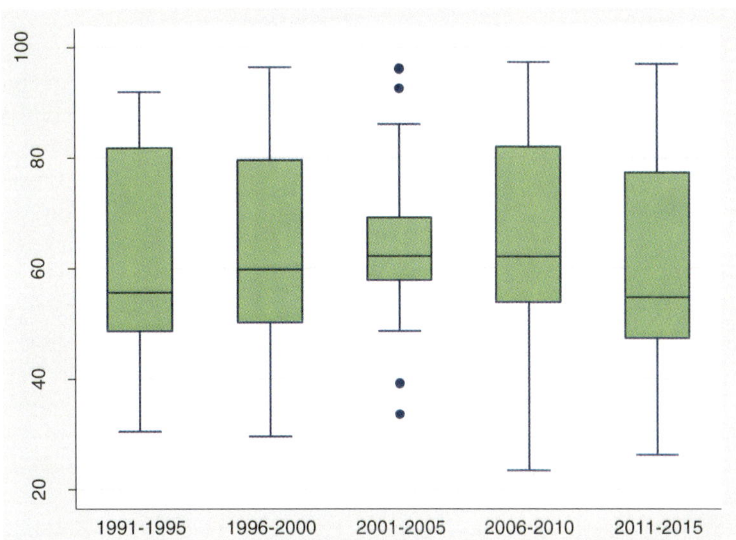

Fig. 1 Box and whisker plot showing trend (1991–2015) in the percentage of single women aged 15–24 years who reported no sexual experience

Table 1 Medians and 95%CIs for primary abstinence (virginity), secondary abstinence (no sex in past 3 months), current use of modern contraception and condom use at last sex: crude and adjusted percentages, by period

Period	No of surveys	Crude		Adjusted	
		Median	(95%, CI)	Median	(95%, CI)
Primary abstinence					
1991–1995	15	55.6	(48.8, 81.2)	55.6	(48.8, 81.2)
1996–2000	25	59.8	(52.8, 73.0)	59.8	(52.7, 72.9)
2001–2005	21	62.3	(57.9, 68.7)	62.6	(57.7, 71.4)
2006–2010	23	62.1	(54.3, 73.2)	61.0	(56.9, 77.2)
2011–2015	28	54.8	(49.1, 67.9)	58.4	(51.7, 68.6)
Secondary abstinence					
1991–1995	15	51.1	(35.8, 58.9)	51.1	(35.8, 58.9)
1996–2000	23	38.3	(35.1, 48.7)	38.3	(35.1, 50.4)
2001–2005	21	48.4	(42.1, 62.8)	47.2	(41.8, 62.8)
2006–2010	22	44.6	(41.7, 60.3)	45.4	(41.5, 60.5)
2011–2015	26	44.0	(38.7, 56.7)	44.9	(39.9, 57.1)
Current use of modern contraception					
1991–1995	11	14.7	(5.1, 26.5)	14.7	(5.1, 26.5)
1996–2000	22	23.2	(19.1, 29.9)	22.5	(16.0, 28.4)
2001–2005	17	30.2	(23.0, 42.1)	27.9	(19.7, 37.4)
2006–2010	20	31.6	(27.3, 39.6)	29.8	(21.5, 36.7)
2011–2015	24	33.4	(28.5, 46.6)	31.2	(27.0, 41.5)
Condom use last sex					
1991–1995		NE		NE	
1996–2000	21	21.3	(15.3, 26.5)	21.9	(13.2, 25.1)
2001–2005	17	33.6	(25.4, 42.5)	29.2	(26.2, 37.1)
2006–2010	20	40.5	(29.5, 50.6)	37.4	(23.9, 44.9)
2011–2015	24	41.9	(34.8, 49.7)	39.6	(29.7, 48.4)

NE Not Estimated due to few number of surveys

and Sierra Leone (Additional file 5). At the time of the most recent survey, current use of a modern method exceeded 50% in several West African countries (Cameroon, Nigeria, Sierra Leone) and several Southern African countries (Lesotho, Namibia, Republic of South Africa and Swaziland).

Examination of method-specific use, including traditional methods, revealed large temporal changes (Table 2). In 1991–1995, periodic abstinence was the most commonly reported method, accounting for 45.9% (95%CI: 20.0–69.7) of all reported use, but its contribution to protection declined sharply and monotonically over the 20 year period; in 2011–2015, the median percentage of users relying on this method was 6.4% (95%CI: 1. 4-15.0). The contribution of condoms to method-mix rose steeply from a median value of 25.9% (95%CI: 6. 2-34.0) in the early 1990s to 61.1% (95%CI: 47. 9-68.4) in 2001–2005 and 58.5% (95%CI: 45. 4-69.5) in the next quinquennium before falling to 51.3% (95%CI: 34. 8-65.9) in the most recent period. The role of oral contraceptives and injectables in contraceptive protection increased steadily, from a median value of 10.4% (95%CI: 5. 7-41.7) in the early 1990s to 24.0% (95%CI: 11.0–33.7) in the recent period. Use of long-acting methods, IUDs and implants, remained negligible.

Condoms and dual protection

The median proportion of sexually active young women who reported condom use at most recent coitus rose significantly from 21.3% (95%CI: 15. 3-26.5) in 1996–2000 to 33.6% (95%CI: 25. 4-42.5) in 2001–5 and further to 40.5% (95%CI: 29. 5-50.6) in 2006–10, with an additional smaller increase to 41.9% (95%CI: 34. 8-49.7) in 2011–15. The IQRs are generally narrower than for other outcomes. The correlation between proportions using condoms and HIV prevalence among young people ages 15-24 years increased from 0.45 ($p = 0.046$) in 1996–2000 to 0.65 ($p = 0.001$) in the most recent period (Additional file 6). In more recent surveys, a question on consistent use was asked; on average, 74% of women who used a condom at last sex reported consistent use (Additional file 7). Reported use at most recent coitus was highest in Lesotho and Namibia, both countries with severe HIV epidemics, but was also over 60% in Burkina Faso, Cameroon and Gabon (Additional file 5). A total of 15 countries recorded significant increases in condom use and, in eight of them, the mean annual increase was 2% or more (Fig. 4).

Information about contraceptive use and condom use at most recent coitus are ascertained at different times in DHS interviews and the question on condom use at last coitus makes no mention of the motive for use. Cross tabulation can thus reveal useful insights into dual method protection and consistency of reported condom use. Table 3 shows the median percentages reporting condom use at most recent coitus by contraceptive use status (no method, condoms and non-barrier method). Among women who reported no contraceptive use, the proportion who used a condom at most recent coitus rose from about 7.9% (95%CI: 4. 8-12.4) in the 1996–2000 to about 30% in the past 10 years. Among users of modern or traditional non-barrier methods, reported use of condoms also rose from 15.3% (95%CI: 11. 3-23.9) in the 1996–2000 to 30.8% (95%CI: 27. 4-36.2) in the most recent period. In all periods the proportion of those stating the use of condoms for contraception who also reported its use at most recent coitus was high, ranging from 84 to 90%.

We also examined the contraceptive status among women reporting condom use at most recent coitus (Additional file 8). The proportions using a non-barrier method of contraception were low in all periods but the proportions using no contraceptive method rose from 19.7% in 1996–2000 to 36.1% in 2011–15. The proportions

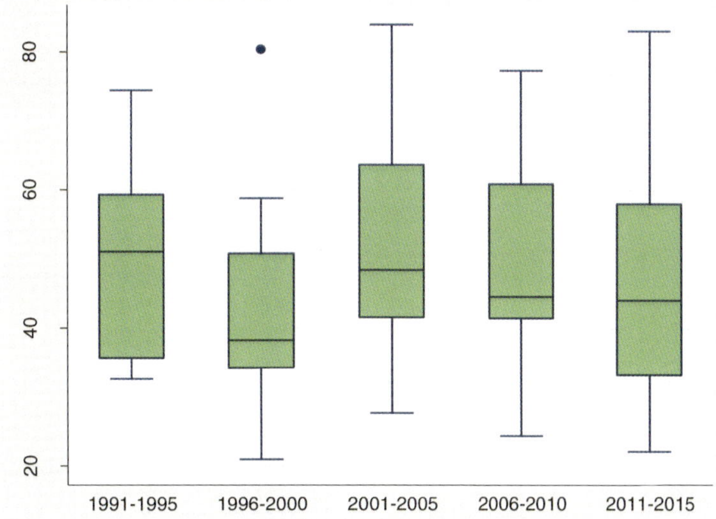

Fig. 2 Box and whisker plot showing trend (1991–2015) in the percentage of sexually experienced single women aged 15–24 years who reported no sex in the 3 months before the survey

reporting condom use for contraception fluctuated between 48 and 61%.

Country ranking by behavioural risk

We defined behavioural risk as having sex in the past 3 months without protection from any contraceptive method nor use of a condom at last sex. The proportion among all single women aged 15-24 years defined thus as at risk are shown in the left-hand columns of Additional file 9 while the right-hand columns exclude virgins. When based on all women, which includes the protective contribution of virginity, the median percent at risk was 7.5%. It was below 2% in six countries and exceeded 20% in Liberia, Cote d'Ivoire and Sierra Leone. When based on sexually experienced women, the median rose to about 20%, with the highest values found in Chad, Liberia and Mali.

Crude versus standardised results

Adjustment of results for age, education and residence makes surprisingly little difference (Table 1). With regards

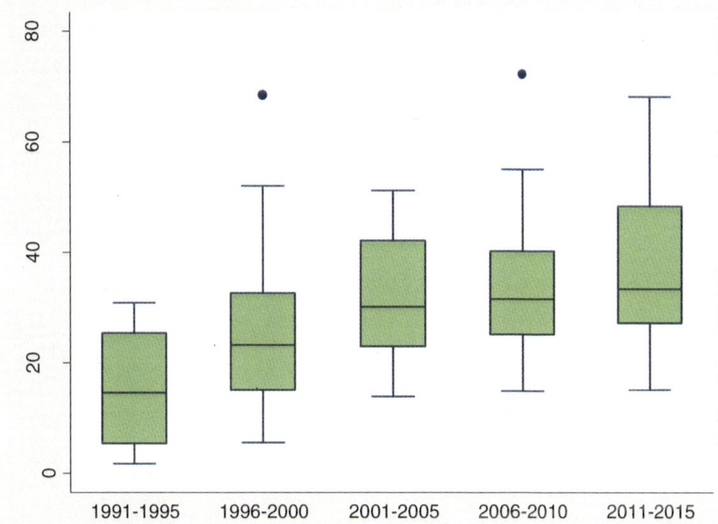

Fig. 3 Box and whisker plot showing trend (1991–2015) in percentage who reported current use of a modern contraceptive method, among single women aged 15–24 who had sex in the last 3 months

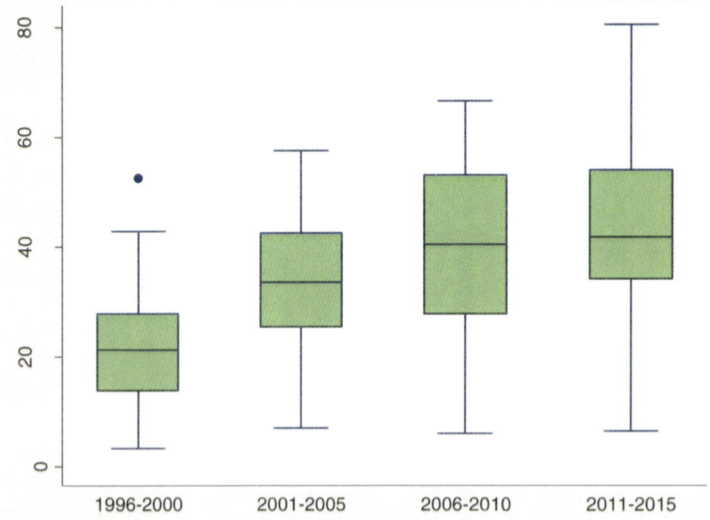

Fig. 4 Box and whisker plot showing trend (1996–2015) in percentage who reported condom use at most recent coitus among single women aged 15–24 who had sex in the last 3 months

to abstinence, the two sets of estimates are closely similar, with the single exception of virginity in the most recent period, where the estimate of 58.4% (95%CI: 51. 7-68.6) was appreciable higher than the crude figure of 54.8% (95%CI: 49. 1-67.9), but did not attain statistical significance. For contraceptive use and condom use at most recent coitus, the sharpness of upward trends was only slightly attenuated.

Discussion

The merit of this paper depends entirely on the credibility of reports by young African women on their behaviour. An extreme sceptic might claim that we have documented no more than the propensities of respondents to give socially desirable answers. We accept that the willingness of young single women to disclose sexual activity may well vary between countries. We checked the potential bias arising from this possibility by repeating the trend analysis for the sub-set of countries with 4 or more surveys but found very similar results to those based on all surveys. Reporting may also be affected by quality of interviewing and mode of data capture. We have minimized this type of uncertainty by relying on a single source, the DHS. The DHS is generally regarded as the gold standard for interview surveys in developing countries and the questions relevant to the topics of this paper are highly standardised across countries and over time.

Nevertheless, in the absence of any practical means of validating responses, interpretation of results needs to be cautious, particularly for reports of sexual behaviour; some country-specific trends are erratic and unconvincing. We are more confident about trends in use of contraceptives and condoms, which are more pronounced and regular than those for sexual abstinence.

We acknowledge a further limitation. The African countries included in this analysis are very diverse in terms of sexual norms, marriage customs, gender relations, disease environment and contraceptive practices. In presenting a regional overview, inevitably we could

Table 2 Median percentages using specific methods among current users of any method: single women aged 15-24 years, sexually active in the past 3 months

Period	Condoms	Oral contraceptives and injectables	Other modern methods	IUDs and implants	Periodic Abstinence	Other traditional methods
	Median (95% CI)	Median (95% CI)	Median (95% CI)	Median (95% CI)	Median (95% CI)	Median (95% CI)
1991–1995	25.9 (6.2, 34.0)	10.4 (5.7, 41.7)	0.3 (0.0, 1.1)	0.0 (0.0, 2.3)	45.9 (20.0, 69.7)	4.2 (1.2, 10.1)
1996–2000	35.2 (27.7, 47.7)	13.2 (10.9, 33.4)	0.0 (0.0, 0.8)	0.0 (0.0, 0.2)	25.2 (14.9, 48.3)	4.7 (2.5, 6.1)
2001–2005	61.1 (47.9, 68.4)	19.9 (12.8, 28.1)	0.4 (0.0, 0.7)	0.0 (0.0, 0.2)	14.0 (4.6, 29.0)	4.1 (1.8, 6.1)
2006–2010	58.5 (45.4, 69.5)	20.9 (15.5, 31.4)	0.4 (0.0, 1.5)	0.0 (0.0, 0.0)	4.9 (0.4, 13.2)	3.7 (1.7, 7.0)
2011–2015	51.3 (34.8, 65.9)	24.0 (11.0, 33.7)	2.4 (0.8, 9.5)	0.8 (0.0, 1.9)	6.4 (1.4, 15.0)	2.1 (1.4, 4.4)

Table 3 Median percentages of using condoms at most recent coitus, by period and current contraceptive use status

Not using any method			Condoms		Non-barrier methods	
Period	Median	(95%, CI)	Median	(95%, CI)	Median	(95%, CI)
1991–1995	NE		NE		NE	
1996–2000	7.9	(4.8, 12.4)	84.4	(77.3, 91.8)	15.3	(11.3, 23.9)
2001–2005	16.1	(9.5, 24.2)	84.1	(78.2, 92.7)	21.1	(16.3, 28.8)
2006–2010	31.5	(13.7, 34.1)	88.9	(83.3, 91.0)	21.9	(10.3, 46.2)
2011–2015	29.0	(17.8, 37.1)	88.2	(84.5, 95.5)	30.8	(27.4, 36.2)

NE Not Estimated due to few number of surveys
[Denominator: single women aged 15-24 years, sexually active in the past 3 months].

not do justice to this diversity. Country-specific results have been presented but it was beyond the scope of this paper to attempt any interpretation of varying trends.

Bearing in mind these caveats, what are the main findings and their implications? The 20 year time period covered in our analyses spans the rapid rise of HIV epidemics in many African countries, the peak incidence in the late 1990s and the subsequent fall in new infections. Despite the emphasis on abstinence of the US President's Emergency Plan for AIDS Relief (PEPFAR) since the early years of this century, we see no evidence of radical changes in sexual behaviour, though it is entirely possible that numbers of sexual partners have fallen. The reported median level of primary abstinence, or virginity, which fluctuates between 55 and 62% is similar to levels observed in Latin America, USA, UK and Australia [15]. The high level of abstinence in the past 3 months among the sexually experienced, varying from 51 to 38% in different periods, is of particular interest because it implies low coital frequency, much lower than for cohabiting women and much lower than for single women in USA or UK [15]. Social disapproval of, or ambivalence about, sexual activity of single girls and young women in Africa is one factor constraining sexual encounters, which often need to be concealed, thus limiting opportunities for sexual encounters [16, 17]. Even after allowance for a degree of possible over reporting, primary and secondary abstinence remain the main way in which single African women protect themselves, as shown by the small proportions at risk in many countries when abstinence is taken into account. Infrequent sex also has implications for choice of contraceptive method, to be discussed below.

While exposure to intercourse has probably changed little over the past 20 years, reported current use of a modern contraceptive method and reported use of a condom at most recent coitus has doubled since the early 1990s among the sexually active. These trends do not reflect changes in the educational, residential and age composition of the study population. The key period of change for contraceptive use was the decade from the early 1990s to early 2000s, when a major and welcome shift from periodic abstinence to condoms occurred. It is of concern that further improvements in modern contraceptive protection since 2001–2005 have been minor. It is also surprising because of the increased commitment to international family planning, and the increased emphasis of the needs of adolescents, leading up to and following the 2012 London Summit on this subject.

Nevertheless, contrary to popular belief, modern method contraceptive use is considerably higher among sexually active single women than among married or cohabiting women, no doubt because of a higher level, and greater intensity, of desire to prevent pregnancy among the single than the married [18]. Method choice also differs radically. Among married African women, injectables are the dominant method, accounting for nearly half of all use, though implants are increasingly popular; condoms are rarely used within marriage except in Southern African countries with particularly severe HIV epidemics [19]. In contrast, the condom is the major method among young single women, though its contribution to overall protection has slipped from 61 to 51% in the past decade. It is encouraging that close to 90% of those reporting condom use as their contraceptive method also reported use of this method at last coitus as this indicator is highly correlated with consistent use [20, 21]. Over the 20 year period, the contribution of orals and injectables to protection has increased from 10 to 24% but use of IUDs and implants remains trivial.

Condom use at most recent coitus was ascertained later in the interview from questions on contraception and made no mention of motive for use. Among those who reported use at last coitus, about half had previously claimed current use of this method for pregnancy-prevention. While the relative importance of the two motives for condom use—prevention of pregnancy and disease—is very difficult to establish, our findings suggest that a contraceptive motive is implicated for about half of all condom users. Double-method protection, simultaneous use of non-barrier contraception and condoms, is commonly regarded as ideal but is a rare form of behaviour [22]. We found encouraging results in that regard: in the most recent period, 31% of users of a non-barrier method reported condom use at last coitus, a level of use similar to that among non-users of contraception.

These findings raise fundamental questions about optimal protective strategies for sexually active young single women in Africa, particularly in settings where risk of infection with HIV or classical sexually transmitted diseases is high. Should we welcome the recent observed shift away from condoms to oral and injectable contraceptives and the strategic emphasis, so far apparently unsuccessful, on encouraging the use of long-acting methods for adolescents [23]? The strongest justification for hormonal method use by single women is that their use does not depend on the cooperation of male partners. Particularly when the male partner is much older, a young woman's urgency to enforce the use of a condom may be weak. It is also true that consistent condom use requires more foresight and discipline than non-coital methods and becomes more problematic as relationships develop and the frequency of sex increases [24]. Clearly, no single method can meet the diverse needs and circumstances of sexually active young women and, of course, ultimately their freedom to choose must be respected.

Another common reason for welcoming increased use of hormonal methods by single women, that they are more effective than condoms, is less well founded. The failure rates of condoms and oral contraceptives are very similar both in East and West Africa [25]. Condom failure rates also tend to be lower for single than married women, probably because of differences in coital frequency [25]. Injectable users have lower failure rates but discontinuation of this method because of side effects and health concerns is high in married women and may be even higher in single women [26]. Moreover, the recognition by the World Health Organization that injectable use may increase the risks of HIV acquisition, and the consequent change in the Medical Eligibility Criteria, could limit future acceptability [27]. Failure and discontinuation rates for highly effective long-acting methods such as implants are low and this method is suitable for single women in countries such as USA and UK because of the long gap between sexual initiation and cohabitation or marriage and the relatively low risk of sexually transmitted infections. In Africa, the need for long term contraceptive protection from implants (or intrauterine devices) is lower than in USA or UK because marriage or cohabitation, and the desire for a child, typically occurs at young ages. We acknowledge that implants are well suited to the needs of young African women in committed long term, albeit non-cohabiting, relationships. In such circumstances, double method protection (ie implant together with condom use) remains the ideal.

From a pregnancy-prevention perspective, however, the condom remains the most suitable option for the large number, probably a majority, of young women who are not in a committed long term relationship and for whom coitus is infrequent. For them, permanent protection from daily use of oral contraceptives, injectables or implants probably seems excessive. The advent of emergency contraception and the rapid proliferation of medical abortion provide a back-up for occasions when condoms, for whatever reason, are not used or break during use.

The recent neglect of condoms by both the family planning and HIV communities, in our judgment, is regrettable. From a disease-prevention perspective, frequent HIV testing and treatment, pre-exposure prophylaxis for very high risk individuals, and male circumcision can make valuable contributions. Yet, condoms remain the major, and most cost effective, component of prevention [28, 29].

In our view the ideal contraceptive package for many young women comprises condoms, emergency contraceptives, pregnancy-testing kits, and advice, where legally possible, on medical abortion. A large majority of young people who use condoms obtain supplies from commercial sources [30]. Thus we urge a re-vitalisation of condom social marketing. The evidence on the effectiveness of mass media promotion and condom social marketing is generally positive [31, 32]. We further suggest that social marketing may be more successful with a pregnancy-prevention emphasis than with an HIV prevention one, for two reasons. First, the association of condoms with promiscuity and disease limits its use [33]. Second, it is obviously easier for a young woman to negotiate use to prevent pregnancy than to prevent HIV.

Conclusions

Our paper complements the extensive existing literature in several ways. We believe that this paper presents the clearest chronological record of changes in key protective behaviours in young single women, thus far published. Drawing on all 112 surveys in sub-Saharan Africa that used the same protocol we document trends at regional and country level over a 20 year period. While trends in contraceptive use and condom use are well known, joint analyses of both outcomes are rare and most omit consideration of abstinence. We pay equal attention to all three behaviours, including shifts in type of contraceptive method used. Questions on contraception and on condom use at most recent coitus are posed at different times in the interview and thus may be regarded as semi-independent items of information. This allows us to measure the extent of dual protection and to estimate the approximate contribution of a contraceptive motive to overall condom use. Lastly, we estimate the effect of structural shifts in the study population, namely age, education and rural-urban residence, on reported behavioural change.

The protective role of sexual abstinence has not changed but remains strong. The high level of abstinence in the past 3 months among sexually experienced women indicated that coitus is infrequent for many. Mixed messages can be drawn from the analysis of trends in current contraceptive use and condom use at most recent coitus. In the past 20 years levels of both indicators have doubled but the pace of change has slowed in the past decade. The central policy lesson concerns the continuing centrality of the condom, both for prevention of pregnancy and disease. Condoms remain the dominant contraceptive method for single women in Africa and pregnancy-prevention is at least part of the motive for half of those reporting its use at last coitus. In our view, the condom is the optimal choice for women who have infrequent sex and live in settings where HIV risk is high. The advent of emergency contraception and medical abortion as back-ups further justifies use of this method. Displacement of condoms by promotion of hormonal methods of contraception for this population is a danger. Rather we urge a re-invigoration of condom social marketing with a strong contraceptive emphasis. Together with a continued HIV testing and treatment and promotion of male circumcision, such re-invigoration should further accelerate the decline in HIV incidence in African youth.

Additional files

Additional file 1: Analysis population (unweighted numbers), by survey, fieldwork date and period. The year of fieldwork, the analysis period, the number of all women (aged 15–49), number of young (aged 15–24), number of young and single, number of young, single and ever had sex, number of young, single and had sex in last 3 months, number of young, single and had sex in last 3 months, and currently using modern contraceptives, and number of young, single and used condom in last coitus.

Additional file 2: Comparisons of the 4 outcomes between all countries and countries with 4+ surveys. The results of the sensitivity analysis comparing the rates of Primary abstinence, Secondary abstinence, Current use of modern contraception, and Condom use last sex between all countries and countries with 4 and more surveys.

Additional file 3: Trends in Primary and Secondary Abstinence (crude and adjusted) within country trends in primary and secondary abstinence, and mean annual rate of change.

Additional file 4: Correlation between education level (secondary or higher) and current use of modern methods at national level, All single women aged 15–24 who had sex in the last 3 months. Pearson correlation coefficients of education and current use of modern methods with *p*-values, by analysis period.

Additional file 5: Trends in current use of modern contraception and condom use last coitus. Trends in crude and adjusted Current use of modern contraception and condom use last coitus, mean annual rate of change with (*p*-values), by country.

Additional file 6: Correlation between percent condom use last coitus and HIV prevalence among 15–24 years old, by sex and period. Pearson correlation coefficients of condom use last coitus and HIV prevalence with p-values, by analysis period.

Additional file 7: Percent reporting consistent condom use with last partner, among women who used a condom at most recent coitus. Lower quartile, median, upper quartile and IQR of consistent condom use with last sexual partner, among Single women aged 15-24 years, sexually active in the past 3 months and reported condom use last coitus.

Additional file 8: Median percentages of current contraceptive use among those who reported condoms use at most recent coitus, by period and method type. Median percentages of current contraceptive use among those who reported condoms use at most recent coitus, by period and method type, among Single women aged 15–24 years, sexually active in the past 3 months and reported condom use last coitus.

Additional file 9: Ranking of countries according to risk among women aged 15-24. Percentage at risk among all women and women who had sex aged 15-24.

Acknowledgements
We would like to acknowledge Dr. James Kiarie and Dr. Moazzam Ali for their helpful comments on an earlier draft.

Funding
This work was funded by the UNDP-UNFPA-UNICEF-WHO-World Bank Special Programme of Research, Development and Research Training in Human Reproduction (HRP), a cosponsored programme executed by the World Health Organization (WHO), Project HQRHR1815140.

Authors' contributions
JC and MMA jointly planned this paper. MMA was primarily responsible for the statistical analysis and JC for drafting and interpretation. All authors read and approved the final manuscript.

Competing interests
The authors declare that they have no competing of interests.

Author details
[1]UNDP-UNFPA-UNICEF-WHO-World Bank Special Programme of Research, Development and Research Training in Human Reproduction (HRP), World Health Organization, 20 Avenue Appia, 1211 Geneva, Switzerland.
[2]Department of Population Health, Faculty of Epidemiology and Population Health, London School of Hygiene and Tropical Medicine, Keppel Street, London WC1E 7HT, UK.

References

1. United Nations Secretary-General. The Global Strategy for Women's, Children's and Adolescents' Health (2016-2030). Available on http://www.who.int/life-course/publications/global-strategy-2016-2030/en/.
2. UNFPA. The power of 1.8 billion: Adolescents, youth and the transformation of the future. 2014.

3. Nove A, Matthews Z, Neal S, Camacho AV. Maternal mortality in adolescents compared with women of other ages: evidence from 144 countries. Lancet Glob Health. 2014:e155–64.
4. Sedgh G, Bearak J, Singh S, et al. Abortion incidence between 1990 and 2014: global, regional, and subregional levels and trends. Lancet. 2016; 388(10041):256–67.
5. Clark S, Koski A, Smith-Greenaway E. Recent trends in premarital fertility across sub-Saharan Africa. Stud Fam Plan. 2017;48(1):3–22.
6. Koski A, Clark S, Nandi A. Has child marriage declined in sub-Saharan Africa? An analysis of trends in 31 countries. Pop Dev Rev. 2017;43(1):7–29.
7. Bongaarts J, Mensch BS, Blanc AK. Trends in the age at reproductive transitions in the developing world: the role of education. Popul Stud. 2017; 71(2):130–54.
8. Mensch B, Grant M, Blanc A. The changing context of sexual initiation in sub-Saharan Africa. Pop Dev Rev. 2006;32(4):699–727.
9. Blanc AK, Tsui AO, Croft TN, Trevitt JL. Patterns and trends in adolescent's contraceptive use and discontinuation in developing countries and comparisons with adult women. Int Persp Sexual Repr Health. 2009;35(2):63–71.
10. Chandra-Mouli V, McCarraher DR, Phillips SJ, Williamson NE, Hainsworth G. Contraception for adolescents in low and middle income countries: needs, barriers, and access. Repr Health. 2014;11:1.
11. UNAIDS Prevention Gap Report 2016. Available on http://www.unaids.org/sites/default/files/media_asset/2016-prevention-gap-report_en.pdf
12. DHS STATcompiler available http://www.statcompiler.com/en/
13. Cleland J, Boerma JT, Carael M, Weir SS. Monitoring sexual behaviour in general populations: a synthesis of lessons of the past decade. Sex Transm Infect. 2004;80(Suppl 2):ii1–7.
14. Cleland J, Ali MM. Sexual abstinence, contraception and condom use by young African women: a secondary analysis of survey data. Lancet. 2006; 368(18):1788–93.
15. Wellings K, Collumbien M, Slaymaker E, Singh S, Hodges Z, Patel D. Sexual behaviour in context: a global perspective. Lancet. 2006;368(9548):1706–28.
16. Harrison A. Hidden love: sexual ideologies and relationship ideals among south African adolescents in the context of HIV/AIDS. Cult Health Sex. 2008; 10(2):175–89.
17. Wight D, Plummer ML, Mshana G, Wamoyi J, Shigongo ZS, Ross DA. Contradictory sexual norms and expectations for young people in rural northern Tanzania. Soc Sci Med. 2006;52:987–97.
18. Tsui AO, Brown W, Li Q. Contraceptive practice in sub-Saharan Africa. Pop Dev Rev. 2017;43(S1):188–91.
19. United Nations, Department of Economic and Social Affairs, population division. World contraceptive use 2016. POP/DB/CP/Rev2016. N.Y.: United Nations; 2016.
20. Lagarde E, Auvert B, Chege J, et al. Condom use and its association with HIV/sexually transmitted diseases in four urban communities of sub-Saharan Africa. AIDS. 2001;15(suppl 4):71–8.
21. Myer L, Mathews C, Little F. Measuring consistent condom use: a comparison of cross-sectional and prospective measurements in South Africa. Int J STD AIDS. 2002;13:62–3.
22. ESHRE Capri Working Group. Simultaneous prevention of unintended pregnancy and STIs: a challenging compromise. Hum Reprod Update. 2014; 20(6):852–963.
23. USAID, Bill and Melinda Gates Foundation, UKAID, et al. Global Consensus Statement for Expanding Contraceptive Choice for Adolescents and Youth to Include Long-Acting Reversible Methods available on: http://www.familyplanning2020.org/youth-larc-statement. Accessed 13 Apr 2018.
24. Mmari K, Herbert A, Van Lith L, et al. What are the Social and Emotional Factors that Influence Adolescent Condom Use in LMIC? Findings from a Rapid Literature Review. Baltimore: Johns Hopkins Bloomberg School of Public Health, Health Communication Capacity Collaborative; 2014.
25. Polis CR, Bradley SEK, Bankole A, Onda T, Croft T, Singh S. Typical-use contraceptive failure rates in 43 countries with demographic and health survey data: summary of a detailed report. Contraception. 2016;94:11–7.
26. Ali MM, Cleland J, Shah IH. "Causes and consequences of contraceptive discontinuation: Evidence from 60 Demographic and Health Surveys". Geneva: World Health Organization; 2012.
27. World Health Organization. Hormonal Contraceptive Eligibility for Women at High Risk of HIV. Geneva: Guidance Statement; 2017.
28. UNFPA, WHO and UNAIDS. Position statement on Condoms and the Prevention of HIV, other Sexually Transmitted Infections and Unintended Pregnancy. 2015.
29. UNAIDS. Consultation on HIV Prevention Cascades: December 2016. Report from Consultations. Organised by UNAIDS. Geneva; 2016.
30. Radovich E, Dennis ML, Wong KLM, Ali M, Lynch CA, Cleland J, Owolabi O, Lyons-Amos M, Benova L. Who meets the contraceptive needs of young women in sub-Saharan Africa? J Adolesc Health. 2018;62(3):273–80. https://doi.org/10.1016/j.jadohealth.2017.09.013.
31. Bertrand JT, Anhang R. The effectiveness of mass Media in Changing HIV/AIDS related behaviour among young people in developing countries. World Health Organ Tech Rep Ser. 2006;938:205–41. 317-341
32. Sweat MD, Denison J, Kennedy C, Tedrow V, O'Reilly K. Effect of social marketing on condom use in developing countries: a systematic review and meta-analysis. WHO Bull. 2012;90:613–22.
33. Williamson LM, Parkes A, Wight D, Petticrew M, Hart GJ. Limits to modern contraceptives among young women in developing countries: a systematic review of qualitative research. Reprod Health. 2009;6:3.

Trends in adolescent first births in five countries in Latin America and the Caribbean: disaggregated data from demographic and health surveys

Sarah Neal[1*], Chloe Harvey[1], Venkatraman Chandra-Mouli[2], Sonja Caffe[3] and Alma Virginia Camacho[4]

Abstract

Background: Adolescents in the Latin American and Caribbean region continue to experience poor reproductive health outcomes, including high rates of first birth before the age of 20 years. Aggregate national level data fails to identify groups where progress is particularly poor. This paper explores how trends in adolescent births have changed over time in five countries (Bolivia, Colombia, Dominican Republic, Haiti, and Peru) using data disaggregated by adolescent age group, wealth and urban / rural residence.

Methods: The study draws on Demographic and Health Survey data from five countries where three surveys are available since 1990, with the most recent after 2006. It examines trends in adolescent births by wealth status and urban/rural residence.

Results: There has been little progress in reducing adolescent first births over the last two decades in these countries. Adolescent first births continue to be more common among the poorest and rural residents, and births among the youngest age-group (< 16 years) are particularly concentrated among these populations.

Conclusion: Adolescent first births continue to be a major issue in these five countries, including amongst the youngest group (< 16 years), although the contexts in which it is occurring are changing over time. Efforts are needed to expand sexual education and services for adolescents and young people, as well as introduce and enforce legislation to provide effective protection from abuse or exploitation. Greater disaggregation of adolescent fertility data is needed if we are to measure progress towards the attainment of the Sustainable Development Goals to "leave no-one behind".

Keywords: Adolescent, Sexual health, Pregnancy, Latin America and the Caribbean

Plain English summary

Adolescent girls in Latin America and the Caribbean continue to be at risk of poor reproductive health and have a high risk of giving birth before the age of 20 years. This study analyses survey data from Bolivia, Colombia, Dominican Republic, Haiti, and Peru to examine trends in the percentage of adolescents giving birth before age 20 years.

We find that little progress has been made in reducing adolescent first births in these countries. Births to young women are much more common among the poorest and those living in rural areas, and this is particularly true for young women who give birth at very young ages (e.g. before 16 years).

Our study highlights the need to improve sexual health education and services for adolescents and young people, as well as ensure legal frameworks to protect them.

* Correspondence: S.Neal@soton.ac.uk
[1]Department of Social Statistics and Demography, University of Southampton, Southampton, UK
Full list of author information is available at the end of the article

Background

Young people in Latin America and the Caribbean (LAC) continue to face significant barriers to their sexual and reproductive health, including adolescent pregnancy. Around 15% of all births in this region are to women below the age of 20 years [1], with an adolescent fertility rate (15–19 years) of 65 per 1000 in 2014 [2]. Teenage pregnancy is associated with a number of adverse health outcomes for both mother and child [3, 4], as well as social and economic disadvantages for individuals and families [5]. The associated loss of productivity and negative impacts on development at the national level [6] has led policy-makers to identify it as an important area for intervention. Sexual behaviour for both male and female adolescents is underpinned by complex socio-economic, educational, cultural, geographical and service-availability factors, and contexts, patterns, and trends may vary markedly for different populations within countries. However, anaysis of data disaggregating populations by socio-economic and other characteristics is rarely carried out, meaning it is difficult to identify those groups who may be making poor progress. Disaggregated data that examines patterns and trends for different groups is valuable in enabling programmes to target those most at risk, and to ensure that the ambition of the Sustainable Development Goals to "leave no-one behind" is achieved. In particular, greater focus on younger adolescents is important, as they face greater health disadvantages for both mother and infant [4, 7, 8] and may require specific approaches and strategies to address pregnancies in this particularly vulnerable group [9–11].

Overall, adolescent pregnancies in LAC are higher than for other regions with similar levels of development, and the relatively poor progress is at odds with the sharp decline in overall fertility. While the age specific fertility rate (ASFR) 15–19 years fell somewhat from 84 per 1000 in 1990 to 65 per 1000 in 2015, total fertility rate (TFR) had fallen sharply in the same period from 3.2 to 2.1 births per woman [12]. In addition, reliance on the adolescent fertility rate does not fully illustrate the issue: while it has fallen somewhat, the percentage of women who enter motherhood before the age of 20 years has actually increased since 1990 [13]. The reduction in adolescent fertility is driven by young mothers having fewer subsequent births, rather than fewer adolescent women becoming mothers at all [13]. It is therefore important to identify and highlight patterns in first births as this illustrates more clearly trends in the proportion of young women exposed to the disadvantages of adolescent motherhood.

Existing literature suggests that the persistence of adolescent fertility reflects a range of cultural and socio-economic factors. While much of the region has benefited from increased economic growth and social development, these benefits are not experienced equally. Even though educational opportunities have increased for young people, this is often not reflected in labour market prospects, particularly for young women [14]. This trend means that many young women (particularly within poorer communities) may continue to have low expectations about their futures in terms of employment, which makes avoiding adolescent pregnancy appear less important [15]. While progress has been made in promoting gender equity within many important aspects of life and in particular education, persistent barriers exist for women in expanding their economic opportunities and exercising agency and choice over their lives [14]. Cultural expectations of early motherhood are also often cited as important drivers, and it is stated that adolescent girls in LAC (particularly amongst the poorest groups and indigenous populations), desire and plan for early motherhood, with early partnering and an assumption of childbearing continuing to be the norm [16]. However, more recent discourses suggest that the fertility desire aspect of adolescent pregnancy has been overplayed, and the region has demonstrated a sharp decline in the proportion of adolescents who report they wanted their pregnancy [17].

This paper addresses how patterns of adolescent[1] first births in women have changed in five countries within the LAC region: Bolivia, Colombia, Dominican Republic, Haiti and Peru. It addresses two questions:

- What is the age distribution of first births to adolescents, and have the percentages of women entering adolescent motherhood in each age group changed since 1990?
- How do the socio-economic characteristics (wealth and urban / rural residence) of young women having a first adolescent birth differ between younger and older adolescents and how have these characteristics changed over time?

These five countries represent a considerable geographic spread within the region, with two from the Caribbean region and the rest within South America. ASFR 15–19 years based on the most recent Demographic and Health Survey (DHS) range from 64 per 1000 (Peru) to 90 per 1000 (Dominican Republic).

The persistence of high adolescent fertility and concerns about negative repercussions for both families and wider society in these five countries has led to increased concern among governments, non-governmental organisations and the media [18, 19]. Developing effective interventions requires a nuanced and in-depth understanding of trends and patterns in adolescent births, which involves disaggregation of data by sub-groups, as well as understanding the context in which births are occurring and how this may be changing.

Methods

The analysis is based on Demographic and Health surveys (DHS), which provide nationally representative data comparable across time and place. The five countries were chosen as they had three available surveys carried out since 1990, with the most recent being after 2006. The use of three surveys enabled us to be more confident about the quality of data, as any sharp differences may suggest data inconsistencies. However, rates of change are not presented for each period as originally intended as the change is so small for all countries.

The countries represent markedly different levels of socio-economic development, and Table 1 provides details of their ASFR 15–19 years, TFR, % female literacy and gross national income per capita (GNI). It is interesting to note that while Haiti has by far the lowest GNI and female literacy, it has one of the lowest ASFR 15–19 years (66 per 1000). Conversely, the Dominican Republic has the highest GNI per capita and near-universal female literacy, yet has the highest ASFR 15–19 years. This lack of clear association between wealth at national level and adolescent pregnancy rate has been identified elsewhere [14] and highlights the complex relationship between socio-economic factors and early motherhood within the region. The countries also represent very marked ethnic and cultural diversity. Table 1 also highlights that during the period covered in this study there have been some declines in ASFR 15–19 years in three countries (Bolivia, Dominican Republic and Haiti), a slight increase in Peru, and quite a marked increase in Colombia.

The analysis was based on the cohort aged 20–24 years as they will have been exposed to the whole period of interest in the study. In addition, in some countries there is evidence of under-reporting of very early adolescent births among respondents aged 15–19 years (although this appears to be less of an issue in LAC than other areas) [20]. We examine disaggregated trends by age group (< 16 year, 16–17 years, and 18–19 years), wealth status, urban/rural residence to understand changes in basic characteristics of young first-time mothers. Wealth was measured using wealth quintiles. These are created using the DHS asset index, which is a measure of a household's cumulative living standard based on ownership of selected assets, house construction and access to water and sanitation facilities. Our focus on first births reflects concerns over lack of progress, particularly as it is often masked by more optimistic trends in adolescent fertility rate. Confidence intervals at the 95% level were calculated for the percentage of first births by age group. We recognise the limitations imposed by the use of cross-sectional data: in particularly characteristics are recorded at time of survey not at time of birth, and this is discussed in more detail in the limitations section of the conclusion.

As discussed earlier, here is evidence that pregnancy outcomes for younger adolescents are worse than for older adolescents [4, 7, 8, 21, 22], so it was deemed important that the age groups were disaggregated in order to identify groups that were particularly vulnerable. Because the literature tends to use different age groupings it is difficult to conclusively identify the upper limit for the most vulnerable, but there is some evidence that disadvantage is particularly concentrated among mothers under the age of 16 years [4, 7, 8, 22], so this cut-off was chosen.

Inequalities are presented as ratios of poorest: richest quintile or rural: urban residence.

Results

Trends in adolescent motherhood

Table 2 shows the percentage of women aged 20–24 years at the time of the survey who reported a first birth before age 20 years (with confidence intervals in parentheses) in each age group for all three surveys for the five countries. Overall percentages for births to women under 20 years vary from 41% in the Dominican Republic to 27% in Haiti based on estimates from the most recent surveys. If we examine trends over time, we find that only Haiti has shown any evidence of a modest decline in first births to women under the age of 20 years across all three surveys (although confidence intervals still overlap for the 1994 and 2012 estimates, suggesting this could reflect sampling error). The estimates have remained static in Bolivia and Dominican Republic between the first and most recent survey and have increased in Colombia and Peru from 31 to 37% and 27 to 33% respectively. The Dominican Republic also has the highest percentage of births to women under 16 years at 7%, and again, only Haiti shows any evidence of a small reduction of births among the youngest (< 16 years) group from

Table 1 ASFR 15–19 years, TFR, female literacy and GNI per capita for five study countries

	Age specific fertility rate: 15–19: Baseline (year of survey in brackets)	Age specific fertility rate: 15–19: final survey (year of survey in brackets)	Total fertility rate 15–49[a]	Women who are literate[a] aged 15–49	GNI per capital PPP (current international $)[b]
Bolivia	94 (1994)	88 (2008)	3.5	92.7	6710
Colombia	70 (1990)	84 (2010)	2.1	–	13,550
Dominican Republic	112 (1996)	90 (2013)	2.5	93	13,600
Haiti	76 (1994)	66 (2012)	3.5	73.6	1760
Peru	61 (1991)	64 (2012)	2.6	94.6	12,060

[a]Data from DHS Statcompiler http://statcompiler.com/en/:For Total fertility it is for most recent survey
[b]Data from The World Bank http://data.worldbank.org/indicator/NY.GNP.PCAP.PP.CD: 2015

Table 2 Trends over time in % of women aged 20–24 years reporting first birth before age 20 years, disaggregated by age (CIs at the 95% in parenthesis)

Country	Year of first survey	Year of second survey	Year of third survey	Actual % change between baseline and final survey	Average % annual rate of change baseline to final survey year
Bolivia	1994	2003	2008		
< 16	5.2 (4.2–6.6)	4.5 (3.8–5.4)	5.2 (4.3–6.2)	0.0	0.0
16/17	13.3 (11.6–15.2)	14.5 (13.0–16.0)	14.9 (13.3–16.5)	1.6	0.9
18/19	19.2 (17.1–21.5)	21.8 (20.0–23.8)	17.3 (15.6–19.1)	−1.9	−0.7
Total < 20	37.7 (35.1–40.4)	40.8 (38.7–43.0)	37.3 (35.2–39.5)	− 0.4	− 0.1
Colombia	1990	2005	2010		
< 16	3.7 (2.6–5.2)	5.5 (4.8–6.2)	5.7 (5.1–6.4)	2.0	2.7
16/17	10.0 (8.2–12.1)	14.0 (12.9–15.2)	14.0 (13.0–15.0)	4.0	2.0
18/19	17.0 (14.3–20.1)	16.4 (15.2–17.7)	16.8 (15.8–17.9)	−0.2	−0.1
Total < 20	30.6 (27.4–34.0)	35.9 (34.2–37.6)	36.5 (35.1–37.8)	5.9	1.0
Dominican Republic	1996	2007	2013		
< 16	6.5 (5.3–8.0)	8.5 (7.4–9.7)	6.8 (5.2–8.7)	0.3	0.3
16/17	15.2 (13.2–17.3)	16.3 (14.8–18.0)	17.0 (14.7–19.5)	1.8	0.7
18/19	17.6 (15.5–19.9)	16.9 (15.3–18.6)	17.1 (14.9–19.7)	−0.5	−0.2
Total < 20	39.3 (36.5–42.1)	41.7 (39.5–43.9)	40.9 (37.7–44.0)	1.6	0.2
Haiti	1994	2005	2012		
< 16	4.6 (3.5–6.1)	4.3 (3.2–5.6)	3.2 (2.5–4.1)	−1.4	−1.7
16/17	10.4 (8.7–12.4)	10.8 (9.2–12.7)	9.7 (8.5–11.2)	−0.7	−0.4
18/19	16.5 (14.4–18.9)	15.1 (13.2–17.1)	14.4 (13.0–16.0)	−2.1	−0.7
Total < 20	31.6 (28.8–34.4)	30.1 (27.6–32.7)	27.3 (25.4–29.4)	−4.3	−0.8
Peru	1991	2007	2012		
< 16	3.3 (2.8–4.0)	3.5 (3.0–4.1)	3.5 (2.8–4.2)	0.2	0.3
16/17	9.1 (8.1–10.1)	10.3 (9.4–11.3)	11.1 (9.9–12.4)	2.0	1.2
18/19	14.5 (13.3–15.9)	14.9 (13.8–16.0)	17.1 (15.5–18.8)	2.6	0.9
Total < 20	26.9 (25.3–28.6)	28.7 (27.2–30.2)	31.6 (29.7–33.6)	4.7	0.9

4.6–3.2%. The Dominican Republic and Colombia have the highest proportion of all adolescent first births occurring in the < 16 years age group (16% for Colombia and 17% for Dominican Republic, based on the most recent survey), and in Colombia this proportion has actually increased over time. Due to the small changes over time, it is not really possible to make any firm comments about whether trends are markedly different for the periods from the baseline to the mid survey compared with between the mid and final survey, but there are no obvious generalizable patterns.

Table 3 illustrates the percentage of women aged 20–24 years at time of survey reporting a first birth before age 20 years, disaggregated by age at first birth grouping and urban/rural residence for the baseline and final survey. If we examine the most recent surveys only, we find a higher proportion of adolescent first births occur in rural areas for all age groups in all countries. In some cases, these differences are quite marked: in Peru, women are twice as likely to give birth before 20 years in rural areas as in urban areas. In all five countries, the rural / urban differential is greater for the < 16 age group than for the 18–19 age group. This suggests that younger adolescent first births are particularly concentrated in rural areas. If we examine trends over time based on annual percentage rate of change for first births to women < 20 years, we see no consistent pattern. Percentages have risen in both urban and rural areas in Colombia. Conversely, percentages have risen in urban areas but fallen in rural areas in the Dominican Republic and Peru. However, in both these countries the rise in urban areas has been greater than the reduction in rural areas: in urban areas, adolescent first births rose at an annual percentage rate of change of 1.0 and 1.2 respectively for the Dominican Republic and Peru, whereas they only fell by − 0.7% and − 0.2%. Additionally, adolescent first births have risen in rural areas but fallen in urban areas in Bolivia, and have fallen for both areas in Haiti (from 28 to 22% in urban areas and from 35 to 32% in rural areas). In the Dominican Republic

Table 3 % of women aged 20–24 years reporting a first birth before 20 years disaggregated by age and urban/rural residence: baseline and final survey

	Bolivia 1994				Bolivia 2008				% point change	Average annual % rate of change < 20
	< 16	16/17	18/19	< 20	< 16	16/17	18/19	< 20		< 20
Urban	4.3	10.7	19.0	34.0	3.9	11.4	14.4	29.7	−4.3	−0.9
Rural	7.1	18.5	19.5	45.2	8.2	23.5	24.3	55.9	10.7	1.7
Ratio rural/urban	1.7	1.7	1.0	1.3	2.1	2.1	1.7	1.9		
	Colombia 1990				Colombia 2010					Annual % rate of change
	< 16	16/17	18/19	< 20	< 16	16/17	18/19	< 20		< 20
Urban	3.0	8.5	15.3	26.8	4.5	12.8	15.1	32.4	5.6	1.0
Rural	5.8	14.3	22.1	42.2	10.7	19.0	23.9	53.5	11.3	1.3
Ratio rural/urban	1.9	1.7	1.4	1.6	2.4	1.5	1.6	1.7		
	Dominican Republic 1996				Dominican Republic 2013					Annual % rate of change
	< 16	16/17	18/19	< 20	< 16	16/17	18/19	< 20		< 20
Urban	5.0	12.7	15.2	32.9	5.5	16.6	16.8	39.0	6.1	1.0
Rural	9.7	20.3	22.7	52.7	10.7	18.1	18.0	46.9	−5.8	−0.6
Ratio rural/urban	1.9	1.6	1.5	1.6	1.9	1.1	1.1	1.2		
	Haiti 1994				Haiti 2012					Annual % rate of change
	< 16	16/17	18/19	< 20	< 16	16/17	18/19	< 20		< 20
Urban	4.9	10.2	12.5	27.6	2.5	7.6	12.2	22.4	−5.2	−1.0
Rural	4.4	10.6	20.4	35.3	3.9	11.7	16.5	32.1	−3.2	−0.5
Ratio rural/urban	0.9	1.0	1.6	1.3	1.6	1.5	1.4	1.4		
	Peru 1991				Peru 2012					Annual % rate of change
	< 16	16/17	18/19	< 20	< 16	16/17	18/19	< 20		< 20
Urban	2.3	6.1	11.4	19.8	2.4	8.4	14.8	25.6		1.2
Rural	7.1	20.1	26.1	53.4	6.8	19.7	24.4	50.9		−0.2
Ratio rural/urban	3.1	3.3	2.3	2.7	2.8	2.3	1.6	2.0		

and Peru, the urban/rural differential has reduced for births to women < 20 years, whereas it has increased in Haiti, Bolivia and Colombia.

Table 4 shows the percentage of first births to women aged 20–24 years at time of survey that occurred < 20 years, disaggregated by age at first birth and wealth quintile. There is a strong wealth gradient for all age groups in all five countries: women in the poorest quintile are at least twice as likely to report a first birth at age < 20 years as those in the richest quintile. Bolivia has the greatest differential for births under the age of 20 years: 66% of women in the poorest quintile have given birth by this age compared with only 12% of women in the richest quintile. The ratio between poorest and richest quintile tends to be smaller for the 18–19 age group and greater for the < 16 age group and can be extremely large in the youngest age group: in Colombia, the ratio of poorest to richest quintiles is 30 in Colombia and 13 in Bolivia. It is difficult to ascertain clear patterns over time by quintile, which may partly be due to limited sample size. However, in two countries, the ratio of richest to poorest quintile for births to women < 20 years has remained static, the ratio has increased in two countries (Bolivia and Haiti), and the ratio has decreased in one country (Peru).

Discussion

Our study set out to answer two questions:

(1) What is the age distribution of first births to adolescents, and have the percentages of younger and older adolescent girls (10–14 and 15–19 years respectively) changed since 1990?
(2) How do the socio-economic characteristics (wealth and urban / rural residence) of young women having a first adolescent birth differ between younger and older adolescents and how have these characteristics changed over time?

Regarding the first question, our study finds very little evidence of marked progress in reducing adolescent first births in any of the countries. Indeed, in two countries (Colombia and Peru) there has been an increase and in a

Table 4 Trends in % of women aged 20–24 years reporting first birth < 20 years disaggregated by age group and wealth quintile

	Bolivia 1994				Bolivia 2008			
	< 16	16/17	18/19	< 20	< 16	16/17	18/19	< 20
Lowest	11.3	18.6	17.5	47.3	10.0	28.5	27.1	65.6
Second	6.2	14.6	26.7	47.4	9.3	19.5	25.1	54.0
Middle	5.5	18.0	21.7	45.2	6.2	18.1	20.6	44.9
Fourth	4.6	12.2	18.5	35.3	3.2	13.2	14.5	30.8
Highest	0.9	5.6	13.7	20.3	1.1	3.7	7.2	11.9
Ratio poorest/richest	12.6	3.3	1.3	2.3	9.1	7.7	3.8	5.5
	Colombia 1990				Colombia 2010			
	< 16	16/17	18/19	< 20	< 16	16/17	18/19	< 20
Lowest	11.8	16.7	24.4	52.9	13.7	22.0	23.5	59.1
Second	2.3	15.8	21.8	39.9	7.1	18.2	22.5	47.8
Middle	4.9	8.8	18.0	31.7	5.0	14.4	16.5	35.9
Fourth	1.7	8.4	13.3	23.4	3.8	9.7	14.8	28.2
Highest	0.4	3.4	10.9	14.6	0.8	7.5	8.2	16.4
poorest/richest	29.5	4.9	2.2	3.6	17.1	2.9	2.9	3.6
	Dominican Republic 1996				Dominican Republic 2013			
	< 16	16/17	18/19	< 20	< 16	16/17	18/19	< 20
Lowest	11.6	31.4	25.8	68.8	10.6	28.9	23.6	63.0
Second	9.9	17.5	24.7	52.2	10.3	21.9	20.7	52.9
Middle	7.7	16.9	17.0	41.6	6.3	16.9	16.9	40.1
Fourth	2.9	9.6	17.4	29.8	4.5	10.9	13.5	28.9
Highest	3.0	6.6	8.4	18.1	2.4	7.4	11.7	21.4
poorest/richest	3.9	4.8	3.1	3.8	4.4	3.9	2.0	2.9
	Haiti 1994–95				Haiti 2012			
	< 16	16/17	18/19	< 20	< 16	16/17	18/19	< 20
Lowest	7.6	12.8	21.4	41.8	4.2	13.6	19	36.8
Second	5.7	12.8	24.8	43.3	4.1	10.2	22.2	36.5
Middle	4.5	10.7	18.5	33.7	3.5	12.8	17.2	33.5
Fourth	5.8	10.6	16.5	32.8	4.0	10.6	12.3	26.8
Highest	1.7	7.6	8.7	18.1	1.3	4.4	7.4	13.0
poorest/richest	4.5	1.7	2.5	2.3	3.2	3.1	2.6	2.8
	Peru 1991–92				Peru 2012			
	< 16	16/17	18/19	< 20	< 16	16/17	18/19	< 20
Lowest	7.6	24.1	28.5	60.2	7.7	23.3	25.2	56.2
Second	5.8	13.6	23.1	42.6	6.4	18.5	25.0	50.0
Middle	3.8	8.9	16.2	29.0	2.3	9.4	16.2	27.9
Fourth	0.7	4.4	9.4	14.5	1.7	6.9	15.2	23.8
Highest	1.3	1.9	4.5	7.7	1.4	3.1	8.0	12.5
poorest/richest	5.8	12.7	6.3	7.8	5.5	7.5	3.2	4.5

further two countries (Dominican Republic and Bolivia) the percentage has stagnated. It is particularly concerning to note the persistence, and in the case of Colombia increase, in births to young women under the age of 16 years. The implications of this are underlined by evidence that the risks of ill health and mortality to the mother and child associated with adolescent births are most concentrated within this age-group [4, 8].

Regarding the second question, our study clearly shows that adolescent first births remain concentrated among poorer and rural women, and in some countries these differentials have increased over time. Inequities between both wealth and place of residence have only decreased in Peru (although because wealth is measured at the time of survey, it is impossible to state categorically whether poverty is a cause or a result of adolescent motherhood). Younger adolescent mothers are also more likely to be poor and live rurally when compared to their older counterparts [4, 8], which further adds to their vulnerability [23].

Our finding of the limited reduction in adolescent first births in the five countries studied are consistent with those from other studies in the LAC regions, which describe stagnation or increases in the levels of teenage motherhood. For instance, a study by Rodriguez-Vignoli [17] found stagnation or increases in the proportion of women aged 15–19 years who were pregnant or had had a first child in a number of countries within the region during a similar period. It is interesting to note that stagnation in Dominican Republic and Bolivia occurs within the context of overall decline in ASFR 15–19 years . This gives further support to Rodriguez-Vignoli's argument that such declines in LAC are driven by a reduction in the number of births to each adolescent, not the proportion of young women who become adolescent mothers in the first place [13]. Batyra's study in Colombia [24] also demonstrates how successive cohorts of women are increasing the timing of subsequent births.

This lack of progress is clearly concerning: not only does this negatively impact the health and wellbeing of young women and their children [4, 7], it will have wider repercussions for families and communities and will also hinder progress towards the Sustainable Development Goals (SDGs). The adolescent fertility rate is an indicator for the third SDG: Ensure healthy lives and promote well-being at all ages. However, reducing adolescent pregnancies will also potentially contribute more widely to the SDGs through reducing the cycle of deprivation, as well as positively impacting on the goals focussing on poverty, hunger, quality education, gender equality and decent work and economic growth [5, 25–28].

The concentration of adolescent births to poorer mothers identified in this study is also in line with other work from the region [29, 30] that finds socio-economic inequalities persist in adolescent pregnancies. Bozon et al. [29] reflects that the traditional feature of marked inequality within Latin American societies translates into gross inequities in sexual experiences and outcomes. Further, our finding that younger adolescent mothers are also more likely to be poor and rural residents compared to their older counterparts are in line with similar findings in the East African context [23].

Our study clearly indicates the need for increased efforts to address adolescent births within these countries. As adolescent pregnancy is often underpinned by social, economic and cultural factors, it is increasingly understood that individual-level focused interventions are likely to have limited impact, and that it is vital to involve families, communities, and wider society [31]. As Caffe et al. have noted, addressing the issue of adolescent first births in LAC is likely to require a broad and multisectoral approach, and strategies that address both the proximal and the distal determinants of adolescent fertility within the LAC context have been widely supported [32].

Education is seen as a key component of multisectoral approaches to reducing adolescent births, and attempts to increase school enrolment through conditional cash transfers have had some success in both Colombia and Peru: both have improved school enrolment and there is some indication of reduced adolescent pregnancy [14]. However, there are no simple solutions. The relationship between education and adolescent pregnancy in LAC is complex, and advances in education coverage in some LAC countries have failed to reduce teenage pregnancies. Rogriguez-Vignoli and Cavenaghi's study [33] found that the impact of education on adolescent pregnancy was not linear, and the threshold for impact increased from 5 years in the 1990s to 7 years in more recent periods. They highlight problems in the educational system whereby inequalities in quality persist, and where educational thresholds for employment have increased as much as, or more than, increases in average education, meaning many more disadvantaged young people are still excluded from the job market. In addition, complex social and cultural factors mitigate the relationship between education and adolescent pregnancy in LAC, including gender relationships and low aspirations.

In addition, adolescents need sexuality education that provides information and skills to protect themselves and avoid adverse health and social outcomes. The social and cultural aspects of adolescent pregnancy underline the importance of a holistic approach to sexuality education that addresses social and cultural norms including gender inequality and relationship dynamics [31]. Within the five countries there is wide variation in approaches to adolescent sexuality education: while Colombia has adopted many of the principles of comprehensive sexuality education (CSE), Peru and the Dominican Republic continue to focus on a much narrower curriculum [34].

Thirdly, adolescents need to be able to obtain contraceptive information and services, including emergency contraception. Rodriguez-Vignoli [13] highlights that lower rates of adolescent pregnancies in other countries with high rates of adolescent sexuality are driven by increased access to contraception and abortion. The First Latin American and Caribbean Regional Conference on Population and Development, held in Montevideo in August 2013 provided a forward-looking consensus, which agreed to the implementation of:

"...comprehensive, timely, good-quality sexual health and reproductive health programmes for adolescents and young people, including youth-friendly sexual health and reproductive health services with a gender, human rights, intergenerational and intercultural perspective, which guarantee access to safe and effective modern contraceptive methods, respecting the principles of confidentiality and privacy, to enable adolescents and young people to exercise their sexual rights and reproductive rights, to have a responsible, pleasurable and healthy sex life, avoid early and unwanted pregnancies, the transmission of HIV and other sexually transmitted infections, and to take free, informed and responsible decisions regarding their sexual and reproductive life and the exercise of their sexual orientation") [35].

However, despite promising moves towards improving sexual and reproductive rights and services in the region, barriers remain for marginalized populations, including adolescents. Socio-economic inequalities in access remain problematic [36], and our findings relating to persisting socio-economic differences highlight the importance of improving access for the poorest and rural residents.

Finally, gender based violence (GBV) needs to be addressed effectively. GBV is a significant problem in much of LAC, and many of the adolescent births may result from coerced sexual contact or abuse from an adult male [28]. It is estimated that between 18% (Dominican Republic) and 43% (Bolivia) of women aged 15–19 years have experienced intimate partner violence (IPV) in the five countries within our study [37]. In all five countries, adolescent respondents aged 15–19 years had an increased risk of experiencing IPV in the previous 12 months than women aged 30–39 years [37]. Additionally, in some countries, reports of forced sexual debut are common. The link between IPV and adolescent pregnancy is clearly recognised in a number of strategies within the region, including the Mexican Adolescent Pregnancy Strategy [38], and most countries in the region now have national commissions to address violence against women. Some countries face particular challenges: in Haiti, where 21% of women aged 15–24 described their first experience of intercourse as "forced" or "rape" [37], a number of reports and studies point to increased SGBV, transactional sex and adolescent pregnancies among displaced communities and populations most affected by the earthquake in 2010 [39, 40]. Additionally, in Colombia many women are still suffering the effects of conflict and displacement, which creates specific problems and hinders progress [41].

Latin American countries have made strides in strengthening legislation around this issue, and there have been promising initiatives to promote change among law enforcement agencies, as well as developing interventions to support victims. A number of community- and school-based programmes have demonstrated success in changing violence-related attitudes and behaviours, and the gender norms that underpin this problem [42], which must be viewed as a vital component of strategies to reduce adolescent births.

Our study has a number of limitations, which reflect constraints in the data on which the analysis is based. Our study only relates to live births, and does not cover spontaneous or induced abortion. An estimated four million induced abortions take place in Latin America each year, despite the fact that it is highly restricted in all countries [43]. The vast majority of these abortions are likely to be unsafe. There is limited understanding on adolescents' use of abortion in this region, and while data are collected in DHS (albeit without distinguishing induced abortion from other pregnancy loss) it is of very poor quality [44] so has not been included in this study.

As mentioned in the methodology section, there are a number of limitations associated with cross-sectional data that influence the interpretation of the findings. In particular, the characteristics of place of residence and wealth are measured at the time of the survey rather than at the time of the birth. This creates problems in interpretation: poverty could be either a driver or a result of adolescent motherhood. Furthermore, young women may migrate following a birth (either to live in a different household or to find employment) which also means the analysis of urban / rural residence should be interpreted with some caution.

It must also be noted that our data is somewhat dated, and may not reflect recent improvements resulting from efforts to address this issue or from wider social and economic changes. The adolescent births identified in the 20–24 year age group could have occurred up to about 10 years before the date of the survey, and some of the surveys themselves are already somewhat dated. At the time of writing the data had not been released for the Colombia 2015 DHS, but the preliminary report suggests that the proportions of women aged 15–19 at the time of survey who have either begun childbearing or are pregnant have fallen [45]. It is vital that new survey data is comprehensively analysed as it is published and additional sources are explored to ensure a contemporaneous picture of ongoing trends in the region.

Conclusion

Adolescent motherhood continues to be an issue for concern in the countries we studied, with little or no progress in reducing the percentage of women who give birth before the age of 20 years. This not only puts the health of many women and their children at risk and limits their educational and economic opportunities, but also impacts more broadly on families, communities, and national development as a whole. Adolescent births continue to be concentrated amongst the poor and those living in rural areas. Additionally, there is a concerning persistence in births to very young adolescents under 16 years of age, who are likely to experience the most severe risks and disadvantages. Efforts to provide sexual health information and services for young people need to accelerated, along with strategies to improve education and employment opportunities and further strengthen legal frameworks to protect those at risk of abuse and exploitation. Additionally, greater efforts need to be made to disaggregate adolescent pregnancy and sexual health data in order to measure progress in vulnerable groups and ensure that the SDG intention that no one is left behind becomes a reality.

Abbreviations

DHS: Demographic and health survey; LAC: Latin America and the Caribbean; PLANEA: Andean plan to prevent teen pregnancy

Acknowledgements

We would like to thank Marina Pleasons and Javiera Fanto Garrido for comments made on earlier drafts.

Funding

SN received funding from a British Academy Postdoctoral Fellowship (grant number 511537101) and the group received further funding from an ESRC Impact Acceleration Account award (number 514695112).

Authors' contributions

SN Jointly conceived the concept, oversaw the analysis and wrote the first draft. CH carried out the analysis. VCM, SC and AVC jointly conceived the concept and contributed to drafts. All authors read and approved the final manuscript.

Competing interests

The authors declare that they have no competing interests.

Author details

[1]Department of Social Statistics and Demography, University of Southampton, Southampton, UK. [2]Human Reproduction Programme/ Department of Reproductive Health and Research, World Health Organization, Geneva, Switzerland. [3]Pan American Health Organization, 525 23rd Street, NW, Washington DC, USA. [4]SRH Team, Latin America and the Caribbean Regional Office, United Nations Population Fund, Panama City, Panama.

References

1. UN Department of Economic and Social Affairs. World Fertility Patterns 2015 [Internet]. New York; 2015. Available from: http://www.un.org/en/development/desa/population/publications/pdf/fertility/world-fertility-patterns-2015.pdf
2. UNdata Adolescent fertility rate (births per 1,000 women ages 15–19) [Internet]. [cited 2016 Aug 16]. Available from: http://data.un.org/Data.aspx?d=WDI&f=Indicator_Code%3ASP.ADO.TFRT
3. Chen X-K, Wen SW, Fleming N, Demissie K, Rhoads GG, Walker M. Teenage pregnancy and adverse birth outcomes: a large population based retrospective cohort study. Int J Epidemiol [Internet] 2007;36(2):368–73. Available from: http://ije.oxfordjournals.org/content/36/2/368.abstract
4. Conde-Agudelo A, Belizán JM, Lammers C. Maternal-perinatal morbidity and mortality associated with adolescent pregnancy in Latin America: Cross-sectional study. Am J Obstet Gynecol [Internet]. 2005 Feb [cited 2013 mar 18];192(2):342–9. Available from: http://www.ncbi.nlm.nih.gov/pubmed/15695970.
5. Glassman A, Silverman R, McQueston K. Adolescent Fertility in Low- and Middle-Income Countries: Effects and Solutions. Cent Glob Dev Work Pap No 295. 2012;(May 2012).
6. Temin M, Levine R, Stonesifer S. Start with a girl a new agenda for global health. Issues Sci Technol. 2010;26(3):33–40.
7. Ganchimeg T, Ota E, Morisaki N, Laopaiboon M, Lumbiganon P, Zhang J, et al. Pregnancy and childbirth outcomes among adolescent mothers: a World Health Organization multicountry study. BJOG [Internet] 2014;121 Suppl:40–8. Available from: https://obgyn.onlinelibrary.wiley.com/doi/abs/10.1111/1471-0528.12630.
8. Sharma V, Katz J, Mullany LC, Khatry SK, LeClerq SC, Shrestha SR, et al. Young maternal age and the risk of neonatal mortality in rural Nepal. Arch Pediatr Adolesc Med. 2008;162(9):828–35.
9. USAID. Reaching very young adolescents (VYAs): advancing Programme, Research and Evaluation Practices. Washington DC: Institute for Reproductive Health, Georgetown University; 2010.
10. UNFPA WHO UNAIDS. Seen but not heard: very young adolescents aged 10–14 years. . Geneva; 2004.
11. Igras SM, Macieira M, Murphy E, Lundgren R. Investing in very young adolescents' sexual and reproductive health. Glob Public Health [Internet]. 2014 Jan [cited 2016 Jan 19];9(5):555–69. Available from: http://www.pubmedcentral.nih.gov/articlerender.fcgi?artid=4066908&tool=pmcentrez&rendertype=abstract
12. UN. UN Data statistics [Internet]. 2014 [cited 2016 Oct 30]. Available from: http://data.un.org/Data.aspx?q=adolescent+fertility&d=WHO&f=MEASURE_CODE%3aasfr1.
13. Rodriguez-Vignoli J. Adolescent fertility in Latin America and the Caribbean. nIUSSP [Internet]. 2016;May. Available from: http://www.niussp.org/article/adolescent-fertility-in-latin-america-and-the-caribbeanla-fecondite-des-adolescentes-en-amerique-latine-et-dans-les-antilles/
14. Azevedo J, Favara M, Haddock S, Lopez-Calva L, Muller M, Perova E. Teenage pregnancy and opportunities in Latin America and the Carribean. Washington DC: World Bank;2012.
15. ECLAC. Social Panorama of Latin America. Population (English Edition). 2014.
16. Rodríguez J. High Adolecent fertility in the context of declining fertility in Latin America. Paper presented at the United Nations expert group meeting on Adolecents, youth and development, 21-22 July 2011. New York: United Nations Expert Group Meeting on Adolecents, Youth and Development, 21–22 July 2011. 2011.
17. Rodríguez-Vignoli J. La reproduccion en la adolescencia y sus desigualdades en America Latina. In Santiago de Chile: United Nations; 2014. http://lac.unfpa.org/sites/default/files/pub-pdf/La%20reproduccion%20en%20la%20adolescencia_0.pdf.
18. Mendoza W, Subiría G. [Adolescent pregnancy in Peru: its current situation and implications for public policies]. Rev Peru med Exp Salud Publica [internet]. 2013;30(3):471–9. Available from: http://www.ncbi.nlm.nih.gov/pubmed/24100825.
19. Alzate MM. Adolescent pregnancy in Colombia: The price of inequality and political conflict. In: International handbook of adolescent pregnancy: Medical, psychosocial, and public health responses; 2014. p. 241–55.
20. Neal S, Hosegood V. Reporting of early adolescent reproductive and sexual health events in household surveys: Do women provide consistent responses? Int Perspect Sex Reprod Health. 2015;December.

21. Chen LC, Gesche MC, Ahmed S, Chowdhury AI, Mosley WH. Maternal mortality in rural Bangladesh. Stud Fam Plann. 1974;5(11):334–41. [cited 2013 may 9]. Available from: https://www.jstor.org/stable/pdf/1965185.pdf?refreqid=excelsior%3A78a8aed351cb29fe9f2f441e0d070c51.
22. Phipps MG, Sowers M. Defining early adolescent childbearing. Am J Public Health. 2002;92(1):125–8.
23. Neal SE, Chandra-Mouli V, Chou D. Adolescent first births in East Africa: disaggregating characteristics, trends and determinants. Reprod Health [Internet]. 2015 Jan [cited 2015 Oct 1];12(1):13. Available from: http://www.pubmedcentral.nih.gov/articlerender.fcgi?artid=4429933&tool=pmcentrez&rendertype=abstract
24. Batyra E. Fertility and the changing pattern of the timing of childbearing in Colombia. Demogr Res. 2016;35(46):1343–72.
25. Capanzana MV, Aguila DV, Javier CA, Mendoza TS, Santos-Abalos VM. Adolescent pregnancy and the first 1000 days (the Philippine situation). Asia Pac J Clin Nutr. 2015;24(4):759–66.
26. Oke YF. Poverty and teenage pregnancy: the dynamics in developing countries. Int J Sustain Dev. 2010;02(05):63–6.
27. Pendse R, Mcclure K, Mouli V, Health A, Mathai M, Portela A. Adolescent Pregnancy. WHO MPS Notes. 2008;1(1):1–4.
28. UNICEF. Challenges: Teenage motherhood in Latin America and the Caribbean Trends, problems and challenges [Internet]. 2007. Available from: https://repositorio.cepal.org/bitstream/handle/11362/36002/1/desafios_4_eng_Final_en.pdf.
29. Bozon M, Gayet C, Barrientos J. A life course approach to patterns and trends in modern Latin American sexual behavior. J Acquir Immune Defic Syndr. 2009;51(Suppl 1):S4–12.
30. Jimenez M, Rodriguez-Vignoli J. Evaluating the millennium development goal target on universal access to reproductive health: a view from Latin America and the Caribbean. In: Population Association of America [Internet]. Detroit; 2009. Available from: http://www.alapop.org/alap/SerieInvestigaciones/InvestigacionesSI1aSi9/DemogTransformations_PartelI-4.pdf
31. Córdova Pozo K, Chandra-Mouli V, Decat P, Nelson E, De Meyer S, Jaruseviciene L, et al. Improving adolescent sexual and reproductive health in Latin America: reflections from an International Congress. Reprod Health [Internet]. 2015;12:11. Available from: http://www.pubmedcentral.nih.gov/articlerender.fcgi?artid=4320614&tool=pmcentrez&rendertype=abstract
32. Caffe S, Pleason M, Camacho A, Brumana L. Looking back and moving forward: can we accelerate progress on adolescent pregnancy in the Americas? Reprod Health. 2017;14:83.
33. Rodriguez-Vignoli J, Cavenaghi S. Adolescent and youth fertility and social inequality in Latin America and the caribbean: what role has education played? Genus. 2014;70(1):1–25.
34. Frayssinet F. Comprehensive Sex Education: A Pending Task in Latin America. Terraviva ICPD@20 Track Progress, Explor Potential Post-2015'. 2013;13.
35. UN E. Montevideo Concensus on population and development. In: First session of the Regional Conference on Population and Development in Latin America and the Caribbean. Montevideo; 2013.
36. Abracinskas L, Corrêa S, Galli B, Garita A. The 'unexpected' Montevideo consensus. Glob Public Health [Internet] 2014;9(6):631–8. Available from: http://www.tandfonline.com/doi/abs/10.1080/17441692.2014.922596
37. Bott S, Guedes A, Goodwin M, Mendoza JA. Violence Against Women in Latin America and the Caribbean: A Comparative Analysis of Population-based data from 12 countries. Pan Am Heal Organ Centers Dis Control Prev [Internet]. 2013;1–16. Available from: http://www.paho.org/hq/index.php?option=com_docman&task=doc_view&gid=21426&Itemid
38. Estrategia Nacional para la Prevención del Embarazo en Adolescentes [Internet]. [cited 2016 Aug 17]. Available from: http://conapo.gob.mx/work/models/CONAPO/Publicaciones/ENAPEA/HTML/files/assets/basic-html/index.html#1
39. Krause S, Heller L, Tanabe M. Priority reproductive health activities in Haiti - an inter-agency MISP assessment conducted by CARE, International Planned Parenthood Federation, Save the Children and Women's Refugee Commission. Reprod Health. 2011;
40. Sloand E, Killion C, Yarandi H, Sharps P, Lewis-O'Connor A, Hassan M, et al. Experiences of violence and abuse among internally displaced adolescent girls following a natural disaster. J Adv Nurs. 2017;73(12):3200–8.
41. ABC Colombia. Colombia: Women, conflict-related sexual violence and the peace process [internet]. London. 2013. Available from: https://reliefweb.int/sites/reliefweb.int/files/resources/ABColombia_Conflict_related_sexual_violence_report.pdf.
42. Chandra-Mouli V, Camacho AV, Michaud PA. WHO guidelines on preventing early pregnancy and poor reproductive outcomes among adolescents in developing countries. J Adolesc Heal [Internet] 2013;52(5):517–22. Available from: https://doi.org/10.1016/j.jadohealth.2013.03.002
43. Kulczycki A. Abortion in Latin America: changes in practice, growing conflict, and recent policy developments. Stud Fam Plan. 2011;42(3):199–220.
44. Stanton C, Lawn JE, Rahman H, Wilczynska-Ketende K, Hill K. Stillbirth rates: delivering estimates in 190 countries. Lancet. 2006;367(9521):1487–94.
45. ENDS. Encuesta Nacional de Demografia y Salud Colombia 2015. Bogota: Resumen ejecutiva encuesta nacional de demografia y salud 2015; 2016.

Contraception determinants in youths of Sierra Leone are largely behavioral

Aline Labat[1*], Marta Medina[2], Mohammed Elhassein[4], Afrina Karim[4], Mohammad B. Jalloh[3], Michèle Dramaix[1], Wei-Hong Zhang[1], Sophie Alexander[1] and Kim E. Dickson[4]

Abstract

Background: Sexual initiation occurs early in Sierra Leone. This study aims to analyze the determinants of condom and/or contraceptive use among a representative sample of young persons (10 to 24 years) in Sierra Leone.

Methods: This is a secondary analysis of data from a study conducted to monitor the implementation of a UNFPA package of interventions directed to improve SRH in young people of Sierra Leone. This assessment was conducted in 2016 at the end of the Ebola outbreak. In consequence, determinants linked to healthy lifestyle behaviors and UNFPA interventions were explored in addition to the usual determinants: socio demographic and sexual lifestyle. This study is a household quantitative survey with open ended questions used to illustrate and complete the analysis.

Results: A total of 1409 young people were interviewed: of these, 216 boys and 381 girls were sexually active. Those who were pregnant or wished for pregnancy were excluded, leaving 194 boys and 268 girls for the analysis of determinants. The proportion of young people using neither condom nor other contraception at their last sexual intercourse in the whole sample was 40.5% and there was no statistically significant difference between boys and girls (42.3 vs 39.2; $P = 0.504$). Determinants were assessed and, after multivariable analysis, results differed between boys and girls and showed the importance of behavioral aspects. Four determinants were common to boys and girls: literacy, distance, negotiation capacity and hand washing. However, the distance factor for girls was to the health facility and for boys it was to school. Three more determinants remained in the boy's model: sleeping under a bednet, number of sexual partners and knowledge of contraceptive methods. Opinions about condoms and contraception revealed important barriers; opposition to contraceptive use was the main reason for non-use for both boys and girls, while lack of access was an important reason for boys.

Conclusion: There is a need to reach out to the 40% of young people who are sexually active and neither pregnant nor with pregnancy desire, and are not using condom or contraception.

Keywords: Adolescent, Youth, Behavior, Condoms, Contraception, Determinants, Gender, Health promotion, Sierra Leone

Plain English summary

One of the most effective interventions to decrease maternal and child deaths is to ensure adequate access to family planning; and one of the most effective ways of avoiding the transmission of sexually transmitted diseases including HIV-AIDS is appropriate provision and use of condoms. However, access and use of both condoms and contraception is low in young people, and specifically in sub-Saharan Africa. To address the issue, this study explored what determined the use of contraception and condoms in a sample of young people between 10 and 24 years in Sierra Leone, through a population based survey. Of the 1409 respondents, 462 were sexually active, and neither pregnant nor wishing to be pregnant. More than 40% used neither condom nor contraception during their last sexual encounter. After multivariable analysis, four determinants were common to boys and girls: distance to school or the health facility, literacy, capacity to "negotiate" (asking not to have sex and asking for condom use), and hand

* Correspondence: aline.labat@ulb.ac.be
[1]Université Libre de Bruxelles, Ecole de Santé Publique, Research Center: Policies and Health Systems - International Health, 808, Route de Lennik, 1070 Brussels, Belgium
Full list of author information is available at the end of the article

washing. For boys only, three additional determinants remained: knowledge of contraceptive methods, number of lifetime sexual partners and sleeping under a bednet. Many non-users were opposed to condoms and contraception for subjective motives. In conclusion, specific actions are needed to reach out to this underserved population.

Background

In sub-Saharan West Africa, maternal, neonatal and under-five-mortality remain high; key strategies to address this situation include increased family planning utilization and delayed first pregnancy [1]. Adolescent pregnancy in Sierra Leone is particularly frequent at an estimated 28% of all pregnancies [2], with 40% of maternal deaths occurring among adolescents [3, 4].

Two important issues of adolescent reproductive and sexual health are teenage pregnancy and risk of STIs HIV [5]. To avoid both, the safest option for sexually active unmarried youths is dual protection, and the least safe is neither. For women aged 15 to 24, the 2013 Sierra Leone demographic and health survey (SLDHS) showed condom use to be 1.0%, and any modern contraception to be 23% [2]. There is only limited information about the sexual and reproductive health (SRH) behaviors of younger adolescents (10–14 years), because in the DHSs, only adolescents above 15 years are interviewed.

Factors influencing youths' utilization of condoms and contraception include inadequate sexual knowledge and risk perceptions, lack of skills and power to negotiate safer sex options [6].

The current study came about following the second of three planned population based surveys of young people. These were commissioned by UNFPA Sierra Leone, and performed by the consortium hera/Université Libre de Bruxelles/FOCUS 1000. The aim of the surveys was to monitor the implementation of the UNFPA component of a UK Department for International Development (DFID) funded project to "improve awareness of, access to, and uptake of, family planning, reproductive and maternal health services across Sierra Leone with a focus on young people". This included improved access to family planning commodities, health provider training and community based interventions. Three community interventions were implemented, aimed at behavior change: (i) a national serial radio drama 'Saliwansai,' (ii) the placement of Volunteer Peer Educators (VPEs) in communities, and, (iii) the enhancement of existing Community Wellness Advocacy Groups (CAGs). These interventions focused on topics such as delaying marriage, staying on at school, safe sex, or giving birth at a health facility. Because of the Ebola outbreack the third survey was not performed.

Beyond the monitoring aspects of the survey, available in the report [7], the aim of the present study was to better characterize determinants of utilization, in particular, behavioral aspects, as well as possible effect of gender or age. This assessment was conducted in 2016 at the end of the Ebola outbreak. In consequence, determinants linked to healthy lifestyle behaviors were also explored. The study was restricted to those interviewed youths who declared they were sexually active and neither they nor their partner was pregnant or wished to get pregnant. These were then classified into four mutually exclusive groups: dual protection, condom only, modern contraception other than condom, and non-users. The underlying assumption is that better characterization of "non-users" will contribute to better understanding and the development of targeted recommendations for further intervention.

Methods

Households survey

The monitoring survey was conducted in three provinces of Sierra Leone, deliberately excluding the Western Area with the capital Freetown, because it was known from the SLDHS that contraception and condom utilization was highest in this region.

Households were selected using a stratified three stage cluster sampling. The 149 chiefdoms in the three provinces were allocated to four strata representing the UNFPA intervention areas. In each chiefdom (primary sampling unit), four clusters of 25 households each, were selected with "Probability Proportional to Size", and using the enumeration areas from the 2004 Sierra Leone Population and Housing Census. In total, the sample included 48 clusters. The sample size was computed, based on the expected time trend, between the planned first and last survey, for three indicators: contraceptive prevalence, condom use, and unmet need for family planning (FP).

A household questionnaire was administered to the head of the household, followed by an individual questionnaire to the males and females aged 10 to 24 years. For this questionnaire, in each household, a maximum of two persons were interviewed (one male and one female). Those of male sex are referred to as "boys" and those of female sex as "girls". The household questionnaire described the composition and assets. The individual questionnaire included 74 items concerning: (1) socio-demographic characteristics; (2) SRH knowledge, attitude, and practice: sexual activity, negotiation, condom use, contraception; (3) exposure to UNFPA supported SRH promoting interventions and; (4) health and use of health services. Most of the questions were similar to those used in the DHS [8] and in the global school-based student health survey (GSHS) [9] to allow valid comparisons.

Ethical considerations

Ethical approval was obtained from Ethical Research Committee of Université Libre de Bruxelles and by the Sierra Leone Ethics and Scientific Review Committee. Each head of household and each individual young person were asked whether they wished to participate. For those under 15 years of age, parental consent was also obtained.

Variables for the study

Having sex with neither condom nor contraception was defined as: the last time the responder had sex, neither he/she, nor his/her partner used a condom or any modern method of contraception, and neither was pregnant nor wished to get pregnant.

Negotiation capacity was defined by combining two questions, which were different for boys and girls. For the girl the two questions were: (i) "can you ask the boy not to have sex" (consent), and (ii) "can you ask your partner to use a condom". For the boys, the two questions were: (i) "is it acceptable if the girl asks not to have sex", and (ii) "is it acceptable if the girl asks you to use a condom". The two variables were combined and produced the following scale: 2 = responded yes to both questions; 1 = responded yes to one question only; and; 0 = responded no to both questions.

Literacy was defined by combining two questions: (i) "what was the highest year of studies you attained?" and, (ii), if they had responded "primary instruction" or "less" they were given a card with a sentence and asked to read it. The two variables were combined and produced the following scale: 1 = reads the entire sentence and/or has secondary, or higher education and; 0 = unable to read, whether the boy/girl had formal education or not.

Sexually active was used as an equivalent to "ever had sex".

Contraception is used for "utilization of modern contraceptive commodities".

"Condom or contraception use" is used for individuals using any of the following: (i) dual protection; (ii) condom alone; (iii) contraception alone.

In total 18 (19) determinants were explored. Nine determinants were socio demographic: age, province, two for distance (distance to school and distance to health facility), two for literacy-education, and three for status of household. In addition, two determinants reflected UNFPA interventions: exposure to enhanced CAGs and to VPEs; five (six) determinants indicated sexual lifestyle: negotiation, age at 1st sex, number of lifetime partners, parity (girls only), in union, and number of FP methods heard about; finally two determinants were considered to be markers of "healthy life style behaviors": sleeping under a bednet and hand washing.

Analysis

The primary outcome was "having sex with neither condom nor contraception" as defined above. All variables were categorical and were summarized with numbers and proportions. Pearson's Chi^2 test or Chi^2 for trend where appropriate, were applied to compare proportions. Odds Ratios (OR) and their 95% Confidence Interval (CI) were used to measure the strength of the associations. Logistic models were built using a stepwise forward selection based on Wald's test; all the considered independent variables except province were proposed for selection. The Hosmer and Lemeshow's test was applied to the final models to check goodness of fit. Adjusted OR's, their 95% CI and *P*-value from Wald's test were derived from the final models. Significance level was 0.05 for all analyses and these were performed with STATA® v14.2.

Additionally, the data in responses and comments to open ended questions in the household survey questionnaire were used for illustration of the quantitative findings.

The full methodology for the survey is described in the reports of surveys 2014 and 2016 [7].

Results

Survey data

A total of 1172 heads of household agreed to participate in the survey and 1409 young people were interviewed, of which 587 (41.6%) reported they had ever had a sexual encounter. These heads of households were mainly farmers, half (49.3%) did not have access to improved water, and over a third had no access to a radio (37.6%) or a mobile phone (36.2%). In the 15 to 19 age group, 70% of girls and 45% of boys declared they were sexually active; while in the 10 to 14 year age group, it was respectively 8 and 4.5%).

Table 1 distribution of behaviors in relation to contraception in sexually active categorized into 5 mutually exclusive categories

Type of method used ("you or your partner")	Sexually Active					
	Boys		Girls		Total	
	n	%	n	%	n	%
Dual	45	22%	25	7%	70	12%
Condom alone	12	6%	9	2%	21	4%
FP alone	55	27%	129	34%	184	31%
Pregnant or wishes to	12	6%	113	30%	125	21%
None of the above	82	40%	105	28%	187	32%
All	206	100%	381	100%	587	100%

Table 2 Determinants of having sex with neither condom nor contraception in boys: bivariate analysis

Variable (n = 194 unless otherwise specified)	Boys			
	n (%)	% neither condom nor contraception	Crude OR (95%CI)	P
Age (years)				0.519[a]
10–14	15 (7.7%)	46.7%	1.33 (0.44–4.00)	
15–19	96 (49.5%)	43.8%	1.18 (0.65–2.14)	
20–24	83 (42.8%)	39.8%	1	
Province				< 0.001
Eastern	61 (31.0%)	54.1%	6.33 (2.56–15.69)	
Northern	82 (42.3%)	50.0%	5.38 (2.25–12.83)	
Southern	51 (26.3%)	15.7%	1	
Distance to school (n = 191)				0.004
< 30 min	142 (74.3%)	35.9%	1	
≥ 30 min	49 (25.7%)	59.2%	2.59 (1.33–5.03)	
Distance to health facility (n = 191)				0.031
< 30 min	94 (49.2%)	34.0%	1	
≥ 30 min	97 (50.8%)	49.5%	1.90 (1.06–3.40)	
Education				< 0.001[a]
None	31 (16.0%)	71.0%	6.26 (2.54–15.44)	
Primary attended	74 (38.1%)	47.3%	2.30 (1.20–4.40)	
Primary completed or superior	89 (45.9%)	28.1%	1	
Literacy				< 0.001
Cannot read/only parts	47 (24.2%)	72.3%	5.39 (2.61–11.15)	
Able to read	147 (75.8%)	32.7%	1	
Source water* (n = 191)				0.058
Unimproved	92 (48.2%)	48.9%	1.75 (0.98–3.13)	
Improved	99 (51.8%)	35.4%	1	
Size of household (n = 193)				0.133
1–5	48 (24.8%)	45.8%	1.63 (0.79–3.37)	
6–8	85 (44.0%)	34.1%	1	
≥ 9	60 (31.0%)	50.0%	1.93 (0.98–3.80)	
Profession head (n = 191)				0.257
Farmer	120 (62.8%)	45.0%	1.42 (0.78–2.59)	
Other	71 (37.2%)	36.6%	1	
Met VPE				0.016
No	94 (48.5%)	51.1%	2.02 (1.14–3.61)	
Yes	100 (51.5%)	34.0%	1	
Met enhanced CAG				0.660
No	152 (78.4%)	41.5%	0.86 (0.43–1.70)	
Yes	42 (21.6%)	45.2%	1	
Negotiation (condom & refusal)				< 0.001[a]
Neither option	60 (30.9%)	60.0%	4.83 (2.31–10.12)	
One out of two options	58 (29.9%)	48.3%	3.01 (1.44–6.29)	
Both options	76 (39.2%)	23.7%	1	
Age at 1st sex (years)				0.340
< 15	69 (35.6%)	49.3%	1.55 (0.81–3.00)	
15	47 (24.2%)	38.3%	0.99 (0.47–2.09)	
16–24	78 (40.2%)	38.5%	1	
Lifetime partners (n = 192)				< 0.001
1	66 (34.4%)	53.0%	6.21 (2.54–15.20)	

Table 2 Determinants of having sex with neither condom nor contraception in boys: bivariate analysis *(Continued)*

Variable (n = 194 unless otherwise specified)	Boys			
	n (%)	% neither condom nor contraception	Crude OR (95%CI)	P
2–4	74 (38.5%)	50.0%	5.50 (2.28–13.27)	
≥ 5	52 (27.1%)	15.4%	1	
In a union				0.666
Yes	49 (25.3%)	44.9%	1.15 (0.60–2.22)	
No	145 (74.7%)	41.4%	1	
Heard of FP methods				< 0.001
0–3	31 (15.9%)	80.7%	7.75 (3.00–20.00)	
4–8	163 84.0%)	35.0%	1	
Slept under bednet				< 0.001
Yes	123 (63.4%)	30.1%	1	
No	71 (36.6%)	63.4%	4.02 (2.17–7.46)	
Hand wash < 4 h				< 0.001
Yes	124 (63.9%)	26.6%	1	
No	70 (36.1%)	70.0%	6.43 (3.37–12.30)	

[a]= chi^2 for trend; VPE = Volunteer Peer Educator; CAG = Community wellness Advocacy Group; FP = Family Planning
*Improved water according to DHS definition

The analysis pertains solely to the respondents who reported they had previously had sexual activity. It was considered acceptable to equate "sexually active" with "ever had sex", because among those who reported ever having sex, 88.2% of boys and 72.4% of girls reported a sexual encounter in the last 3 months.

Respondents were assigned into five mutually exclusive groups based on the use of condom or contraception at the last sexual encounter: (i) dual protection (n = 70), (ii) condom alone (n = 21), (iii) contraception alone (n = 184), (iv) pregnant, or whose partner was pregnant or who wished to become pregnant (n = 125), and (v) neither contraception nor condom nor pregnancy desire (n = 187) (see Table 1).

This leaves for analysis of determinants, after exclusion of those pregnant or wishing to get pregnant, a sample of 462 young people: 187 who used neither condom nor modern contraception and 275 who used one or both.

Among the 125 pregnant or wishing to get pregnant, 52 were adolescents (10 to 19 years), 2 boys and 50 girls.

Bivariate analysis of survey data

Our sample included 462 young people, 194 boys and 268 girls. The proportion of young people using neither condom nor contraception in the whole sample was 40. 5%. There was no statistically significant difference between boys (42.3%) and girls (39.2%) (P = 0.504).

For boys (Table 2), the following characteristics were significantly associated with using a condom or contraception: province, distance to school, distance to health facility, education, literacy, meeting a VPE, capacity to negotiate, number of life time partners, number of FP methods heard about, sleeping under a bednet and hand washing.

For girls, the following characteristics were significantly associated with using a condom or contraception: age, distance to health facility, education, literacy, capacity to negotiate (Table 3).

Statistically significant interactions were observed between sex of the respondent (boy or girl) and five of the determinants: province, distance from school, number of FP methods heard about, having slept under a bednet and having washed hands in the previous 4 h. For all these variables, the association with the outcome was stronger in boys than in girls.

Multivariable analysis of survey data

A multivariable model has been developed for boys and girls; results are presented in Tables 4 and 5.

Only four variables remained in the girls' model, whereas seven remained in the boys'. Three variables were common to the girls' and boys' models: hand washing in the previous 4 h, literacy and capacity to negotiate. However, in boys, hand washing in previous 4 h was the first variable to enter the model, while it was negotiation for the girls' model. Literacy was the second variable to enter in both models; however the corresponding adjusted OR was higher in the boys' model. Distance appears in both models, though it is to the health facility for girls and to school for boys. In addition to these four variables, in the boys' model, number of partners, number of FP methods heard about, and sleeping under a bednet remained significant after adjusting for all other included in the model.

Table 3 Determinants of having sex with neither condom nor contraception in girls: bivariate analysis

Variable (*n* = 268 unless otherwise specified)	Girls			
	N (%)	% neither condom nor contraception	OR (95%CI)	P
Age (years)				0.022[a]
10–14	24 (9.0%)	62.5%	3.25 (1.30–8.09)	
15–19	129 (48.1%)	39.5%	1.27 (0.76–2.15)	
20–24	115 (42.9%)	33.9%	1	
Province				0.953
Eastern	72 (26.9%)	40.3%	1.10 (0.58–2.09)	
Northern	109 (40.7%)	39.5%	1.07 (0.60–1.90)	
Southern	87 (32.5%)	37.9%	1	
Distance to school				0.592
< 30 min	189 (70.5%)	40.2%	1	
≥ 30 min	79 (29.5%)	36.7%	0.86 (0.50–1.48)	
Distance to health facility				0.033
< 30 min	134 (50.0%)	32.8%	1	
≥ 30 min	134 (50.0%)	45.5%	1.71 (1.04–2.81)	
Education				0.023[a]
None	57 (21.3%)	54.4%	2.28 (1.18–4.43)	
Primary attended	109 (40.7%)	35.8%	1.07 (0.61–1.88)	
Primary or superior	102 (38.1%)	34.3%	1	
Literacy				< 0.001
Cannot read/ only parts	110 (41.0%)	54.6%	3.01 (1.81–5.02)	
Able to read	158 (59.0%)	28.5%	1	
Source water*				0.532
Unimproved	134 (50.0%)	41.0%	1.17 (0.72–1.91)	
Improved	134 (50.0%)	37.3%	1	
Size of household				0.613
1–5	95 (35.4%)	43.2%	1.30 (0.73–2.30)	
6–8	103 (38.4%)	36.9%	1	
≥ 9	70 (26.1%)	37.1%	1.01 (0.54–1.90)	
Profession head				0.333
Farmer	151 (56.3%)	41.7%	1.28 (0.78–2.10)	
Other	117 (43.7%)	35.9%	1	
Met VPE				0.059
No	139 (51.9%)	44.6%	1.61 (0.98–2.64)	
Yes	129 (48.1%)	33.3%	1	
Met enhanced CAG				0.623
No	153 (57.1%)	37.9%	0.88 (0.54–1.45)	
Yes	115 (42.9%)	40.9%	1	
Negotiation (condom & refusal)				< 0.001[a]
Neither option	86 (32.1%)	61.6%	6.78 (3.46–13.29)	
One out of two options	88 (32.8%)	38.6%	2.66 (1.36–5.19)	
Both options	94 (35.1%)	19.2%	1	
Age at 1st sex (years) (*n* = 266)				0.116
< 15	131 (49.2%)	43.5%	1.84 (1.01–3.35)	
15	57 (21.4%)	42.1%	1.74 (0.85–3.56)	
16–24	78 (29.3%)	29.5%	1	
Lifetime partners (*n* = 266)				0.353
1	140 (52.6%)	43.6%	1.39 (0.44–4.36)	

Table 3 Determinants of having sex with neither condom nor contraception in girls: bivariate analysis *(Continued)*

Variable (*n* = 268 unless otherwise specified)			Girls	
	N (%)	% neither condom nor contraception	OR (95%CI)	P
2–4	112 (42.1%)	34.8%	0.96 (0.30–3.07)	
≥ 5	14 (5.3%)	35.7%	1	
Parity				0.573
0	139 (51.9%)	38.1%	1	
1	81 (30.2%)	37.0%	0.95 (0.54–1.68)	
≥ 2	48 (17.9%)	45.8%	1.37 (0.71–2.66)	
In a union				0.335
Yes	128 (47.8%)	42.2%	1.27 (0.78–2.08)	
No	140 (52.2%)	36.4%	1	
Heard of FP methods				0.155
0–3	27 (10.1%)	51.9%	1.78 (0.80–3.95)	
4–8	241 (89.9%)	37.8%	1	
Slept under bednet				0.654
Yes	203 (75.7%)	38.4%	1	
No	65 (24.3%)	41.5%	1.14 (0.64–2.01)	
Hand wash < 4 h				0.033
Yes	214 (79.9%)	36.0%	1	
No	54 (20.1%)	51.9%	1.91 (1.05–3.50)	

a= chi^2 for trend; HF = health facility, VPE = Volunteer Peer Educator; CAG = Community Wellness Advocacy Group
*Improved water according to DHS definition

Except for literacy and distance, all other determinants are behavioral, whereas the more classic determinants like economic assets or occupation do not remain in the multivariable model.

Additionally, we explored reasons given for not using a condom or contraception (Table 6). All reasons which were given by more than 5% of respondents for condoms, and by more than 15% for contraception are presented.

Opposition of the partner was the most frequent reason for not using condom or contraception for both boys (46.8%) and girls (70.2%). Interestingly, both boys and girls put the responsibility of the opposition on their partner. Non availability of condoms was also among the top reasons mentioned. Lack of access to contraception was one of the top three mentioned by boys but not by girls.

Comments made by youths in the individual survey

Some of the comments about not using condoms or modern contraception, in open ended questions in the household survey, warrant further thought from planners and educators.

Two girls explained that they had used neither condom nor family planning because their previous intercourse had been a rape (2 out of 105 non-users). Eight boys and girls believed the condom constituted a health risk: one believed it could kill, one other that it brings on "death and illness", one mentioned it brought on infection, three mentioned it was harmful for health, one girl mentioned that it would corrupt her milk, and two more were worried that it would stick in the vagina. Further comments included: "shameful", "forbidden", "inconvenient", "lack of knowledge about utilization", and "waste of time".

Discussion

The overall contraceptive prevalence rate (condom alone, or contraception alone or both) was 55% for boys and 43% for girls. Dual protection was observed in a higher number of boys (22%) than girls (7%). In addition, globally 6% of boys and 30% of girls declared that their partners or themselves were pregnant or wished to be. Among these, 42% (17% of the boys and 44% of the girls) were in the 10–19 age group, which is in opposition with the National Strategy for the reduction of teen-age pregnancy [10].

In the multivariable model, four determinants of condom or contraception use were common to boys and girls: literacy, distance, negotiation and hand washing. The distance which remained in the model for girls was to the health facility, while for boys it was to school. This could be due to the fact that girls most commonly obtain contraception from health providers at facilities while with boys this is not critical to access condoms.

In the bivariate model there was significant gender interaction for five determinants of condom or contraception use. One of the two UNFPA interventions, the

Table 4 Multivariable analysis of utilization of condom/contraception at last intercourse: 189 sexually active boys

Variable (in order of inclusion)	Adjusted OR (95%CI)	P
Hand wash < 4 h		< 0.001
Yes	1	
No	6.57 (2.63–16.45)	
Literacy		< 0.001
Cannot read/only parts	8.50 (2.90–24.94)	
Able to read	1	
Heard of FP methods		0.018
0–3	4.37 (1.28–14.88)	
4–8	1	
Lifetime partners		0.004
1	5.86 (1.59–21.70)	
2–4	9.55 (2.51–36.36)	
≥ 5	1	
Distance to school		0.004
< 30 min	1	
≥ 30 min	5.16 (1.71–15.55)	
Slept under bednet		0.009
Yes	1	
No	3.27 (1.35–7.91)	
Negotiation (condom & refusal)		0.030
Neither option	3.81 (1.37–10.62)	
One out of two options	2.50 (0.90–6.91)	
Both options	1	

H-L test: $P = 0.684$ – Pseudo $R^2 = 0.435$; FP = Family Planning
Not included (NS): age, age 1st sex, distance to HF, education, union, met VPE, met CAG, type water, size household, occupation head household

Table 5 Multivariable analysis of utilization of condom/contraception at last intercourse: 268 sexually active girls

Variable (in order of inclusion)	Adjusted OR (IC95%)	P
Negotiation (condom & refusal)		< 0.001
Neither option	6.88 (3.34–14.20)	
One out of two options	2.73 (1.35–5.50)	
Both options	1	
Literacy		0.004
Cannot read / only parts	2.28 (1.30–3.99)	
Able to read	1	
Distance to health facility)		0.008
< 30 min	1	
≥ 30 min	2.16 (1.23–3.79)	
Hand wash < 4 h		0.047
Yes	1	
No	2.00 (1.01–3.98)	

H-L test: $P = 0.846$ – Pseudo $R^2 = 0.167$; FP = Family Planning
Not included (NS): age, age 1st sex, distance to school, education, number of partners, union, heard PF methods, met VPE, met CAG, parity, type water, size household, occupation head household, slept under bednet

VPE placements was a determinant for boys and there was a strong trend for girls. The enhanced CAGs on the other hand showed no effect. However, there are various possible explanations: (i) the likelihood of meeting a VPE is higher than for a CAG; (ii) in general, the core content of VPE messages is more related to sexual health; and (iii) CAG messages may have been more modulated in relation to the EVD outbreak, with a greater focus on prevention of infection dissemination and hand washing in particular. This hypothesized change may be reflected in the strong association with hand washing found for both boys and girls.

The open questions show serious misgivings about condoms and contraception. Two girls explained the motive for non use as being raped; though this is not numerically important this needs to be kept in mind.

The study has many strengths. Data were collected with electronic tablets which enhanced the quality and the completeness of data. It has been suggested that electronic tablets might be one of the greatest advances of the 21st century, because they contribute to good monitoring in Low and Middle Income Countries (LMICs) [11]. Boys and girls answered the same questions, including questions about barriers or negotiation, this has allowed to show strong gender differences. The behavioral determinants showed significant gender interaction, with effects systematically stronger in boys. In a recent UK study, gender and age were determinants of contraception intention, supporting the need for tailored sex education [12].

Using, to a large extent, the same questions as in the DHS and the GSHS allows for comparisons with these data sets. Regarding descriptive data such as economic assets, distance or education the fact that the results of this survey are essentially in the same direction and of the same order of magnitude as the results from the 2013 SLDHS provides a certain degree of data validation.

The study also has some weaknesses: the sample size is small, especially for sexually active youngsters of less than 15, decreasing power, and the data pertain to the post EVD outbreak in Sierra Leone, decreasing external validity.

A number of the study results are similar to published results from other countries; however this study provides unique information for the Sierra Leone context. Determinants which remain in the final models both for boys and girls: literacy and distance to school and health facilities are well described in four recent systematic reviews of contraception use determinants in LMICs in general [13] or specifically in sub-Saharan Africa [14–16]. Distance presumably functions in two manners: directly as the time it takes in terms of reduced access, and probably also as an indicator of populations difficult to reach out to, with less opening to the modern world. Literacy

Table 6 Reasons given for not using condom or contraception

Most frequent reasons in boys (*n* = 79)	n (%)	Most frequent reasons in girls (*n* = 104)	n (%)
For not using condom			
1.Partner doesn't want	37 (46.8%)	1.Partner doesn't want	73 (70.2%)
2.Condoms not available	31 (39.2%)	2.Faithful	39 (37.5%)
3.Don't know where to get	25 (31.7%)	3.Condoms not available	25 (24.0%)
4.Faithful	22 (27.9%)	4.Don't know where to get	16 (15.4%)
5.Religious	21 (26.6%)	5.Religious	13 (12.5%)
For not using contraception			
1.Partner opposed	33 (41.8%)	1.Partner opposed	40 (38.5%)
2.Not married	18 (22.8%)	2.Others opposed	25 (24.0%)
3.Lack of access	17 (21.5%)	3.Knows no method	18 (17.3%)
4.Respondent opposed	15 (19.0%)	4.Knows no source	18 (17.3%)
5.Knows no method	14 (17.7%)	5.Respondent opposed	16 (15.4%)
6.Knows no source	14 (17.7%)	6.Religious	14 (13.5%)

Three boys and one girl did not answer

remained in the present model; whereas age and education, which are ubiquitous in studies of determinants of contraception use, and which were present in the bivariate analysis, did not remain in the multivariate. A possible explanation is that literacy is a direct resultant of both age and exposure to education and might be a better reflection of the causal pathway of non-utilization of contraception. An argument in this direction can be found in a quasi-experimental study; Leon et al. implemented, in India, a three-year community intervention to globally promote woman's empowerment. They observed, in the intervention area, a significant change on beliefs about the decision to have children, but only in the illiterate women [17]. The results of Leon generate the hypothesis that literacy acts not only as a determinant of utilization, but possibly needs to be taken into account for choice of interventions.

Two other determinants were common to boys and girls and are essentially behavioral: the first is related to sexual behavior and includes a composite of "sexual consent" and "condom negotiation". This determinant is not found in many studies. However, in a qualitative study in young high school girls in Ghana, all who were using condoms considered they were able to require their partner to use it [18].

Two more behavioral determinants warrant some discussion, hand washing, which remained in both the girls' and boys' model, and bednet utilization which remained for boys only. Unsurprisingly, no data on contraception and either hand washing, or bednet utilization, could be found in the literature. However it can be hypothesized that determinants could be similar, as all of these are desirable behaviors. Two such examples follow. A study in Nigeria on school children assessed which canals were most effective in increasing hand washing during the EVD outbreak; the two most effective were the church and television, the second being once more, a marker of more affluent households [19]. For bednet utilization, in a recent survey of determinants in Cameroon, knowledge of utility and educational level remain in the final model suggesting again, that these are more global determinants of healthy behavior [20]. Two more determinants were specific to boys only: theoretical knowledge of contraception, and number of partners, which appear in most systematic reviews such as those mentioned above.

The open questions revealed, among others, two issues: coerced sex in teen-agers and severe misconceptions about condoms and contraception. Both these are documented in previously published studies, as in deprived populations of Kampala for coercion where 25% of the interviewed had been raped [21] or urban Cameroon for misconceptions about contraception [22].

This study has direct implications. The first two pertain to the content of SRH messages for adolescents. Should there be a shift towards a clear recommendation of "dual protection" or "safe sex"? A stronger emphasis on promotion of dual protection for young, unmarried people would be beneficial, even in a country with a relatively low HIV prevalence like Sierra Leone (1.5% of 15–49 years), to avoid other forms of STIs (13.4% for males and 10.5% for females), self reported, in the same age group [2].

The other major implication is about reaching out to underserved populations. In a study in Senegal, on "harder to reach" populations, these are defined as "less exposed to external influence and at risk of being underserved despite their high level of need", and considered to belong to the three categories: adolescents, unmarried and rural poor [23]. Changing attitudes in communities which are far from everything is a true challenge [24].

Conclusions

This study shows that sexually active young people who use condoms or contraception are generally better educated, easier to reach and have safer health behaviors.

Our study reinforces the notion that interventions need to be targeted specifically, taking into account characteristics such as gender, age, marital status, literacy and outreach issues.

This study suggests that a truly comprehensive vision of sexual health is warranted, including topics apparently not systematically addressed at present, such as coercion, intra partner violence, negotiation, consent, and avoiding teen-age pregnancy. This can theoretically be best addressed through school programs such as the PREPARE in South Africa [25].

Abbreviations

CAG: Community Wellness Advocacy Groups; CI: Confidence interval; DFID: Department for International Development (UK AID); DHS: Demographic and Health Survey; EVD: Ebola virus disease; FP: Family planning; GSHS: Global School-based student Health Survey; HIV-AIDS: Human Immunodeficiency Virus - Acquired Immune Deficiency Syndrome; IRMNH: Improving Reproductive Maternal and Newborn Health; IUD: Intrauterine device; LMIC: Low and middle income countries; OR: Odds ratios; SLDHS: Sierra Leone Demographic and Health Survey; SRH: sexual and reproductive health; STI: Sexually Transmitted Infection; UNFPA: United Nations Population Fund; UNICEF: United Nations International Children's Emergency Fund; VPE: Volunteer Peer Educators

Acknowledgements

Thanks to: heads of household and young people who responded the questionnaires; supervisors, enumerators, drivers; the Ministry of Health and Sanitation and the district health management teams in Kenema, Kono, Kambia, Koinadugu, Bonthe, Moyamba, Kailahun and Pujehun; Restless Development for information on VPE work; Lilas Weber for developing, and implementing the first monitoring survey in 2014, as well as backup support in survey 2016; Paul Sengeh for coordination of the field work for the household survey; Samuel Pratt for coordination of the health facility survey; Mohamed F Jalloh and Ibrahim Tucker supervisor of focus group discussions; Ingeborg Jille Traas for constructive discussions of earlier drafts, Safiatu Foday for support for the coordination of the study implementation; and for administrative support, hera in Reet and FOCUS 1000 in Freetown.

Funding

The survey was commissioned to hera Reet, Belgium by UNFPA Sierra Leone in response to RFP N° SLE/2013/07/02 through financial support from DFID.

Authors' contributions

AL implemented the survey in the field, was responsible for the 1st analysis and prepared the manuscript. MM and SA contributed to the design of the study and were co-responsible for all aspects. ME and AK contributed at all times to the survey, the analysis, and preparation of the paper. MJ was responsible for the implementation of the survey. MD and WZ contributed to the design of the population survey and performed the secondary analysis for this study. KD reviewed all drafts and provided substantial contributions to the writing of the paper. All authors read and approved the final manuscript.

Competing interests

The authors declare that they have no competing interests.

Author details

[1]Université Libre de Bruxelles, Ecole de Santé Publique, Research Center: Policies and Health Systems - International Health, 808, Route de Lennik, 1070 Brussels, Belgium. [2]hera, Right to Health and Development, Reet, Belgium. [3]FOCUS 1000, NGO, Freetown, Sierra Leone. [4]UNFPA, Freetown, Sierra Leone.

References

1. Black RE, Levin C, Walker N, Chou D, Liu L, Temmerman M, DCP3 RMNCH Authors Group. Reproductive, maternal, newborn, and child health: key messages from disease control priorities 3rd edition. Lancet. 2016;3(388): 2811–24. https://doi.org/10.1016/S0140-6736(16)00738-8. Epub 2016 Apr 9. Review. PubMed PMID: 27072119
2. Statistics Sierra Leone (SSL) and ICF International. Sierra Leone demographic and health survey 2013. Freetown and Rockville: SSL and ICF International; 2014.
3. Nove A, Matthews Z, Neal S, Camacho AV. Maternal mortality in adolescents compared with women of other ages: evidence from 144 countries. Lancet Glob Health. 2014;2(3):e155–64.
4. November L, Sandall J. 'Just because she's young, it doesn't mean she has to die': exploring the contributing factors to high maternal mortality in adolescents in eastern Freetown; a qualitative study. Reprod Health. 2018; 15(1):31.
5. Chandra-Mouli V, Svanemyr J, Amin A, Fogstad H, Say L, Girard F, Temmerman M. Twenty years after international conference on population and development: where are we with adolescent sexual and reproductive health and rights? J Adolesc Health. 2015;56:1–6.
6. Yakubu I, Salisu WJ. Determinants of adolescent pregnancy in sub-Saharan Africa: a systematic review. Reprod Health. 2018;15(1):15.
7. Multi-Year Annual Survey to Monitor Programme Effectiveness of the "Improving Reproductive Maternal and Newborn Health" (IRMNH) Programme; Survey 2016: http://sierraleone.unfpa.org/en/publications/multi-year-annual-survey-monitor-programme-effectiveness-improving-reproductive Accessed 30 June 2017.
8. ICF International. Demographic and health survey Interviewer's manual. MEASURE DHS basic documentation no. 2. Calverton: ICF International; 2012.
9. Global School based Student Health Survey Sierra Leone (no results available) http://www.who.int/chp/gshs/sierraleone/en/. Accessed 24 Apr 2017.
10. National Strategy for the reduction of teen-age pregnancy – Let girls be girls http://hivhealthclearinghouse.unesco.org/sites/default/files/resources/Sierra_Leone_National_Strategy_for_the_Reduction_of_Teenage_Pregnancy.pdf. Accessed 30 June 2017.
11. Costello A. Irreverent, melancholic, dogged. BMJ. 2016;353:i3550. https://doi.org/10.1136/bmj.i3550. PubMed PMID: 27358256
12. Bayley JE, Baines D, Brown KE. Developing the evidence base for gender- and age-relevant school sex education: questionnaire findings from an adolescent sample using an augmented theory of planned behaviour. Sex Health. 2017;14(6):548–57.
13. Wulifan JK, Brenner S, Jahn A, De Allegri M. A scoping review on determinants of unmet need for family planning among women of reproductive age in low and middle income countries. BMC Womens Health. 2016;16:2.
14. Blackstone SR, Nwaozuru U, Iwelunmor J. Factors influencing contraceptive use in sub-Saharan Africa: a systematic review. Int Q Community Health Educ. 2017;37(2):79–91.
15. Ayanore MA, Pavlova M, Groot W. Unmet reproductive health needs among women in some west African countries: a systematic review of outcome measures and determinants. Reprod Health. 2016;13:5. https://doi.org/10.1186/s12978-015-0104-x. Review. PubMed PMID: 26774502; PubMed Central PMCID: PMC4715869

16. Emina JB, Chirwa T, Kandala NB. Trend in the use of modern contraception in sub-Saharan Africa: does women's education matter? Contraception. 2014;90(2):154–61.
17. León FR, Lundgren R, Sinai I, Sinha R, Jennings V. Increasing literate and illiterate women's met need for contraception via empowerment: a quasi-experiment in rural India. Reprod Health. 2014;11(1):74.
18. Krugu JK, Mevissen FE, Prinsen A, Ruiter RA. Who's that girl? A qualitative analysis of adolescent girls' views on factors associated with teenage pregnancies in Bolgatanga, Ghana. Reprod Health. 2016;13:39.
19. Ilesanmi OS, Alele FO. The effect of Ebola virus disease outbreak on hand washing among secondary school students in Ondo state Nigeria, October, 2014. Pan Afr Med J. 2015;22(Suppl 1):24. https://doi.org/10.11694/pamj.supp.2015.22.1.6614. eCollection 2015. PubMed PMID: 26740852; PubMed Central PMCID: PMC4695531
20. Fokam EB, Kindzeka GF, Ngimuh L, Dzi KT, Wanji S. Determination of the predictive factors of long-lasting insecticide-treated net ownership and utilisation in the Bamenda Health District of Cameroon. BMC Public Health. 2017;17(1):263.
21. Renzaho AM, Kamara JK, Georgeou N, Kamanga G. Sexual, reproductive health needs, and rights of young people in slum areas of Kampala, Uganda: a cross sectional study. PLoS One. 2017;12(1):e0169721.
22. Ajong AB, Njotang PN, Kenfack B, Yakum MN, Mbu ER. Knowledge of women in family planning and future desire to use contraception: a cross sectional survey in urban Cameroon. BMC Res Notes. 2016;9:347.
23. Cavallaro FL, Benova L, Macleod D, Faye A, Lynch CA. Examining trends in family planning among harder-to-reach women in Senegal 1992-2014. Sci Rep. 2017;7:41006.
24. Victora CG, Barros AJ, França GV, da Silva IC, Carvajal-Velez L, Amouzou A. The contribution of poor and rural populations to national trends in reproductive, maternal, newborn, and child health coverage: analyses of cross-sectional surveys from 64 countries. Lancet Glob Health. 2017;5(4):e402–7.
25. Mathews C, Eggers SM, Townsend L, Aarø LE, de Vries PJ, Mason-Jones AJ, De Koker P, McClinton Appollis T, Mtshizana Y, Koech J, Wubs A, De Vries H. Effects of PREPARE, a multi-component, school-based HIV and intimate partner violence (IPV) prevention Programme on adolescent sexual risk behaviour and IPV: cluster randomised controlled trial. AIDS Behav. 2016; 20(9):1821–40. https://doi.org/10.1007/s10461-016-1410-1. PubMed PMID: 27142057; PubMed Central PMCID: PMC4995229

Client and provider factors associated with integration of family planning services among maternal and reproductive health clients in Kigoma Region

M. M. Dynes[1*], E. Bernstein[1], D. Morof[1], L. Kelly[1], A. Ruiz[2], W. Mongo[3], P. Chaote[4], R. N. Bujari[5] and F. Serbanescu[1]

Abstract

Background: Integration of family planning (FP) services into non-FP care visits is an essential strategy for reducing maternal and neonatal mortality through reduction of short birth intervals and unplanned pregnancies.

Methods: Cross-sectional surveys were conducted across 61 facilities in Kigoma Region, Tanzania, April–July 2016. Multilevel, mixed effects logistic regression analyses were conducted on matched data from providers ($n = 330$) and clients seeking delivery ($n = 935$), well-baby ($n = 272$), pregnancy loss (PL; $n = 229$), and other routine (postnatal, HIV/STI, other; $n = 69$) services. Outcomes of interest included receipt of FP information and a modern FP method (significance level $p < 0.05$).

Results: Clients had significantly greater odds of receiving FP information if the primary reason for seeking care was for PL versus (vs) any other types of care (aOR 1.97), had four or more pregnancies vs fewer (aOR 1.78), and had had a FP discussion with their partner vs no FP discussion (aOR 1.73). Clients had lower odds of receiving FP information if they were aged 40–49 vs 15–19 (aOR 0.50) and reported attending religious services at least weekly vs less frequently (aOR 0.61). Clients of providers who perceived that in-service training had helped vs had not helped job performance (aOR 2.27), and clients of providers having high vs low recent FP training index scores (aOR 1.58) had greater odds of receiving FP information.

Clients had greater odds of receiving a modern method when they received information on two or more vs fewer methods (aOR 7.13), had had a FP discussion with their partner vs no discussion (aOR 5.87), if the primary reason for seeking care was for PL vs any other types of care (aOR 4.08), had zero vs one or more live births (aOR 3.92), made their own FP decisions vs not made own FP decisions (aOR 3.17), received FP information from two or more vs fewer sources (aOR 3.12), and were in the middle or high vs the low wealth tercile (aOR 1.99 and 2.30, respectively). Well-baby care clients, Other routine services clients, and married clients had significantly lower odds of receiving a method (aOR 0.14; aOR 0.08; and aOR 0.41, respectively) compared to their counterparts.

Conclusions: Strategies that better integrate FP into routine care visits, encourage women to have FP discussions with their partners and providers, increase FP training among providers, and expand FP options and sources of information may help reduce the unmet need for FP, and ultimately lower maternal and neonatal mortality.

Keywords: Family planning, Family planning counseling, Family planning integration, Contraception, Contraceptive methods, Sub-Saharan Africa, Tanzania, Multilevel modeling

* Correspondence: mdynes@cdc.gov
[1]Centers for Disease Control and Prevention, Division of Reproductive Health, Atlanta, USA
Full list of author information is available at the end of the article

Plain English summary

Integrating family planning (FP) services into non-FP care visits is an important approach to reduce maternal and newborn deaths through reduction of short birth intervals and unplanned pregnancies. Analyses of matched interviews with 1505 clients and 330 providers in Kigoma Region, Tanzania identified key factors for clients receiving FP information and a modern method. Clients were more likely to receive FP information if they were at the facility for pregnancy loss, had four or more pregnancies, and had discussed FP with their partner. Clients were less likely to receive FP information if they were 40 to 49 years old and attended religious services at least weekly. Providers were more likely to provide FP information if they perceived in-service training had helped their job performance, and had received more recent FP training. Clients were more likely to receive a FP method if they received information on two or more FP methods, had discussed FP with their partner, were at the facility for pregnancy loss, had no live births, made their own FP decisions, received FP information from two or more sources, and were in the middle or high wealth groups. Well-baby care clients, Other services clients, and married clients were less likely to receive a FP method compared to others. FP services need to be better integrated into well-baby and other routine outpatient services. Interventions are needed that encourage women to have FP conversations with their partners and providers, expand FP options and sources of information, and encourage providers to ask about reproductive health goals at each client encounter.

Introduction

Sub-Saharan Africa experiences disproportionately high maternal mortality in comparison to other regions, contributing to two-thirds of the world's total maternal deaths in 2015 [1]. Tanzania had an estimated 8200 maternal deaths in 2015, the fourth highest number of maternal deaths in sub-Saharan Africa and the sixth highest number in the world [1]. Family planning (FP) can reduce the risk of maternal and neonatal mortality by reducing the number of short birth intervals, as well as unplanned and high-risk pregnancies [2–7]. In 2016, the total fertility rate (TFR) in Tanzania's Western Zone, which includes Kigoma Region, was 6.7 births per woman – the highest TFR in all of Tanzania [8].

Research in Western and African clinical settings has found that quality FP counseling—identified as six distinct elements by the Bruce Framework [9]—has a significant impact on FP knowledge and use [10, 11]. To increase postpartum FP uptake and reduce unmet need, FP counseling and provision are routinely recommended for integration into antenatal, labor and delivery, and postnatal care services [12–17]. However, evidence varies on whether the increase in FP use relates to the type of care services in which FP services are being integrated [13, 23, 27], number of times counseling is provided [17–20], whether the FP counseling is provided during the antenatal versus postpartum period [15, 17–21], and whether modern contraceptive supplies are available at the time/onsite. Moreover, some studies have found positive effects while others have found no effect [16, 21, 22].

Furthermore, many factors may influence FP uptake even when services are integrated. Necessary infrastructure improvements, increased staff resources, and availability of FP supplies rarely accompany the integration of FP services into other health services [14, 19]. Long wait times, unclear pathways to FP providers, and lack of privacy deter women from accepting a FP referral [23]. In health facility assessments in Kigoma Region, Tanzania in 2015, only 57% of dispensaries had implants and only 39% had intrauterine devices (IUD) available to clients [24].

Client predictors of FP use

Women's individual, sociodemographic characteristics, and life circumstances also influence FP uptake. Partner communication and support, self-efficacy, intensity of antenatal care visits, and previous FP use have been found to be positively associated with FP uptake [16, 20, 25]. Lower wealth and history of physical intimate partner violence have been associated with nonuse of FP methods [12, 17, 25, 26]. Women's reasons for not using FP include wanting to talk with their partner first [23], waiting until their current baby is older [23], waiting until their menses return [27], and fearing side effects and health risks [28].

Provider predictors of FP use

Health providers' perceptions and biases may influence provision of services and subsequent likelihood of client FP uptake. Providers may counsel clients against using certain methods or impose medically unfounded barriers to FP methods based on perceived client characteristics including age, partner consent, marital status, and parity [7, 23, 29, 30]. Providers' personal biases have been found to be more commonly imposed for long-term or permanent methods [29], for condoms and pills depending on client age [29] and parity [7], and among providers in private facilities [8] or those with less FP in-service training [7, 29]. In contrast, provider willingness to share personal experiences of FP use [31] and perception of client characteristics, such as education and ability to understand FP options [29], may be positively associated with provider engagement in more directed FP counseling, and may result in greater client satisfaction with services [32].

Reproductive health in Kigoma region Tanzania

In 2016, Kigoma Region's TFR was 6.5 births per woman, the modern FP prevalence rate among women in union was 20%, and the unmet need for FP among women in union was 36% [33]. There are several national Ministry of Health, Community Development, Gender, Elderly, and Children (MoHCDGEC) ongoing efforts to improve maternal health in Tanzania that have particularly targeted Kigoma Region. These include the *National Roadmap Strategic Plan to Accelerate Reduction of Maternal, Newborn and Child Deaths in Tanzania 2008–2015; the Big Results Now* (BRN) initiative; and Wazazi Nipendeni ("Parents Love Me"), a mobile health initiative that includes FP and safe motherhood text messages. Since 2006, the *Project to Reduce Maternal Deaths in Tanzania* has worked in the region with the aim of decreasing maternal mortality through strengthening emergency obstetric and neonatal care and improving access to and use of FP. As part of monitoring and evaluation activities conducted for the Bloomberg Philanthropies-funded *Project to Reduce Maternal Deaths in Tanzania*, the Centers for Disease Control and Prevention (CDC) has been providing technical assistance to document the integration of FP into health facilities providing maternity care in Kigoma.

Gaps in literature

Previous studies have explored outcomes of FP counseling and service provision into non-FP services or have described the influence of provider or client characteristics on FP uptake. However, the literature reflects inconsistent associations between receipt of FP information and uptake in methods, and further inconsistencies in the role of client and provider factors in FP integration. Furthermore, there are no published studies on the influence of both client and provider characteristics as predictors of FP integration. This study helps to fill these gaps in the evidence by considering both client and provider characteristics associated with receipt of FP information and modern method among non-FP clients in Kigoma, Tanzania. This information will provide the Tanzanian MoHCDGEC, as well as other stakeholders, with evidence needed to make informed decisions about programmatic and policy implementation for FP integration into maternal and reproductive health services.

Methods

Study setting and design

Kigoma Region covers 45,066 km^2 and is located in the northwestern Tanzania. In 2012, the region had a population of 2,127,930; approximately 83% of the population is designated as rural with farming as the primary economic activity. Nine out of 10 people in Kigoma have attained a primary school education and 76% of the adult population is literate. [34]

We conducted cross-sectional surveys consisting of facility-based client exit interviews and provider interviews across 61 facilities (6 hospitals, 25 health centers, and 30 dispensaries) in Kigoma Region, Tanzania from April 30 to July 1, 2016.

Sampling and data collection

Facility sampling

All governmental and private hospitals ($n = 6$) and health centers (excluding those in refugee camp settings) ($n = 25$) in Kigoma Region were included. A sample of 30 dispensaries (of the 198 in the region providing delivery services) was selected to maximize geographic distribution and meet the following inclusion criteria: 1) have an estimated 180 or more births per year; 2) have two or more onsite health providers; 3) be a site for national or project partner facility improvements, and 4) refer patients to one of the 25 health centers.

Provider and client sampling

Convenience sampling was used to enroll providers and clients within selected facilities; all providers and clients providing/seeking care on study days were invited to participate if they met inclusion criteria. All types of providers who routinely conducted labor and delivery, pregnancy loss (PL; defined as spontaneous or induced abortion), FP, or postnatal care services were eligible, except for medical doctors and specialists who had limited numbers and availability. Clients were eligible if they were 15 to 49 years of age and received delivery, PL, and routine out-patient (FP, antenatal care [ANC], well-baby, and other) care services at the facility. Clients were excluded if they were younger than 15 or older than 49 years of age, delivered at home or on the way to the facility, had a cesarean section delivery, or experienced a stillbirth or neonatal death.

We determined that 189 provider interviews were sufficient to detect a 5% relative mean change in key variables of interest related to their knowledge and practice with 90% power and an alpha of 0.05. A sample of 908 client interviews was needed to detect a 15% absolute difference in the variables of interest with 90% power and an alpha of 0.05 (assuming a 50% reference proportion). We aimed to interview between two and six delivery and outpatient clients per provider per care type to reduce provider-specific bias; this selection rule was not applied to PL interviews due to the limited availability of PL clients and providers.

Interview procedures

Questionnaires were pre-tested in January 2016. Final questionnaires were translated from English to Swahili and back-translated to English. Providers were interviewed if they met inclusion criteria and consented to participate. Their clients were approached for participation as they exited care services; clients were asked which care service they received and the corresponding interview guide was administered. All interviews were administered face-to-face by an interviewer in Swahili.

Study tools

For client exit interviews, three separate questionnaires were used that were tailored to client service provision type. Questionnaires captured sociodemographic characteristics, perceptions of and satisfaction with services, facility experiences, receipt of FP information and uptake by method, and pregnancy history and intention. Providers completed a questionnaire and knowledge test designed to capture information about provider demographic characteristics, education, training, clinical knowledge, and practices related to labor and delivery care, newborn care, PL, and FP care.

Outcome variables

In this analysis, we examined two binary outcome variables based on women's self-report: 1) *Receipt of FP information* (0, did not receive FP information; 1, received FP information); and 2) *Receipt of a modern FP method* (pill, injection, intrauterine device [IUD], implant, male or female condom, male or female sterilization, or emergency contraception: 0, did not receive a modern FP method; 1 received a modern FP method).

Independent variables

Client-level

The client-level variables of interest included:

- *Client age* (15 to 19, 20 to 29, 30 to 39, 40 to 49),
- *Delivery care was the primary service sought* (yes, no),
- *PL care was the primary service sought* (yes, no),
- *Well-baby care was the primary service sought* (yes, no; [immunization, growth]),
- *Other routine services was the primary service sought* (yes, no; [postnatal care, HIV testing and management, STI]),
- *Literacy* (able to read and write, able to read or write/neither read nor write),
- *Highest education attended* (no formal education, primary, secondary, university),
- *Number of prior pregnancies* (zero to three, four or more),
- *Number of live births* (zero, one to two, three to five, six or more),
- *Marital status* (not in union, in union),
- *Frequency of attendance at religious services* (less than once a week, once a week or more often),
- *Wealth* (low, middle, high wealth),
- *Has heard family planning messages in the last three months* (yes, no),
- *Desired timing of future childbearing* (wants a child in the next two years, wants a child in more than two years/does not want),
- *FP discussion with partner* (no discussion, has discussed FP with partner),
- *FP decision-making* (does not make own FP decisions, able to make own FP decisions),
- *FP information index* (received information about zero or one FP method, received information about two or more FP methods; variable only used for the *Receipt of a modern FP method* model), and
- *FP information source index* (received FP information from zero or one source, received FP information from two or more sources; variable only used for the *Receipt of a modern FP method* model).

The variable *Wealth* was developed using principal components analysis (PCA) where household assets and characteristics were weighted based on their contribution to the first component and summed to create an index [35]. Each household was given a wealth index score categorized into terciles representing low, middle, and high levels of relative household wealth.

Provider-level

The provider-level variables of interest included:

- *Provider age* (younger than the mean of 38 years of age, 38 years or more),
- *Sex* (male, female),
- *Highest education completed* (primary, secondary, university),
- *Cadre* (clinicians [Assistant Medical Officers/Clinical Officers/Assistant Clinical Officers/Clinical Assistants], nurses/midwives [Nurse Officers/Assistant Nurse Officers/Registered Nurses/Midwives/Enrolled Nurses], other staff [Medical Attendants/Maternal and Child Health Aides]),
- *Years in cadre* (less than the mean of 11 years, 11 or more years),
- *Years at the facility* (less than the mean of eight years, eight years or more),
- *Work hours per week* (less than the mean of 56 h per week, 56 or more hours per week),
- *Job satisfaction* (a little/very satisfied, a little/very dissatisfied/neither satisfied nor dissatisfied),
- *Perceptions of fairness in pay* (feels he/she is not paid fairly, feels paid fairly),
- *Perceptions of adequacy of training* (feels training is inadequate for job duties, feels training is adequate),
- *Regularly provides FP services* (yes, no),
- *FP bias* (reports no bias against providing FP service, bias reported on one or more client characteristics[1]),
- *FP recent-training PCA score* (low [below mean], high [mean or higher]),
- *FP ever-training PCA score* (low [below mean], high [mean or higher]),
- *FP practice PCA score* (low [below mean], high [mean or higher]),

- *Perceptions of helpfulness of in-service training* (feels in-service training has not been helpful, feels in-service training has been helpful),
- *Electronic mentoring opportunities* (no access to e-learning/ emergency call system/ teleconference, has access to one or more electronic mentoring activities).

The variables for *FP recent-training PCA score* (FP training in 2015 or in the first half of 2016), *FP ever-training PCA score* (FP pre- or in-service training at any time), and *FP practice PCA score* (current provision of FP services) were developed with PCA using 14 items that cover a range of FP topics.[2] Elements for recent-training, ever-training, and current practice were weighted based on their contribution to the first principal component and summed to create three separate indices.

Analytic approach

Client and provider data were linked. Due to the focus of this study on FP integration into non-FP services, FP clients ($n = 214$), current FP users ($n = 128$), and providers who only gave care to FP clients ($n = 38$), were excluded from analyses. ANC ($n = 225$) and other pregnant clients ($n = 40$) were also excluded due to lack of data on desire for future childbearing and FP decision-making.

Data analyses were conducted using Stata 14. Bivariate analyses were conducted to identify client and provider variables associated with the outcome variables of interest. Client and provider variables with an unadjusted association with the outcomes of interest at a level of $p < 0.10$ were included in multivariate modeling. A multilevel mixed-effects logistic regression model was used to examine the effects of patient and provider characteristics on either receipt of FP information or receipt of a modern FP method, with random intercepts for each provider. A *p*-value of less than 0.05 was considered statistically significant for multilevel models. We included facility-clustered standard errors to account for unobserved heterogeneity within facilities.

Results

From April 30–July 1, 2016, 2155 female clients (delivery $n = 960$, PL $n = 230$, outpatient $n = 965$ [inclusive of antenatal, postnatal care, HIV testing and management, STI, and other) and 361 providers were interviewed. Following removal of data from non-linked clients and providers, FP clients, pregnant clients, and current FP users, data from 1505 clients (primary reasons for visit: delivery $n = 935$, PL $n = 229$, well-baby $n = 272$, other routine services $n = 69$) and 330 providers (clinicians $n = 69$, nurses/midwives $n = 176$, other staff $n = 85$) were used in the analysis.

Client and provider characteristics

Descriptive characteristics of the clients included in the analyses are displayed in Table 1. The majority of clients were in a union (90.4%), had attended religious services at least weekly (85.8%), were able to read and write (71.1%), and had attended primary school education (65.8%). About half of clients were 20 to 29 years of age (49.8%) and received care at a health center (48.9%). Two-thirds of clients came to the facility for the purpose of delivery services (62.1%), while less than one-fifth came for the purpose of well-baby (18.1%), PL (15.2%), and other services (4.6%). Whereas 59.4% of clients reported having a FP discussion with their partner, less than one-fifth of clients (17.9%) reported feeling they are able to make their own FP decisions.

Descriptive characteristics of the providers included in the analyses are displayed in Table 2. The majority of providers included in the study were female (63.3%), college/ university educated (66.7%), worked in a health center (55.2%), and were in the nurse/midwife cadre (53.3%). About two-thirds of providers have worked for more than 10 years in the cadre (61.5%) and more than 7 years at their current facility (70%). Providers worked an average of 54 h per week, with 57.9% working more than this average. Less than half of providers were a little or very satisfied with their job (44.9%), and less than one-fifth of providers reported feeling they were paid fairly for their job duties (17.0%). Three-quarters routinely provided FP services (75.5%), and nearly two-thirds of providers displayed at least one type of FP bias related to age, parental consent, spousal consent, or parity (62.3%).

Receipt of FP information

Descriptive characteristics for receipt of FP information

About half of clients reported receiving FP information during their non-FP visit (51.7%). Among those who reported receiving FP information, the provider speaking with the client was the most common source of FP information (98.5%). The most commonly discussed methods were injection (80.1%), implant (78.7%), and intrauterine device (70.6%) (Table 1). More than half of clients reported wanting to wait for more than two years before having another child (56.6%), and 19.1% of clients reported not desiring to have any more children. More than half of PL (60.3%) and delivery (52.7%) care clients reported receiving FP information, compared to 45.6% of well-baby care and 33.3% of other routine services clients (Fig. 1).

Bivariate analyses

Results of bivariate analyses for *Receipt of FP information* are displayed in the Appendix. Client covariates with a significant positive association with receipt of FP information included *Client age, PL care was the primary service sought, Highest education attended, Wealth, Number of prior pregnancies, Has had FP discussion with partner,* and *Heard FP messages in the last 3 months.*

Table 1 Characteristics of Women Included in the Family Planning Integration Study Sample—Kigoma Region, Tanzania, April to July 2016 (n = 1505)

	Women, n (%)	95% CI
Age in years		
15–19	214 (14.2)	12.5–16.0
20–29	750 (49.8)	47.3–52.4
30–39	427 (28.4)	26.1–30.7
40–49	93 (6.2)	5.0–7.4
Don't know	21 (1.4)	0.8–2.0
Delivery care was primary service sought		
Yes	935 (62.1)	59.7–64.6
No	570 (37.9)	35.5–40.4
Well-baby care was primary service sought		
Yes	272 (18.1)	20.5–24.8
No	1233 (81.9)	79.9–83.8
Pregnancy loss (PL) care was primary service sought		
Yes	229 (15.2)	13.4–17.0
No	1276 (84.8)	82.9–86.5
Other routine services (postnatal care, HIV testing and management, STI, other) was primary service sought		
Yes	69 (4.6)	3.5–5.6
No	1436 (95.4)	94.2–96.4
Facility type		
Hospital	421 (28.0)	25.7–30.2
Health center	736 (48.9)	46.4–51.4
Dispensary	348 (23.1)	21.0–25.3
Highest education attended		
No education	325 (21.6)	19.5–23.7
Primary	990 (65.8)	63.4–68.2
Secondary or higher	190 (12.6)	10.9–14.3
Literacy		
Can read and write	1070 (71.1)	68.8–73.4
Cannot read or write	360 (23.9)	21.7–26.1
Can either read or write, but not both	64 (4.3)	3.2–5.3
Missing or refused	11 (0.7)	0.3–1.2
Wealth		
Low wealth	478 (31.8)	29.4–34.1
Middle wealth	514 (34.2)	31.8–36.6
High wealth	513 (34.1)	31.7–36.5
Number of live births		
None	43 (2.9)	2.0–3.7
1 to 2	662 (44.0)	41.5–46.5
3 to 5	504 (33.5)	31.1–35.9
6+	293 (19.5)	17.5–21.5
Missing	3 (0.2)	0.0–0.4

Table 1 Characteristics of Women Included in the Family Planning Integration Study Sample—Kigoma Region, Tanzania, April to July 2016 (n = 1505) *(Continued)*

	Women, n (%)	95% CI
Number of prior pregnancies		
0 to 3	832 (55.3)	52.8–57.8
4+	673 (44.7)	42.2–47.2
Marital status		
In a union	1361 (90.4)	88.8–91.8
Not in a union	144 (9.6)	8.2–11.2
Has had FP discussion with partner		
Yes	894 (59.4)	56.9–61.9
No or don't know	603 (40.1)	37.6–42.5
Missing	8 (0.5)	0.2–0.9
Able to make own FP decisions		
Yes	270 (17.9)	16.0–19.9
No or don't know	1231 (81.8)	79.8–83.7
Missing	4 (0.3)	0.0–0.5
Received FP information during non-FP visit		
Yes	778 (51.7)	49.2–54.2
No	727 (48.3)	45.8–50.8
Number of FP methods information was received about during non-FP visit		
0 or 1 FP method	798 (53.0)	50.5–55.5
2 or more FP methods	707 (47.0)	44.5–49.5
Modern FP methods information received about among women who reported receiving information about 1 or more methods (*n* = 778)[a]		
Injection	623 (80.1)	77.1–82.7
Implant	612 (78.7)	75.6–81.4
Intrauterine device	549 (70.6)	67.3–73.7
Pills	528 (67.9)	64.5–71.1
Male condom	262 (33.7)	30.4–37.1
Female condom	117 (15.0)	12.7–17.7
Tubal ligation	100 (12.9)	10.7–15.4
Vasectomy	28 (3.6)	2.5–5.2
Emergency Contraception	25 (3.2)	2.2–4.7
Number of sources FP information was received from during non-FP visit		
0 or 1 source of FP information	1349 (89.6)	88.0–91.1
2 or more sources of FP information	155 (10.3)	8.9–11.9
Missing	1 (0.1)	0.0–0.5
Sources that FP information received from among women who reported receiving information from 1 or more sources (*n* = 777)[a]		
Provider spoke to client	766 (98.5)	97.3–99.1
FP educational talk	89 (11.3)	9.3–13.8
FP educational flyer	67 (8.6)	6.8–10.8
Client asked provider	50 (6.3)	4.8–8.3

Table 1 Characteristics of Women Included in the Family Planning Integration Study Sample—Kigoma Region, Tanzania, April to July 2016 (n = 1505) *(Continued)*

	Women, n (%)	95% CI
FP educational video	10 (1.3)	0.7–2.4
Received modern FP method during non-FP visit		
No	1378 (91.6)	90.0–92.9
Yes	127 (8.4)	7.1–10.0
Modern FP method received among women who reported receiving a modern method (*n* = 127)[a]		
Injection	43 (33.9)	26.1–42.6
Implant	39 (30.7)	23.2–39.4
Male condom	18 (14.2)	9.1–21.5
Intrauterine device	14 (11.0)	6.6–17.9
Pill	9 (7.1)	3.7–13.2
Tubal ligation	3 (2.4)	0.8–7.2
Female condom	1 (0.8)	0.1–5.5
Heard FP messages from any source in last 3 months		
Yes	555 (36.9)	34.4–39.3
No or don't know	950 (63.1)	60.7–65.6
Desired timing of future childbearing		
1–2 years	287 (19.1)	17.8–21.1
More than 2 years	852 (56.6)	54.1–59.1
Does not want	288 (19.1)	17.1–21.1
Don't know or refused	78 (5.2)	4.1–6.3
Frequency of attendance at religious services		
Attends at least weekly	1291 (85.8)	84.0–87.5
Attends less often than weekly	214 (14.2)	12.5–16.0

[a]Denotes sum greater than 100% due to multiple methods/sources reported by some clients

Client covariates with a significant negative association with receipt of FP information included *Other routine services was the primary service sought, Frequency of attendance at religious services*, and *Desired timing of future childbearing.*

Provider covariates with a significant positive association with receipt of FP information included *Provider highest education completed, Routinely provides FP services, FP Ever-training PCA score, FP Recent-training PCA score, FP Practice PCA score, Perception in-service training has helped job performance, and Access to electronic mentoring opportunities. Hours worked per week* was the only provider covariate with a significant negative association with receipt of FP information.

Multilevel analyses

Results of multilevel, mixed-effects logistic regression analyses for *Receipt of FP information* are shown in Table 3. The odds of receiving FP information were higher for PL clients vs those seeking any other types of care (aOR 1.97, 95% CI 1.01–3.84), for those with four or more vs fewer pregnancies (aOR 1.78, 95% CI 1.21–2.60), and for those who had, vs had not, had a FP discussion with their partner (aOR 1.73, 95% CI 1.33–2.25).

The odds of receiving FP information were lower for clients aged 40 to 49 years vs those aged 15 to 19 years (aOR 0.50, 95% CI 0.26–0.97) and for clients who reported attendance at religious services weekly or more often vs those who reported less frequent attendance (aOR 0.61, 95% CI 0.44–0.85). Client-level variables found not to have a significant adjusted relationship with receipt of FP information include client *Other services was primary service sought, Highest education attended, Wealth, Desired timing of future childbearing,* and *Heard FP messages in last three months.*

The odds of receiving FP information were higher for clients of providers who perceived that in-service training has vs has not helped their job performance (aOR 2.27, 95% CI 1.35–3.84), and for clients of providers who had high as compared to low FP recent training scores (aOR 1.58, 95% CI 1.11–2.26). Provider-level variables found not to have a significant adjusted relationship with receipt of FP information include *Provider highest education completed, Work hours per week, Routinely provides FP services, FP ever-training PCA score, FP practice PCA score,* and *Access to electronic mentoring opportunities.*

The intraclass correlation (ICC) describes the proportion of the total variance that can attributed to the hierarchal grouping by the provider variable. Net of all predictors included in the final FP information model, about one-quarter of the total variance (ICC = 0.27) occurred between providers.

Receipt of a modern FP method

Descriptive characteristics for receipt of a modern FP method

Less than one in 10 clients (8.4%) reported receiving a modern FP method; among those who reported receiving a modern method, injection (33.9%), implant (30.7%), and male condoms (14.2%) were the most common methods received (Table 1). About one-quarter of PL (23.6%) and 7.3% of delivery care clients reported receiving a modern method, while only 1.5% of well-baby care and other routine services clients reported receiving a method (Fig. 1). Sixteen percent (15.7%) of clients who received information on two or more FP methods reported receiving a modern FP method at their care visit, while only 2.0% of clients who received information on zero or one method reported this (Fig. 2). Similarly, one-fifth of clients (20.0%) who received FP information from two or more sources reported receiving a modern FP method, while only 7.1% of clients who received FP information from zero or one source reported receiving a method (Fig. 2).

Bivariate analyses

Results of bivariate analyses for *Receipt of a modern FP method* are displayed in the Appendix. The client covariates with a significant positive association with receipt of a

Table 2 Characteristics of Providers included in the Family Planning Integration Study Sample—Kigoma Region, Tanzania, April to July 2016 ($n = 330$)

	Providers, n (%)	95% CI
Age in years		
20–29	125 (37.9)	32.6–43.1
30–39	54 (16.4)	12.4–20.4
40–49	74 (22.4)	17.9–26.9
50+	77 (23.3)	18.7–27.9
Sex		
Female	209 (63.3)	58.1–68.6
Male	121 (36.7)	31.4–41.9
Highest education completed		
Primary	15 (4.6)	2.3–6.8
Secondary	95 (28.8)	23.9–33.7
College/university	220 (66.7)	61.6–71.8
Cadre		
Clinician	69 (20.9)	16.5–25.3
Nurse/midwife	176 (53.3)	47.9–58.7
Other staff	85 (25.7)	21.0–30.5
Years in cadre		
0 to 10 years	127 (38.5)	33.2–43.8
11+ years	203 (61.5)	56.2–66.8
Years at the facility		
0 to 7 years	99 (30.0)	25.0–35.0
8+ years	231 (70.0)	65.0–75.0
Facility type		
Hospital	82 (24.9)	20.2–29.5
Health center	182 (55.2)	49.8–60.5
Dispensary	66 (20.0)	15.7–24.3
Work hours per week		
54+ hours per week	191 (57.9)	52.5–63.2
Less than 54 h per week	139 (42.1)	36.8–47.5
Routinely provides FP services		
Yes	249 (75.5)	70.8–80.1
No	81 (24.6)	19.9–29.2
FP ever-training PCA score[a]		
Low	132 (40.0)	34.7–45.3
High	198 (60.0)	54.7–65.3
FP recent-training PCA Score[a]		
Low	227 (68.8)	63.8–73.8
High	103 (31.2)	26.2–36.2
FP Practice PCA Score[a]		
Low	131 (39.7)	34.4–45.0
High	199 (60.3)	55.0–65.6

Table 2 Characteristics of Providers included in the Family Planning Integration Study Sample—Kigoma Region, Tanzania, April to July 2016 ($n = 330$) *(Continued)*

	Providers, n (%)	95% CI
Access to electronic mentoring opportunities		
No access	165 (50.0)	44.6–55.4
Access to at least 1 type (emergency call system, e-learning, teleconference)	165 (50.0)	44.6–55.4
Perception in-service training has helped job performance		
Yes	285 (86.4)	82.6–90.1
No	45 (13.6)	9.9–17.4
Job Satisfaction		
Very or a little satisfied	148 (44.9)	39.5–50.2
Neutral, a little dissatisfied or very dissatisfied	182 (55.2)	49.8–60.5
Perception paid fairly for job duties		
Yes	56 (17.0)	12.9–21.0
No	274 (83.0)	79.0–87.1
Perception of adequacy of training for job duties		
Yes	227 (68.8)	63.8–73.8
No	103 (31.2)	26.2–36.2
Displays at least 1 FP bias[b]		
Yes	207 (62.7)	57.5–68.0
No	123 (37.3)	32.0–42.5

[a]Providers were asked if they had ever received training in, had recently received training in (in the last 18 months), and if they had provided the service in the last 3 months related to the following 14 FP items: 1) counsel women about FP and contraception; 2) give an injectable; 3) insert an IU(C)D; 4) remove an IU(C)D; 5) insert an implant; 6) remove an implant; 7) perform a tubal ligation; 8) perform a vasectomy; 9) provide counseling on FP options; 10) provide counseling on the efficacy of FP methods; 11) provide counseling on the potential side effects of FP methods; 12) provide counseling on the potential warning signs of FP methods; 13) provide clinical management of FP side effects; and 14) provide FP for HIV positive women

[b]Providers were asked if they decide whether or not to provide FP services to clients based on one or more of the following client characteristics: marital status/parental consent/partner consent/age/parity

modern contraceptive method included *PL care was the primary service sought, Client highest education attended, Literacy, Wealth, Number of live births, Has had FP discussion with partner, Able to make own FP decisions, Number of FP methods received information about,* and *Number of sources for FP information.* Client covariates with a significant negative association with receipt of a modern contraceptive method included *Well-baby care was the primary service sought, Other routine services was the primary service sought, Marital status,* and *Desired timing of future childbearing.*

Provider covariates with a significant positive association with receipt of a modern contraceptive method included *FP Practice PCA score* and *Access to electronic mentoring opportunities.* Provider covariates with a significant negative

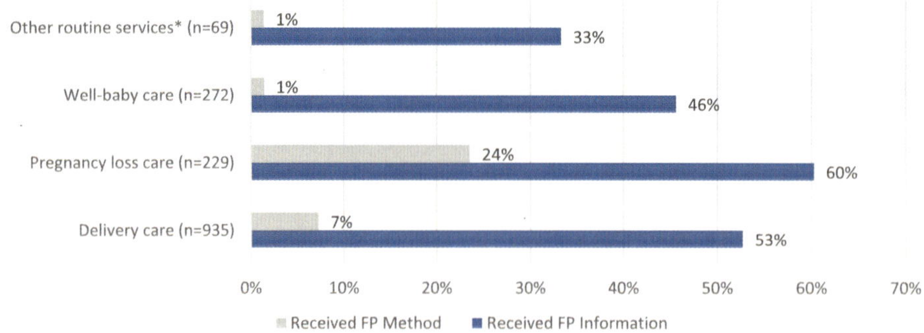

Fig. 1 Receipt of Family Planning Information and a Modern Method by Care Type—Kigoma Region, Tanzania, April to July 2016 (n = 1505). *Other routine services included clients who sought postnatal care, HIV testing and treatment, sexually transmitted infection (STI) care, and others.

association with receipt of a modern contraceptive method included *Provider age, Cadre, and Work hours per week.*

Multilevel analyses

Results of multilevel, mixed-effects logistic regression analyses for receipt of a modern FP method are shown in Table 4. The odds of receiving a modern FP method were higher for clients who received information on two or more vs fewer methods (aOR 7.13, 95% CI 2.13–23.80), for those who had a FP discussion with their partner (aOR 5.87, 95% CI 2.81–12.28), for clients seeking PL care vs those seeking all other types of care (aOR 4.08, 95% CI 1.97–8.44), for those with zero vs one or more live births (aOR 3.92, 95% CI 1.40–10.94), for those who reported they are able to make their own FP decisions (aOR 3.17, 95% CI 1.55–6.49), for clients who received FP information from two or more vs fewer sources (aOR 3.12, 95% CI 1.40–6.92), and for those in the middle and high wealth terciles vs low wealth tercile (aOR 1.99, 95% CI 1.11–3.56; aOR 2.30, 95% CI 1.30–4.07, respectively).

Well-baby care clients, Other services clients, and married clients had significantly lower odds of receiving a FP method compared to clients seeking any other type of services and unmarried clients (aOR 0.14, 95% CI 0.04–0.54; aOR 0.08, 95% CI 0.01–0.87; aOR 0.41, 95% CI 0.18–0.93, respectively). Client-level variables found not to have a significant adjusted relationship with receipt of a FP method include *Highest education attended, Literacy,* and *Desired timing of future childbearing.*

None of the provider-level variables were found to have a significant adjusted relationship with receipt of a modern FP method by a client. Net of all predictor variables included in the FP method model, nearly 30% of the total variance (ICC 0.30) occurred between providers.

Discussion

Integrating FP service provision into other types of healthcare visits can provide an important opportunity to reduce the unmet need for FP and ultimately lower maternal and neonatal mortality. We sought to understand the factors that predicted receipt of FP information and a modern FP method among women attending maternal, child, and reproductive health care services in Kigoma, Tanzania. The results demonstrate the association between the receipt of FP information with both the client and provider characteristics, while receipt of a modern FP method is associated with only client factors. This information will help inform FP training and programming in Kigoma, Tanzania.

First, level of FP integration is not consistent across non-FP care types. Unlike results from a study in Senegal, which found low receipt of FP information among PL clients compared to clients of other care types [16], our study found that women who sought PL services had nearly two times greater odds of receiving FP information and more than four times greater odds of receiving a modern method compared to women seeking other types of services. In contrast, women who sought well-baby care services and other routine care services had 86 and 92% lower odds of receiving a modern FP method, respectively.

Women's self-efficacy, assessed with questions about past FP discussions with partner and ability to make one's own FP decisions, was strongly associated with receipt of information and modern FP methods. Women who reported past FP discussions with their partner as compared with those who did not had nearly two times greater odds of receiving FP information and more than five times greater odds of receiving a FP method. In addition, women who reported the ability to make their own FP decisions had three times greater odds of receiving a method compared to women unable to make their own decisions. These results align with previous studies in India, Senegal, and Turkey, which also found that that partner communication [16, 25] and self-efficacy [20] are positively associated with FP uptake. These findings suggest that women who have had conversations with their FP partners and/or feel they can make their own decisions may be initiating

Table 3 Multilevel Mixed-Effects Logistic Regression Analysis for Receipt of Family Planning (FP) Information—Kigoma Region, Tanzania, April to July 2016 (Clients $n = 1497$, Providers $n = 330$)

	Adjusted OR (95% CI)	*p*-value
FIXED EFFECTS - CLIENT LEVEL VARIABLES		
Client age in years		
15–19 (reference)		
20–29	0.93 (0.66–1.33)	0.707
30–39	0.61 (0.37–1.03)	0.063
40–49	0.50 (0.26–0.97)	0.039
Don't know	4.11 (0.95–17.76)	0.058
Highest education attended		
No education		
Primary	1.25 (0.87–1.79)	0.230
Secondary	1.53 (0.93–2.51)	0.093
College or university	1.03 (0.39–2.74)	0.947
Pregnancy loss (PL) care was primary service sought		
No (reference)		
Yes	1.97 (1.01–3.84)	0.048
Other routine services was primary service sought		
No (reference)		
Yes	0.43 (0.18–1.03)	0.058
Frequency of religious service attendance		
Less often than weekly (reference)		
Weekly or more often	0.61 (0.44–0.85)	0.003
Wealth		
Low wealth (reference)		
Middle wealth	1.24 (0.82–1.88)	0.300
High wealth	1.27 (0.81–1.97)	0.294
Number of prior pregnancies		
0 to 3 (reference)		
4+	1.78 (1.21–2.60)	0.003
Desired timing of future childbearing		
More than 2 years, or does not want (reference)		
1 to 2 years	0.73 (0.51–1.04)	0.079
Heard FP messages in last three months		
No (reference)		
Yes	1.21 (0.88–1.67)	0.233
Has had FP discussion with partner		
No or don't know (reference)		
Yes	1.73 (1.33–2.25)	0.000
FIXED EFFECTS - PROVIDER-LEVEL VARIABLES		
Highest education completed		
Primary (reference)		
Secondary	1.25 (0.60–2.63)	0.552
College/University	2.03 (0.97–4.25)	0.060
Work hours per week		
Less than 54 h per week (reference)		
54+ hours per week	0.68 (0.45–1.01)	0.054
Routinely provides FP services		
No (reference)		
Yes	1.45 (0.85–2.47)	0.170
FP ever-training PCA score[a]		
Low (reference)		
High	1.01 (0.57–1.79)	0.970
FP recent-training PCA score[a]		
Low (reference)		
High	1.58 (1.11–2.26)	0.012
FP Practice PCA Score[a]		
Low (reference)		
High	0.86 (0.48–1.53)	0.606
Access to electronic mentoring opportunities		
No access (reference)		
Access to at least 1 type (emergency call system, e-learning, teleconference)	1.38 (0.85–2.23)	0.191
Perception in-service training has helped job performance		
No (reference)		
Yes	2.27 (1.35–3.84)	0.002
RANDOM EFFECTS		
Provider-level variance (SE)	1.21 (0.28)	
Provider-level variance partition coefficient	0.27 (0.19–0.37)	
Level 1 units	1497	
Level 2 units	330	
Log likelihood	− 921.18412	

[a]Providers were asked if they had ever received training in, had recently received training in (in the last 18 months), and if they had provided the service in the last 3 months related to the following 14 FP items: 1) counsel women about FP and contraception; 2) give an injectable; 3) insert an IU(C)D; 4) remove an IU(C)D; 5) insert an implant; 6) remove an implant; 7) perform a tubal ligation; 8) perform a vasectomy; 9) provide counseling on FP options; 10) provide counseling on the efficacy of FP methods; 11) provide counseling on the potential side effects of FP methods; 12) provide counseling on the potential warning signs of FP methods; 13) provide clinical management of FP side effects; and 14) provide FP for HIV positive women

FP conversations with providers, thereby driving the receipt of information and a method during a care visit.

The quantity of FP information received at the visit, including the number of methods information was received about and the number of sources information came from,

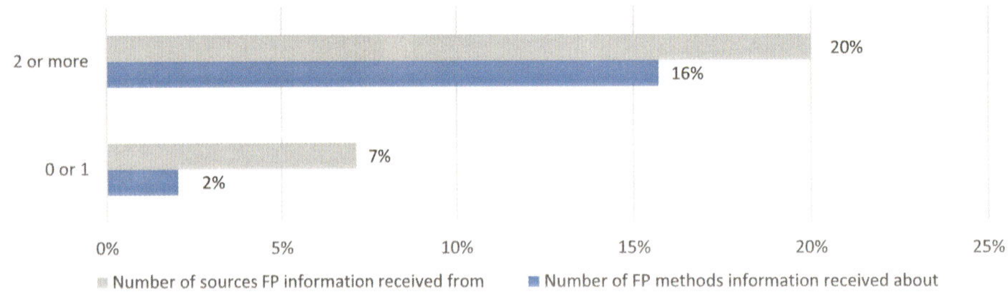

Fig. 2 Percentage of Clients Who Received a Modern Family Planning Method by Number of Methods Information was Received about and Number of Sources Information was Received from—Kigoma Region, Tanzania, April to July 2016 (n = 1505)

was strongly associated with FP method receipt. Women who received FP information about two or more methods had seven times greater odds of receiving a contraceptive method compared to women who received FP information about one or zero methods. Similarly, women who received FP information from two or more sources had nearly three times greater odds of receiving a method compared to women who received FP information from one or zero sources. These findings may inform elements of counseling in clinical practice.

Additional demographic characteristics, including parity, marital status, religiosity, and wealth, were also associated with receipt of FP information and modern FP methods. Women with four or more live births had nearly two times greater odds of receiving FP information compared to women with three or fewer live births. One possible explanation for this is providers' perceptions of women's eligibility for receiving methods. A study on provider-imposed barriers to family planning in Kenya found that women's parity influenced providers' method offerings; specifically, providers reported to impose FP method restrictions on women without children [7]. However, we found that women reporting having no children born alive had nearly four times greater odds of receiving a FP method. This finding may represent a desire to postpone childbearing. Specifically, among this sub-group of clients with no live births, a comparatively higher proportion were teenagers (38.1% vs 13.6%), unwed (25.6% vs 8.9%), and seeking PL care (93.0% vs 13.0%) compared to those with live births. We also found that women with no live births were not more likely to receive FP information, suggesting that this sub-group of clients were driving the requests for receipt of FP methods.

Women who reported more frequent attendance at religious services had 39% lower odds of receiving FP information compared to women with less frequent attendance. This finding suggests that religiosity either influences women's request for FP information or influences provider's perception of client interest in FP. Women in the middle and high wealth categories had two and two and a half times greater odds of receiving a FP method, respectively. This finding aligns with previous findings that poorer women receiving FP counseling and education have lower uptake of FP methods [12]. Given that FP is available at no cost to women in Tanzania, this difference may reflect an inverse relationship between future fertility preferences and wealth. Alternatively, this finding might suggest a provider's bias in offering modern methods to wealthier clients.

Recent in-service training and positive perceptions of in-service training as a whole among providers were important factors for client receipt of FP information. Other studies have found that a greater proportion of providers without in-service FP training imposed parity, age, marital, and other restrictions on provision of FP methods [7, 29, 36, 37]. In our study, clients of providers who had recent in-service training on a higher number of FP topics had one and a half times greater odds of receiving FP information at their visit compared to clients of providers who had recent in-service training on a lower number of FP topics. Similarly, clients of providers who reported that in-service training has helped their job performance had more than two times greater odds of receiving FP information compared clients of providers who reported in-service training has not helped. While we found that provider factors were important for client's receipt of FP information, provider factors were not predictive of client's receipt of a FP method. This suggests that client's desire for adopting a modern method expressed during non-FP visits may be the primary driver of receiving FP methods.

Findings from this study corroborate evidence that women's self-efficacy in FP decision-making [20], women's specific demographic characteristics (e.g., religiosity, wealth) [12], and providers' in-service training [7, 29] influence women's odds of receiving a FP method. This study adds new evidence pertaining to important elements of FP counseling and receipt of a method—namely, the quantity of FP information received at a single care visit (e.g., number of methods described, number of sources of FP information). While many studies address factors associated with receipt of FP methods, this study also adds new insight into factors associated with receipt of FP information, including provider characteristics related to the timing FP in-service training, partner communication, high parity, older age, and lack of religiosity.

Table 4 Multilevel Mixed Effects Logistic Regression Analysis for Receipt of a Modern Family Planning (FP) Method—Kigoma Region, Tanzania, April to July 2016 (Clients $n = 1482$, Providers $n = 330$)

	Adjusted OR (95% CI)	*p*-value
FIXED EFFECTS - CLIENT LEVEL VARIABLES		
Highest education attended		
No education (reference)		
Primary	0.43 (0.17–1.13)	0.088
Secondary or higher	0.85 (0.24–3.03)	0.799
University	1.39 (0.16–11.87)	0.765
Literacy		
Cannot read or write, or can do one (reference)		
read and write	1.89 (0.72–4.91)	0.193
Pregnancy loss (PL) care was primary service sought		
No (reference)		
Yes	4.08 (1.97–8.44)	0.000
Other services was primary service sought		
No (reference)		
Yes	0.08 (0.01–0.87)	0.038
Well-baby care was primary service sought		
No (reference)		
Yes	0.14 (0.04–0.54)	0.004
Marital status		
Not in a union (reference)		
In a union	0.41 (0.18–0.93)	0.034
Wealth		
Low wealth (reference)		
Middle wealth	1.99 (1.11–3.56)	0.021
Highest wealth	2.30 (1.30–4.07)	0.004
Live births		
1 or more (reference)		
None	3.92 (1.40–10.94)	0.009
Has had FP discussion with partner		
No or don't know (reference)		
Yes	5.87 (2.81–12.28)	0.000
Can make own FP decisions		
No or don't know (reference)		
Yes	3.17 (1.55–6.49)	0.002
Number of FP methods received information about during non-FP visit		
0 to 1 (reference)		
2 or more	7.13 (2.13–23.80)	0.001

Table 4 Multilevel Mixed Effects Logistic Regression Analysis for Receipt of a Modern Family Planning (FP) Method—Kigoma Region, Tanzania, April to July 2016 (Clients $n = 1482$, Providers $n = 330$) *(Continued)*

	Adjusted OR (95% CI)	*p*-value
Number of sources FP information received from during non-FP visit		
0 to 1 (reference)		
2 or more	3.12 (1.40–6.92)	0.005
Desired timing of future childbearing		
More than 2 years or does not want (reference)		
1–2 years	0.47 (0.20–1.13)	0.090
FIXED EFFECTS - PROVIDER-LEVEL VARIABLES		
Age in years		
38 years or younger (reference)		
39+ years	0.77 (0.37–1.62)	0.498
Cadre		
Clinician (reference)		
Nurse/midwife	0.81 (0.41–1.59)	0.535
Other staff	0.90 (0.35–2.30)	0.824
Hours worked per week		
55 h or less per week (reference)		
56+ hours	0.63 (0.35–1.15)	0.132
Access to electronic mentoring opportunities		
No access (reference)		
Access to at least 1 type (emergency call system, e-learning, teleconference)	1.27 (0.57–2.82)	0.562
FP Practice PCA Score[a]		
Low (reference)		
High	1.14 (0.60–2.17)	0.685
RANDOM EFFECTS		
Provider-level variance (SE)	1.39 (0.71)	
Provider-level variance partition coefficient	0.30 (0.13–0.53)	
Level 1 units	1482	
Level 2 units	330	
Log likelihood	– 292.07447	

[a]Providers were asked if they had provided the service in the last 3 months related to the following 14 FP items: 1) counsel women about FP and contraception; 2) give an injectable; 3) insert an IU(C)D; 4) remove an IU(C)D; 5) insert an implant; 6) remove an implant; 7) perform a tubal ligation; 8) perform a vasectomy; 9) provide counseling on FP options; 10) provide counseling on the efficacy of FP methods; 11) provide counseling on the potential side effects of FP methods; 12) provide counseling on the potential warning signs of FP methods; 13) provide clinical management of FP side effects; and 14) provide FP for HIV positive women

Strengths and limitations

This study has several strengths. First, the study has matched client and provider data, enabling quantification of the importance of both client and provider level factors for FP integration. In addition, clients of varied care services were included in the analyses, allowing a better understanding of the strengths and limitations of FP integration by care type. Moreover, we operationalized select independent variables in ways that have not been done in previously published work. For example in the model for *Receipt of a modern FP method,* receipt of FP information was operationalized into two distinct independent variables that quantify same-visit access to information: 1) *Number of FP methods information was received about,* and 2) *Number of sources information received from.* Additionally, provider-level *FP ever-training score, FP recent-training score,* and *FP Practice score* variables were operationalized using multiple FP care elements to differentiate the importance of both dose and timing of training and practice to provision of FP integration services.

There are several limitations to this study that are important to consider. First, the study employed a cross-sectional design which limits our ability to make causal inferences between the independent variables and outcomes of interest. We noted wide confidence intervals for some variables in the regression analyses which likely reflect small cell sizes; these results should be interpreted with caution. Ongoing longitudinal data collection and analyses will strengthen the robustness of the potential relationships. We used convenience sampling to recruit providers and clients, limiting the generalizability of the findings within or beyond Kigoma Region. To minimize this limitation, we aimed to interview all providers and clients who met the inclusion criteria and were available for interview during the study period. Data limitations included lack of a rural versus urban variable and information about receipt of FP counselling at multiple points in time. These exclusions eliminated our ability to assess the influence of setting and counselling over time on receipt of FP information and uptake.

Research, programmatic, and policy implications

Our findings highlight areas for future research and have clear implications for programmatic and policy work. Additional research with matched client and provider data is needed to further delineate the relative importance of client and provider factors for FP integration. Studies such as this could be replicated in other areas of Tanzania and eastern Africa, or beyond, to better understand how similar or disparate the determinants of receiving FP information and methods are across regions and countries. Future analyses would benefit from inclusion of interaction terms to better understand how specific client characteristics, such religion, age, and parity, intersect with provider perceptions and potential biases in ways that influence provision of FP services. Observational and descriptive studies are also needed to better understand logistical considerations for integration of services in facilities (e.g., location of FP providers and methods, process for receiving services either directly or through referral, other access barriers).

Increased attention is needed to better integrate FP counseling and service provision routinely into well-baby and other routine care services. Capitalizing on the year post delivery is one strategy that has been effective in other settings [15, 17, 23]. Community- and facility-based strategies are needed that encourage women to have conversations with their partners and to create service environments where women feel they can begin conversations with providers and make their own decisions to initiate FP. Based on our findings, expanding the number of FP method options and sources of information provided at single visits would also likely drive an uptake in FP use. The US-based National Campaign to Prevent Teen and Unplanned Pregnancy's One Key Question is a program that encourages primary care providers to routinely ask women about their reproductive health goals using a simple question: would you like to become pregnant in the next year? [38] This approach, among others, could be piloted in Kigoma, and if deemed effective, incorporated into national policies.

Conclusion

Despite much evidence establishing the salient role of FP counseling to improve reproductive health outcomes, there is less consensus about the relative impact of client or provider attributes on the receipt of FP information or a modern method. We address the question of whether including both client and provider characteristics adds predictive value when analyzing the risk of FP integration or uptake. Our findings demonstrate that both client and provider factors significantly influence FP integration. Improved understanding of the interplay between clients and providers is critical for the effective provision of FP services and should be considered in the design of reproductive health policies and future data collection exercises.

Endnotes

[1]Providers were asked if they decide whether or not to provide FP services to clients based on one or more of the following client characteristics: marital status/parental consent/partner consent/age/parity

[2]Providers were asked if they had ever received training in, had recently received training in (in the last 18 months), and if they had provided the service in the last 3 months related to the following 14 FP items: 1) counsel women about FP and contraception; 2) give an injectable; 3) insert an IU(C)D; 4) remove an IU(C)D; 5) insert an implant; 6) remove an implant; 7) perform a tubal ligation; 8) perform a vasectomy; 9) provide counseling on FP options; 10) provide counseling on the efficacy of FP methods; 11) provide counseling on the potential side effects of FP methods; 12) provide counseling on the potential warning signs of FP methods; 13) provide clinical management of FP side effects; and 14) provide FP for HIV positive women.

Appendix

Table 5 Association between Client and Provider Characteristics and Receipt of Family Planning (FP) Information and a Modern FP Method—Kigoma Region, Tanzania, April to July 2016 (Clients $n = 1505$, Providers $n = 330$)

	Receipt of FP Information		Receipt of Modern FP Method	
	Unadjusted OR (95% CI)	*p*-value	Unadjusted OR (95% CI)	*p*-value
CLIENT LEVEL VARIABLES				
Age in years				
15–19 (reference)				
20–29	1.23 (0.85–1.77)	0.272	1.22 (0.64–2.34)	0.551
30–39	1.22 (0.82–1.81)	0.335	1.18 (0.59–2.38)	0.641
40–49	0.95 (0.51–1.75)	0.862	0.85 (0.28–2.56)	0.771
Don't know	5.82 (1.50–22.54)	0.011	0.28 (0.03–2.90)	0.284
Delivery care was primary service sought				
No (reference)				
Yes	0.96 (0.71–1.29)	0.771	0.68 (0.43–1.08)	0.101
Well-baby care was primary service sought				
No (reference)				
Yes	0.85 (0.59–1.22)	0.377	0 .13 (0.05–0.39)	0.000
Pregnancy loss (PL) care was primary service sought				
No (reference)				
Yes	2.06 (1.32–3.20)	0.001	6.41 (3.74–11.01)	0.000
Other routine services (Postnatal, HIV, STI, other) was primary service sought				
No (reference)				
Yes	0.38 (0.20–0.75)	0.005	0.13 (0.02–1.07)	0.057
Highest education attended				
No education (reference)				
Primary	1.24 (0.91–1.70)	0.178	1.22 (0.68–2.18)	0.509
Secondary	1.55 (0.97–2.47)	0.068	4.26 (2.10–8.64)	0.000
University	1.00 (0.37–2.68)	0.997	4.38 (1.19–16.13)	0.026
Literacy				
Cannot read and write, or can read or write, but not both (reference)				
Read and write	1.15 (0.87–1.53)	0.324	2.40 (1.38–4.17)	0.002
Wealth				
Low wealth (reference)				
Middle wealth	1.31 (0.96–1.79)	0.092	2.12 (1.16–3.88)	0.015
High wealth	1.46 (1.06–2.02)	0.022	3.64 (2.02–6.58)	0.000
Number of live births				
1+ (reference)				
None	0.72 (0.34–1.51)	0.383	3.61 (1.52–8.55)	0.004
Number of prior pregnancies				
0–3 (reference)				
4+	1.38 (1.07–1.77)	0.013	1.11 (0.73–1.68)	0.625
Marital status				
Not in a union (reference)				
In a union	0.95 (0.62–1.45)	0.798	0.44 (0.23–0.83)	0.012

Table 5 Association between Client and Provider Characteristics and Receipt of Family Planning (FP) Information and a Modern FP Method—Kigoma Region, Tanzania, April to July 2016 (Clients $n = 1505$, Providers $n = 330$) *(Continued)*

	Receipt of FP Information		Receipt of Modern FP Method	
Frequency of attendance at religious services				
Attends at least weekly (reference)				
Attends less often than weekly	0.70 (0.49–1.01)	0.056	0.83 (0.48–1.45)	0.512
Has had FP discussion with partner				
No (reference)				
Yes	1.92 (1.48–2.48)	0.000	4.01 (2.35–6.83)	0.000
Able to make own FP decisions				
No (reference)				
Yes	1.10 (0.79–1.53)	0.565	2.93 (1.82–4.73)	0.000
Heard FP messages in last 3 months				
No (reference)				
Yes	1.29 (0.99–1.68)	0.064	1.25 (0.81–1.92)	0.317
Desired timing of future childbearing				
More than 2 years, or does not want (reference)				
1 to 2 years	0.76 (0.57–1.00)	0.050	0.55 (0.33–0.91)	0.020
Number of FP methods received information about during non-FP visit				
None or 1 (reference)				
2+	NA		12.24 (6.48–23.10)	0.000
Number of sources FP information received from during non-FP visit				
None or 1 (reference)				
2+	NA		4.75 (2.62–8.62)	0.000
PROVIDER LEVEL VARIABLES				
Provider age				
39+ years (reference)				
38 years or less	1.00 (0.68–1.46)	0.994	0.55 (0.32–0.95)	0.032
Sex				
Male (reference)				
Female	0.73 (0.49–1.08)	0.115	0.84 (0.48–1.49)	0.555
Highest education completed				
Primary (reference)				
Secondary	2.00 (0.72–5.54)	0.184	1.23 (0.23–6.69)	0.810
College/university	3.00 (1.11–8.06)	0.030	2.20 (0.43–11.29)	0.343
Cadre				
Clinician (reference)				
Nurse/midwife	1.00 (0.62–1.63)	0.990	0.49 (0.26–0.93)	0.029
Other staff	0.87 (0.50–1.52)	0.624	0.40 (0.18–0.88)	0.023
Work hours per week				
Less than 54 h per week (reference)				
54+ hours per week	0.51 (0.35–0.74)	0.000	0.40 (0.23–0.70)	0.001
Years in cadre				
0 to 10 years				
11+ years	1.27 (0.86–1.87)	0.228	0.77 (0.44–1.36)	0.372
Years at the facility				
0 to 7 years				
8+ years	1.32 (0.88–1.99)	0.179	0.95 (0.52–1.72)	0.858

Table 5 Association between Client and Provider Characteristics and Receipt of Family Planning (FP) Information and a Modern FP Method—Kigoma Region, Tanzania, April to July 2016 (Clients $n = 1505$, Providers $n = 330$) *(Continued)*

	Receipt of FP Information		Receipt of Modern FP Method	
Routinely provides FP services				
No (reference)				
Yes	2.02 (1.30–3.13)	0.002	1.19 (0.61–2.33)	0.614
FP ever-training PCA score[a]				
Low (reference)				
High	1.70 (1.16–2.49)	0.007	1.53 (0.85–2.74)	0.153
FP recent-training PCA score[a]				
Low (reference)				
High	1.70 (1.14–2.53)	0.009	1.28 (0.71–2.28)	0.412
FP Practice PCA Score[a]				
Low (reference)				
High	1.64 (1.11–2.41)	0.013	1.72 (0.95–3.09)	0.071
Perception in-service training has helped job performance				
No (reference)				
Yes	2.64 (1.51–4.63)	0.001	1.75 (0.70–4.38)	0.230
Access to electronic mentoring opportunities				
No access (reference)				
Access to at least 1 type (emergency call system, e-learning, teleconference)	1.88 (1.29–0.74)	0.001	2.28 (1.31–3.98)	0.004
Job Satisfaction				
Very or a little satisfied (reference)				
Neutral or a little or very dissatisfied	0 .95 (0.65–1.38)	0.779	0.94 (0.54–1.64)	0.825
Perception of adequacy of training for job duties				
No (reference)				
Yes	1.06 (0.70–1.60)	0.780	1.31 (0.70–2.43)	0.402
Perception in-service training has helped job performance				
No (reference)				
Yes	2.64 (1.51–4.63)	0.001	1.75 (0.70–4.38)	0.230
Perception paid fairly for job duties				
No (reference)				
Yes	1.43 (0.87–2.36)	0.160	0.73 (0.33–1.58)	0.421
Displays at least one FP bias[b]				
No (reference)				
Yes	1.16 (0.78–1.71)	0.468	0.90 (0.51–1.59)	0.709

[a]Providers were asked if they had ever received training in, had recently received training in (in the last 18 months), and if they had provided the service in the last 3 months related to the following 14 FP items: 1) counsel women about FP and contraception; 2) give an injectable; 3) insert an IU(C)D; 4) remove an IU(C)D; 5) insert an implant; 6) remove an implant; 7) perform a tubal ligation; 8) perform a vasectomy; 9) provide counseling on FP options; 10) provide counseling on the efficacy of FP methods; 11) provide counseling on the potential side effects of FP methods; 12) provide counseling on the potential warning signs of FP methods; 13) provide clinical management of FP side effects; and 14) provide FP for HIV positive women

[b]Providers were asked if they decide whether or not to provide FP services to clients based on one or more of the following client characteristics: marital status/parental consent/partner consent/age/parity

Abbreviations

95% CI: 95% Confidence intervals; ANC: Antenatal care; BEmONC: Basic Emergency Obstetric and Neonatal Care; BRN: Big Results Now; CDC: Centers for Disease Control and Prevention; CEmONC: Comprehensive Emergency Obstetric and Neonatal Care; DRH: Division of Reproductive Health; FP: Family planning; ICC: Intraclass correlation; IUD: Intrauterine Device; LAM: Lactational amenorrhea method; MOHCDGEC: Ministry of Health, Community Development, Gender, the Elderly, and Children; NBS: National Bureau of Statistics; OR: Odds Ratios; PCA: Principal Components Analysis; PL: Pregnancy loss; PNC: Postnatal Care; TFR: Total Fertility Rate; WHO: World Health Organization

Acknowledgements

Our sincere gratitude to the clients and providers who so generously gave us their time and shared their experiences. We would also like to thank the

Kigoma Regional Ministry of Health, AMCA Inter Consult, interviewers, and data entry staff for their dedication to this project. The authors would also like to acknowledge the support of CDC colleagues Susanna Binzen, Fernando Carlosama, Jonetta Mpofu, Michelle Schmitz, and intern from Emory University Rollins School of Public Health, Hannah Nguyen.

Funding

This study was funded by Bloomberg Philanthropies and the Fondation H&B Agerup.

Disclaimer

The findings and conclusions in this report are those of the authors and do not necessarily represent the official position of the US Centers for Disease Control and Prevention.

Declarations

The data collection for our project was approved by the National Institute for Medical Research (NIMR) in Tanzania as one activity among a larger set of activities for the *Project to Reduce Maternal Deaths in Tanzania*. Interviewers received one week of training in quantitative interview techniques and best practices in research and ethics. Informed consent was obtained from each participant and confirmed with the participant's thumbprint.

Authors' contributions

MD was responsible for the study design, undertook the fieldwork and data collection, analysis, interpretation, and helped write the manuscript. EB and DM were involved in the literature search, interpretation of findings, and helped write the manuscript. AR supervised data entry, participated in data cleaning, and helped finalize the manuscript. LK participated in data analysis, interpretation of findings, and helped write the manuscript. WM and PC helped interpret findings. RB helped collect data and interpret findings. FS helped with the study design and interpretation of findings. All authors read and approved the final manuscript submitted for publication.

Competing interests

The authors have no competing interests to declare.

Author details

[1]Centers for Disease Control and Prevention, Division of Reproductive Health, Atlanta, USA. [2]Centers for Disease Control and Prevention, Division of Reproductive Health (CDCF Contractor), Atlanta, USA. [3]EngenderHealth, Washington, DC, USA. [4]Regional Medical Officer, Kigoma, Kigoma Region, Tanzania. [5]AMCA Inter Consult, Dar es Salaam, Tanzania.

References

1. WHO. Trends in maternal mortality. 1990 To 2015. Estimates by WHO, UNICEF, UNFPA, the World Bank & the UN population division. Geneva: World Health Organization; 2015.
2. Chola L, McGee S, Tugendhaft A, Buchmann E, Hofman K. Scaling up family planning to reduce maternal and child mortality: the potential costs and benefits of modern contraceptive use in South Africa. PLoS One. 2015;10(6): e0130077. https://doi.org/10.1371/journal.pone.0130077.
3. Ahmed S, Li Q, Liu L, Tsui A. Maternal deaths averted by contraceptive use: an analysis of 172 countries. Lancet. 2012;380(9837):111–25.
4. Collumbien M, Gerressu M, Cleland J. Non-use and use of ineffective methods of contraception. In: Comparative quantification of health risks: global and regional burden of disease attributable to selected major risk factors. Geneva: WHO; 2004. p. 1255–320. ISBN 9241580313.
5. Ganatra B, Faundes A. Role of birth spacing, family planning services, safe abortion services and post-abortion care in reducing maternal mortality. Best Pract Res Clin Obstet Gynaecol. 2016;36:145–55. https://doi.org/10.1016/j.bpobgyn.2016.07.008.
6. Rutstein SO. Effects of preceding birth intervals on neonatal, infant and under-five years mortality and nutritional status in developing countries: evidence from the demographic and health surveys. Int J Gynaecol Obstet. 2005;89(Suppl 1):S7–24.
7. Tumlinson K, Okigbo CC, Speizer IS. Provider barriers to family planning access in urban Kenya. Contraception. 2015;92(2):143–51. ISSN 0010-7824
8. Ministry of Health, Community Development, Gender, Elderly and Children (MoHCDGEC) [Tanzania Mainland], Ministry of Health (MoH) [Zanzibar], National Bureau of Statistics (NBS), Office of the Chief Government Statistician (OCGS), and ICF. 2016. Tanzania Demographic and Health Survey and Malaria Indicator Survey (TDHS-MIS) 2015–16. Dar es Salaam, Tanzania, and Rockville, Maryland, USA: MoHCDGEC, MoH, NBS, OCGS, and ICF.
9. Bruce J. Fundamental elements of quality of care: a simple framework. Stud Fam Plan. 1990;21(2):61–91.
10. Zapata LB, Tregear SJ, Curtis KM, Tiller M, Pazol K, Mautone-Smith N, Gavin LE. Impact of contraceptive counseling in clinical settings: A systematic review. Am J Prev Med. 2015;49(2 suppl 1):S31–45. https://doi.org/10.1016/j.amepre.2015.03.023.
11. Tessema GA, Streak Gomersall J, Mahmood MA, Laurence CO. Factors determining quality of care in family planning services in Africa: a systematic review of mixed evidence. PLoS One. 2016;11(11):e0165627. https://doi.org/10.1371/journal.pone.0165627.
12. Achyut P, Mishra A, Montana L, Sengupta R, Calhoun LM, Nanda P. Integration of family planning with maternal health services: an opportunity to increase postpartum modern contraceptive use in urban Uttar Pradesh, India. J Fam Plann Reprod Health Care. 2016;42(2):107–15. https://doi.org/10.1136/jfprhc-2015-101271.
13. Cleland J, Shah IH, Daniele M. Interventions to improve postpartum family planning in low- and middle-income countries: program implications and research priorities. Stud Fam Plan. 2015;46(4):423–41.
14. Gaffield ME, Egan S, Temmerman M. It's about time: WHO and partners release programming strategies for postpartum family planning. Global Health, Science and Practice. 2014;2:4–9. https://doi.org/10.9745/GHSP-D-13-00156
15. Lopez LM, Grey TW, Hiller JE, Chen M. Education for contraceptive use by women after childbirth (review). Cochrane Database Syst Rev. 2015;7: CD001863. https://doi.org/10.1002/14651858.CD001863.pub4.
16. Speizer IS, Fotso JC, Okigbo C, Faye CM, Seck C. Influence of integrated services on postpartum family planning use: a cross-sectional survey from urban Senegal. BMC Public Health. 2013;13:752.
17. Yadav D, Dhillon P. Assessing the impact of family planning advice on unmet need and contraceptive use among currently married women in Uttar Pradesh, India. PLoS One. 2015;10(3):e0118584. https://doi.org/10.1371/journal.pone.0118584.
18. Adanikin A, Onwudiegwu U, Loto O. Influence of multiple antenatal counselling sessions on modern contraceptive uptake in Nigeria. Eur J Contracept Reprod Health Care. 2013;18(5):381–7.
19. Ayiasi RM, Muhumuza C, Bukenya J, Orach G. The effect of prenatal counselling on postpartum family planning use among early postpartum women in Masindi and Kiryandongo districts, Uganda. Pan Afr Med J. 2015;21(138)
20. Vural F, Vural B, Cakiroglu Y. The effect of combined antenatal and postnatal counselling on postpartum modern contraceptive use: prospective case-control study in Kocaeli, Turkey. J Clin Diagn Res. 2016;10(4):QC04–7.
21. Akman M, Tuzun S, Uzuner A, Basgul A, Kavak Z. The influence of prenatal counselling on postpartum contraceptive choice. J Int Med Res. 2010;38(4):1243–9.
22. Vance G, Janowitz B, Chen M, Boyer B, Kasonde P, Asare G, Kafulubiti B, Stanback J. Integrating family planning messages into immunization services: a cluster-randomized trial in Ghana and Zambia. Health Policy Plan. 2014;29:359–66.
23. Cooper CM, Fields R, Mazzeo CI, Taylor N, Pfitzer A, Momolu M, Jabbeh-Howe C. Successful proof of concept of family planning and immunization integration in Liberia. Glob Health: Sci Pract. 2015;3(2):71–84.
24. Centers for Disease Control and Prevention. Health facility assessment of emergency obstetric and neonatal Care Services in Kigoma Region, Tanzania: selected findings, 2016. Atlanta, GA: centers for disease control and Prevention; 2016.
25. Mody SK, Nair S, Dasgupta A, Raj A, Donta B, Saggurti N, Naik DD, Silverman JG. Postpartum contraception utilization among low-income women seeking immunization for infants in Mumabi, India. Contraception. 2014;89:516–20.

26. Eluwa GIE, Atamewalen R, Odogwu K, Babatunde A. Success providing postpartum intrauterine devices in private-sector health care facilities in Nigeria: factors associated with uptake. Glob Health: Sci Pract. 2016;4(2):276–83.
27. Dulli LS, Eichleay M, Rademacher K, Sortijas S, Nsengiyumva T. Meeting postpartum women's family planning needs through integrated family planning and immunization services: results of a cluster-randomized controlled trial in Rwanda. Glob Health: Sci Pract. 2016;4(1):73–86.
28. Sedgh G, Hussain R. Reasons for contraceptive nonuse among women having unmet need for contraception in developing countries. Stud Fam Plan. 2014;45(2):151–69.
29. Calhoun LS, Speizer IS, Rimal R, Sripad P, Chatterjee N, Achyut P, Nanda P. Provider imposed restrictions to clients' access to family planning in urban Uttar Pradesh, India: a mixed methods study. BMC Health Serv Res. 2013;13:532.
30. Sidze EM, Lardoux S, Speizer IS, Faye CM, Mutua MM, Badji F. Young women's access to and use of contraceptives: the role of providers' restrictions in urban Senegal. Int Perspect Sex Reprod Health. 2014; 40(4):176–83.
31. Benson LS, Perrucci A, Drey EA, Steinauer JE. Contraception. 2012;85(2):198–203. https://doi.org/10.1016/j.contraception.2011.05.021.
32. Tumlinson K, Pence BW, Curtis SL, Marshall SW, Speizer IS. Quality of care and contraceptive use in urban Kenya. Int Perspect Sex and ReproHealth. 2015;41(2):69–79. https://doi.org/10.1363/4106915.
33. Centers for Disease Control and Prevention 2016. Kigoma Reprod Health Survey: Kigoma Region, Tanzania. Atlanta, GA: Centers for Disease Control and Prevention; 2017.
34. National Bureau of Statistics & Office of Chief Government Statistician. The United Republic of Tanzania, Kigoma region: basic demographic and socio-economic profile. In: 2012 population and housing census; 2016.
35. Filmer D, Pritchett LH. Estimating wealth effects without expenditure data--or tears: an application to educational enrollments in states of India. Demography. 2001;38(1):115–32. PubMed PMID: 11227840
36. Rauh-Benoit LA, Tepper NK, Zapata LB, Whiteman MK, Curtis KM, Mandel MG, Marchbanks PA, Jamieson DJ. Healthcare provider attitudes of safety of intrauterine devices in the postpartum period. J Women's Health. 2017; 26(7):768–73. https://doi.org/10.1089/jwh.2016.5985.
37. Schwandt HM, Speizer IS, Corroon M. Contraceptive service provider imposed restrictions to contraceptive access in urban Nigeria. BMC Health Serv Res. 2017;17:268. https://doi.org/10.1186/s12913-017-2233-0.
38. Hipp S, Carlson A, McFarlane E. Improving reproductive life planning in Hawai'i: one key question. Hawaii J Med Public Health. 2017;76(9):261–4.

High and growing disapproval of sex-selection technology in Australia

Rebecca Kippen[1*], Edith Gray[2] and Ann Evans[2]

Abstract

Background: In Australia, the National Health and Medical Research Council has banned the use of assisted reproductive technology for social sex selection, but notes "there is limited research into the question of whether Australians support the use of sex selection for non-medical purposes". This paper investigates Australian attitudes to sex-selection technology by different means (IVF, abortion, and a hypothetical pill), for different reasons (medical, family balancing, any reason), and by differing respondent characteristics (age, sex, education and religiosity).

Methods: In 2007 and 2016, the Australian Survey of Social Attitudes (AuSSA) collected data on the attitudes of Australian adults to sex selection through IVF, abortion, and a hypothetical pill. We calculate population-weighted distributions and 95% confidence intervals of responses, and carry out logistic regressions to investigate the demographic characteristics of Australians who strongly disapprove of IVF or abortion for sex selection.

Results: In 2016, around three-quarters of AuSSA respondents were opposed to legalising sex selection through IVF for any reason, or for family balancing for a second or third child. Thirty-seven per cent were opposed to IVF for medical sex selection. Two-thirds of respondents in both 2007 and 2016 disapproved or strongly disapproved of IVF for sex selection, while the proportion who strongly disapproved increased from 31 to 40%. Disapproval/strong disapproval of abortion for sex selection increased from 74 to 81% from 2007 to 2016, while strong disapproval alone rose from 44 to 55%. More than 70% of respondents in both 2007 and 2016 stated that a hypothetical pill for sex selection should not be legal. Our analysis finds that female, young, more-educated, and more religious respondents are more likely to strongly disapprove of sex selection via IVF or abortion, and that the increase in those who strongly disapprove from 2007 to 2016 is statistically significant.

Conclusions: Australians generally disapprove of the use of sex-selection technology. If legislation is to be guided by community attitudes, then the prohibition against sex selection for non-medical purposes through assisted reproductive technology should be maintained.

Keywords: Sex-selection technology, Australia, Gender, Sex ratio, IVF, Abortion

Plain English summary

In Australia, the use of reproductive technology to choose the sex of children is outlawed for other than medical reasons. Regarding this prohibition, the Australian National Health and Medical Research Council (NHMRC) noted in 2017 that "society's readiness to accept a practice is a relevant and important consideration" and "there is limited research into the question of whether Australians support the use of sex selection for non-medical purposes".

We address this question through analysis of a large nationally representative survey: the 2007 and 2016 Australian Survey of Social Attitudes. We find surprisingly low levels of support for the use of sex-selection technology, with most Australians disapproving of sex selection through IVF, abortion, and a hypothetical pill. This disapproval has strengthened over the period 2007 to 2016, with female, young, more-educated and more religious respondents more likely to strongly disapprove of sex selection via IVF or abortion.

We conclude that if legislation is to be guided by "society's readiness to accept a practice", as noted by the NHMRC, then the prohibition against sex selection for

* Correspondence: rebecca.kippen@monash.edu
[1]School of Rural Health, Monash University, 26 Mercy St, Bendigo, VIC 3552, Australia
Full list of author information is available at the end of the article

non-medical purposes through assisted reproductive technology should be maintained.

Background

In Australia, the use of assisted reproductive technology (ART) to select the sex of children for non-medical reasons has been banned since 2004. In that year, the Australian National Health and Medical Research Council (NHMRC) introduced *Ethical Guidelines on the Use of Assisted Reproductive Technology in Clinical Practice and Research* [1]. These guidelines, under the section heading "Do not select sex for nonmedical purposes" stated:

> Sex selection is an ethically controversial issue. The Australian Health Ethics Committee believes that admission to life should not be conditional upon a child being a particular sex. Therefore, pending further community discussion, sex selection (by whatever means) must not be undertaken except to reduce the risk of transmission of a serious genetic condition.

An Appendix to the 2004 guidelines listed three reasons for and three reasons against the use of sex selection for non-medical reasons, in order to "foster and assist community debate". Reasons for were: family balancing, fulfilment of religious obligations or cultural expectations that require offspring of a particular sex, and the right to individual reproductive autonomy. Reasons against were: incompatibility with unconditional acceptance by parents of their children, possible expression of gender bias against girls, and possible sex ratio distortions leading to a "shortage of women for men to marry" [1].

In practice the sex selection prohibition applied to in vitro fertilisation (IVF) only, with preimplantation genetic diagnosis (PGD) used to determine embryo sex before implantation. At the time the prohibition was introduced in Australia in 2004, the practice of social sex selection via IVF was minimal. Three of the eight Australian states and territories had already legislated against social sex selection using IVF, and only a small number of ART clinics in the other states offered social sex selection [2]. In the year before the NHMRC guidelines came into force, only 90 babies across Australia and New Zealand were born as a result of 'ART involving PGD' (in the context of more than 300,000 total births), with PGD mostly used to test for genetic disorders, rather than for social sex selection [3, 4].

The NHMRC guidelines were revised in 2007 [5], and again in 2017 [6]. The prohibition against sex selection for non-medical reasons remained in place. In their 2017 revised guidelines, the NHMRC noted:

> Many of the issues surrounding ART are as much social and political as they are ethical. With any controversial practice, society's readiness to accept a practice is a relevant and important consideration. At the time of publication, there is limited research into the question of whether Australians support the use of sex selection for non-medical purposes.

This paper adds to debate and knowledge in this area by using a large national survey to assess support by Australians for the use of IVF to choose the sex of a child for medical reasons, for family balancing, or for any reason, since support may vary by the motive for sex selection. The NHMRC and some researchers have previously suggested that social sex selection for family balancing—where parents with children all of the same sex choose to have a child of the opposite sex—may be more socially and ethically acceptable than other motivations for social sex selection, such as choosing to have a first-born son or only sons [7–10].

We also investigate whether support for sex selection in Australia has changed over time, whether it varies by other methods of sex selection (sex-selective abortion or a hypothetical blue pill/pink pill) in contrast to IVF, or by demographic characteristics of the survey respondents. This updates a previous study conducted in 2007 [7].

Data and methods

Data for this study are derived from the Australian Survey of Social Attitudes (AuSSA). AuSSA is an annual national postal survey of adult Australians chosen at random from the Australian Electoral Roll (enrolment on the Roll is compulsory for all Australian citizens aged 18 years and over). The survey is "Australia's main source of data for the scientific study of the social attitudes, beliefs and opinions of Australians, how they change over time, and how they compare with other societies" [11]. In 2007 and 2016, AuSSA included the following questions on sex selection:

1. Do you approve or disapprove of the use of IVF technology to avoid characteristics of children such as: a certain sex?
   Strongly approve/Approve/Neither approve nor disapprove/Disapprove/Strongly disapprove/Don't know
2. Do you approve or disapprove of the use of abortion to avoid having children with characteristics such as: a certain sex?
   Strongly approve/Approve/Neither approve nor disapprove/ Disapprove/Strongly disapprove/Don't know
3. Suppose there was a medication available that enabled parents to choose the sex of their children. Couples simply had to take a blue pill to ensure the

birth of a boy or a pink pill to ensure the birth of a girl. Do you think such a medication should be legally available?
Yes/No/Don't know

4. If you were planning to have children, would you take advantage of such a medication?
Yes/No/Don't know

Questions 3 and 4 were adapted from a question asked by Dahl et al. in a series of studies [12–14] in the early 2000s: "Suppose there was a medication enabling parents to choose the sex of their children. Couples simply had to ingest a blue pill to ensure the birth of a boy or a pink pill to ensure the birth of a girl. Would you take advantage of such a medication?"

Additional questions around whether IVF for sex selection should be legal, and under what circumstances, were asked in 2016 only:

5. Should IVF be legal in Australia for choosing a child's sex for: medical reasons?
Yes/No/Don't know
6. Should IVF be legal in Australia for choosing a child's sex for: family balancing - sex of second child different from first?
Yes/No/Don't know
7. Should IVF be legal in Australia for choosing a child's sex for: family balancing - sex of third child different from first two?
Yes/No/Don't know
8. Should IVF be legal in Australia for choosing a child's sex for: any reason?
Yes/No/Don't know

In 2007, three versions of AuSSA—A, B and C—with different sets of questions were sent out. Version A contained the above questions 1 to 4 on sex selection, and was sent to 6666 people on the Australian Electoral Roll. Responses totalled 2781, or 42% [15]. In 2016, one version of the survey was sent to 5000 people, with a response rate of 25% (1267). Responses are weighted to national counts of the adult citizen population by age, sex, and education.

We calculated population-weighted distributions of sample survey responses to each of the eight questions, shown in Figs. 1, 2 and 3. These figures also show 95% confidence intervals for the population proportion for each response category, shown as error bars for each proportion, and calculated with z-scores on the assumption the data were normally distributed. Non-overlapping confidence intervals indicate that differences between proportions are statistically significant.

We also constructed two logistic regression models, testing whether "Strong disapproval" of IVF for sex selection, or "Strong disapproval" of abortion for sex selection, varies by age, sex, education or religious attendance, and whether the level of "Strong disapproval" changed in the Australian population between 2007 and 2016 (Table 1). These models show odds ratios, 95% confidence intervals, *p*-values, predicted probabilities, and sample n for each category.

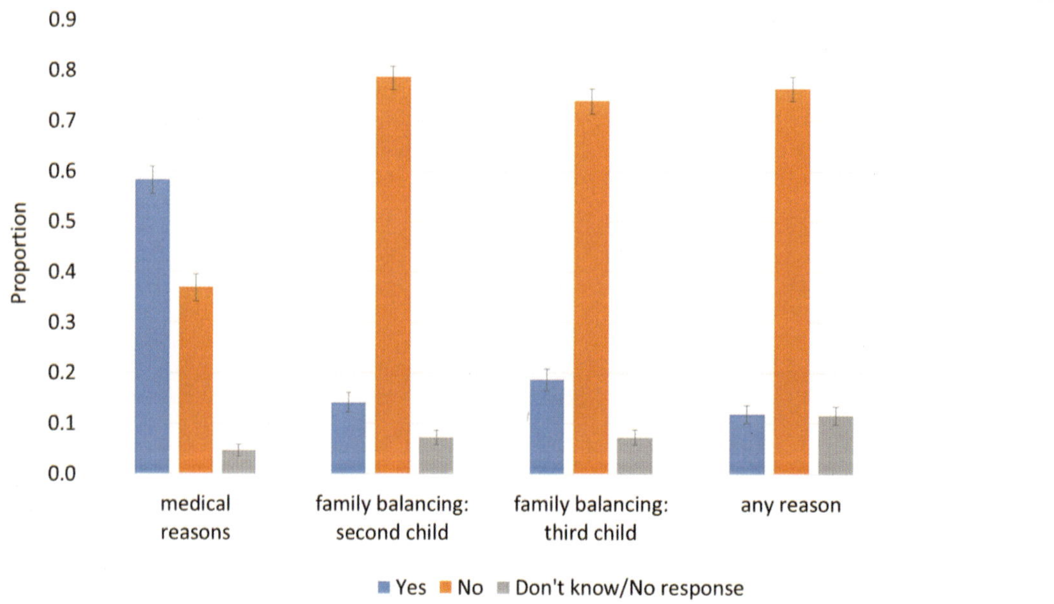

Fig. 1 Responses to "Should IVF be legal in Australia for choosing a child's sex for: medical reasons; family balancing—sex of second child different from first; family balancing—sex of third child different from first two; any reason". Note: Weighted to population characteristics. 95% confidence intervals shown. Source: Australian Survey of Social Attitudes, 2016, $n = 1267$

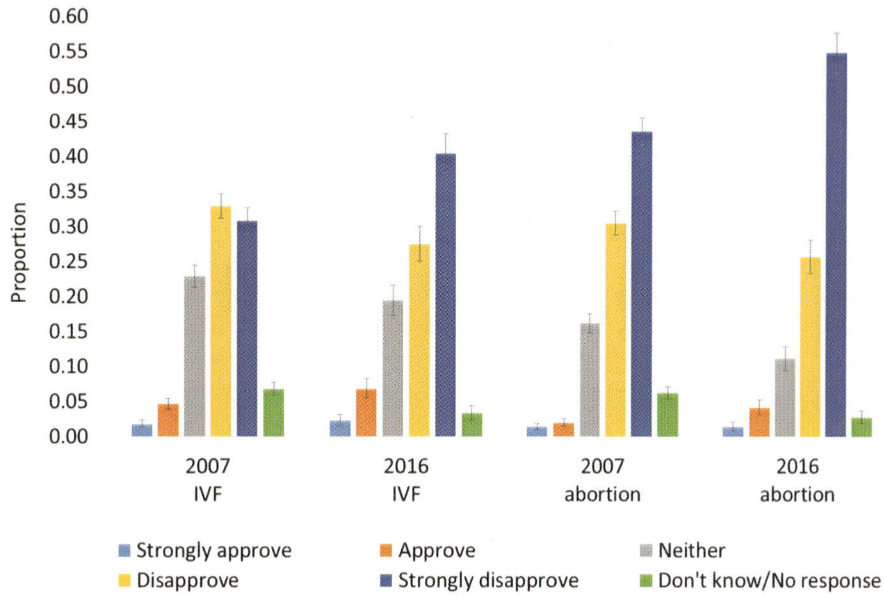

Fig. 2 Responses to "Do you approve or disapprove of the use of IVF technology to avoid characteristics of children such as: a certain sex" and "Do you approve or disapprove of the use of abortion to avoid characteristics of children such as: a certain sex". Note: Weighted to population characteristics. 95% confidence intervals shown. Source: Australian Survey of Social Attitudes, 2007 and 2016, $n = 4048$

Results

Sex selection through IVF for medical reasons, family balancing or any reason

The 2016 Australian Survey of Social Attitudes asked, for the first time, whether IVF should be legal in Australia for choosing a child's sex, and under what circumstances. Results are shown in Fig. 1.

Fifty-eight per cent of Australian adults believe that sex selection through IVF should be legal for medical reasons. Thirty-seven per cent of respondents answered in the negative, while 5% did not know, or did not give a response. In contrast, around three-quarters of Australians are opposed to legalising sex selection through IVF for any reason, for choosing the sex of a second child different

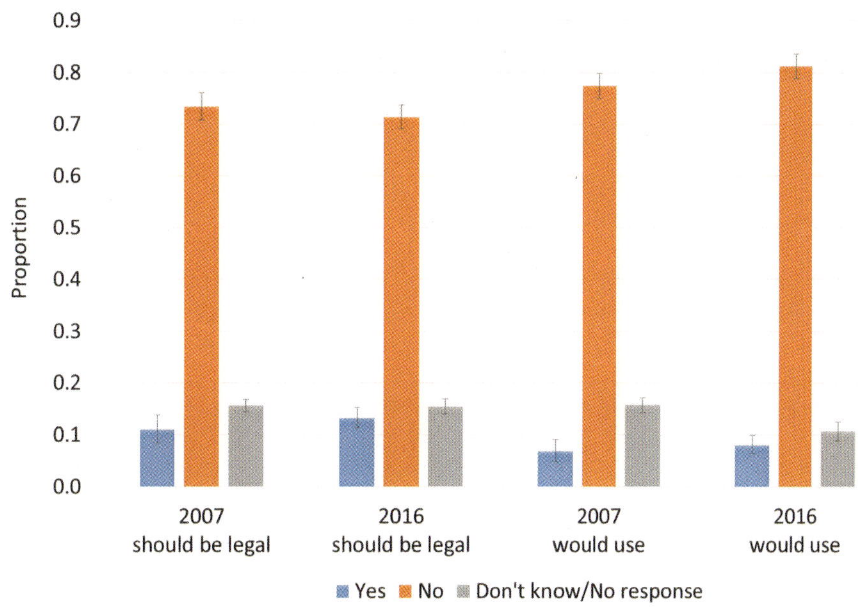

Fig. 3 Responses to "Suppose there was a medication available that enabled parents to choose the sex of their children…Do you think such a medication should be legally available?" and "If you were planning to have children, would you take advantage of such a medication?". Note: Weighted to population characteristics. 95% confidence intervals shown. Source: Australian Survey of Social Attitudes, 2007 and 2016, n = 4048

Table 1 Logistic regressions. Responses to "Do you approve or disapprove of the use of IVF technology [abortion] to avoid characteristics of children such as: a certain sex". Strongly disapprove (vs Disapprove, Neither, Approve, Strongly Approve), by survey year, and respondent sex, age, education and religious attendance

Sample characteristics	IVF					Abortion				
	Odds ratio	95% CI	*p*-value	Pred. prob.	n	Odds ratio	95% CI	*p*-value	Pred. prob.	n
SEX										
Ref: Male	1.00			0.378	1836	1.00			0.506	1845
Female	1.39	(1.21–1.59)	0.000	0.457	1945	1.31	(1.14–1.49)	0.000	0.572	1959
AGE										
Ref: 17–34 years	1.00			0.470	666	1.00			0.686	672
35–49 years	0.95	(0.77–1.16)	0.606	0.457	989	0.77	(0.63–0.94)	0.012	0.627	987
50–64 years	0.95	(0.78–1.16)	0.611	0.457	1215	0.61	(0.50–0.75)	0.000	0.572	1223
65+ years	0.57	(0.46–0.72)	0.000	0.337	878	0.39	(0.31–0.49)	0.000	0.462	886
EDUCATION										
Ref: Bachelor degree or above	1.00			0.536	1030	1.00			0.649	1038
Other post-school qualification	0.73	(0.62–0.86)	0.000	0.457	1588	0.72	(0.62–0.85)	0.000	0.572	1590
Year 12 or equivalent	0.71	(0.55–0.91)	0.007	0.450	377	0.64	(0.50–0.82)	0.000	0.543	380
Year 10/11 or equivalent	0.59	(0.46–0.74)	0.000	0.403	500	0.50	(0.40–0.63)	0.000	0.479	505
Below Year 10	0.56	(0.41–0.77)	0.000	0.393	261	0.41	(0.31–0.56)	0.000	0.433	264
RELIGIOUS ATTENDANCE										
Ref: Never	1.00			0.483	1465	1.00			0.601	1471
Once a year or less frequently	0.90	(0.76–1.07)	0.234	0.457	1074	0.89	(0.75–1.05)	0.157	0.572	1074
Several times a year	0.90	(0.72–1.11)	0.318	0.455	497	0.97	(0.79–1.20)	0.806	0.595	499
Once a month or more	1.29	(1.06–1.57)	0.010	0.547	651	1.27	(1.05–1.54)	0.016	0.656	664
YEAR										
Ref: 2007	1.00			0.365	2596	1.00			0.472	2613
2016	1.47	(1.26–1.70)	0.000	0.457	1216	1.50	(1.29–1.73)	0.000	0.572	1221
Total sample					3812					3834

Source: Australian Survey of Social Attitudes, 2007 and 2016
Ref: Reference category
95% CI: 95% confidence interval for odds ratios
Pred. prob.: Predicted probability. Other characteristics set at Female, 50–64 years, Other post-school qualification, Once or year or less frequently, 2016
Don't know/No response cases for the dependent variable are excluded from analysis
Don't know/Other/No response cases for independent variables are included in the analysis but not shown
p-values of less than 0.05 are considered significant

from the first, or for choosing the sex of a third child different from the first two.

Only 14% believe IVF should be legally available for choosing the sex of a second child different from the first, and 19% for family balancing for a third child. Twelve per cent support the legalisation of sex selection through IVF for any reason, with an equal proportion declining to answer this question or giving a "Don't know" response. For the two family balancing options, 7% of survey participants gave a 'Don't know' response, or did not provide a response (Fig. 1). The differences between the yes/no responses for legalisation of sex selection for medical reasons, and the yes/no responses for legalisation of sex selection for family balancing or for any reason, are statistically significant; Australians are much more likely to be favour of sex selection through IVF for medical reasons, and much more likely to be opposed to sex selection through IVF for other than medical reasons.

Disapproval of IVF and abortion for choosing a child's sex

Questions around approval or disapproval of IVF or abortion for choosing the sex of a child were asked in AuSSA in 2007 and 2016. Population-weighted responses are shown in Fig. 2. For all four groupings, the largest response categories are "Disapprove" and "Strongly disapprove", with "Strongly disapprove" the largest category for IVF in 2016, and abortion in both 2007 and 2016.

Around two-thirds of respondents in both 2007 and 2016 disapproved or strongly disapproved of the use of IVF for sex selection. Those who disapproved or strongly disapproved of the use of abortion for sex selection increased from 74% in 2007 to 81% in 2016.

The combined Approve/Strongly approve category increased for IVF between 2007 and 2016, from 6% to 9%, and for abortion from 3% to 6%. However, these increases were not statistically significant. The proportion who selected "Neither approve nor disapprove" or "Don't know", or who gave no response, fell for both IVF and abortion between 2007 and 2016.

The most significant shift in attitudes to the use of IVF or abortion for sex selection was in the strengthening of the "Strongly disapprove" response between 2007 and 2016. Those who strongly disapprove of the use of IVF for sex selection increased from 31% to 40%, and for abortion, from 44% to 55%, between 2007 and 2016 (Fig. 2). This result is statistically significant, as indicated by the non-overlapping confidence intervals.

Demographic characteristics associated with strong disapproval of the use of sex selection through IVF or abortion

We constructed two logistic regression models to determine whether particular groups of Australians were more likely to strongly disapprove of the use of sex-selective IVF or abortion. Characteristics considered were sex, age, education, and religious attendance (as a proxy for religiosity). In these models, we also included a marker for survey year to assess whether the increase in strong disapproval from 2007 to 2016—seen in Fig. 2—remained after controlling for respondent characteristics.

Results of the two models are shown in Table 1. Odds ratios greater than 1.00 indicate that the population group in question has a higher proportion who strongly disapprove compared to the reference category, while odds ratios of less than 1.00 indicate a lower level of strong disapproval in comparison to the reference category. *P*-values of less than 0.05 are considered significant. The predicted probabilities of a person with the specified characteristics "strongly disapproving" of sex-selective IVF or abortion are also shown.

In the first model, those more likely to strongly disapprove of IVF for sex selection are women (predicted probability = 46%, $p = 0.000$, compare men), young people aged 17–34 years (predicted probability = 47%, $p = 0.000$, compare 65+ years), those with a bachelor degree or above (predicted probability = 54%, $p = 0.000$, compare other education levels), and those who attend religious services once a month or more (predicted probability = 55%, $p = 0.010$, compare never). Levels of strong disapproval are higher for sex-selective abortion than for sex-selective IVF (Model 2) but patterns are similar to those found for IVF. Again, those more likely to strongly disapprove of abortion for sex selection are women (predicted probability = 57%, $p = 0.000$, compare men), young people aged 17–34 years (predicted probability = 69%, $p = 0.000$, compare other age groups), those with a bachelor degree or above (predicted probability = 65%, $p = 0.000$, compare other education levels), those who attend religious services once a month or more (predicted probability = 66%, $p = 0.016$, compare never). Those who strongly disapprove of IVF for sex selection are essentially a subset of those who strongly disapprove of abortion for sex selection (not shown). As in Fig. 2, the proportion of the population who strongly disapprove of IVF or abortion for sex selection increased significantly between 2007 and 2016 (Table 1; $p = 0.000$).

Attitudes to a hypothetical blue pill/pink pill for choosing a child's sex

In the early 2000s, Dahl et al. ran a series of surveys on sex selection in Germany, the United Kingdom, and the United States [12–14]. One of the questions asked was whether the respondent would take advantage of a hypothetical blue pill or pink pill, were such technology available, to ensure the birth of a son or daughter. We employed this question in the Australian Survey of Social Attitudes, and also extended it to ask whether respondents believed this medication should be legal, were it to exist. The rationale for these questions is to separate out those who may be opposed to the *method* of sex selection (such as IVF or abortion), from those opposed to the *motivation* (e.g. gender discrimination) or *outcome* (e.g. sex-ratio imbalance) of sex selection. Weighted responses to these two questions, for 2007 and 2016, are shown in Fig. 3.

As with IVF and abortion for sex selection, most Australians are opposed to a hypothetical blue pill/pink pill option. More than 70% believe that such technology should not be legally available, around 15% did not know or gave no response, and only 12% responded that the medication should be legal. If such a medication *were* available, 8% of respondents stated that they would take advantage of it, and around 80% stated that they would not. Response distributions were similar between 2007 and 2016.

Discussion

This analysis of data from the 2007 and 2016 Australian Survey of Social Attitudes shows high and strengthening disapproval of sex selection via IVF or abortion. Most Australians believe that social sex selection via IVF should not be legal, even if it is for family balancing for a second or third child. However most are in favour of sex selection for medical reasons. In addition, most Australians believe that a hypothetical blue/pink pill for sex selection should not be legal.

From 2007 to 2016, there has been a shift from 'Neither approve nor disapprove' and 'Disapprove' to 'Strongly disapprove' for the use of IVF or abortion to choose the sex of a child. This shift is statistically significant. That is, disapproval of sex selection via IVF or abortion has strengthened in the Australian population over the past decade. This change is not indicative of strengthening opposition to IVF and abortion in general. Other research that we have conducted based on 2007 and 2016 AuSSA data (not shown) indicates low levels and little change in disapproval for IVF and abortion for reasons other than social sex selection, such as to avoid a physical disability. Rather, results of this study are reflective of strengthening opposition to choosing to have a child on the basis of whether that child is male or female.

Those most likely to strongly disapprove of IVF or abortion for sex selection are women, young adults, university educated, and more religious respondents. These would seem to be strange bedfellows. An area for further research is to determine why these groups are more opposed than are others to sex selection. It may be that women, young adults and the university educated see sex selection as problematic because of the perceived implication that the process equates sex with gender, with parents selecting the sex of their offspring because of normative stereotypes of gender. If this is the case, then opposition is likely to continue to strengthen in the future. Conversely, more religious respondents may oppose sex selection because of the methods employed. Other studies in Australia and internationally find that the more religious are more likely to oppose the use of IVF or abortion for any reason, not just for sex selection [16–18].

The findings of high opposition to social sex selection—whatever the means—are in line with international results. A 2006 review of research internationally on "Attitudes towards sex selection for non-medical reasons" [19] identified 21 relevant studies conducted 1971–2005, 16 on US populations, 4 from Germany and 1 from the United Kingdom. All these studies found majority disapproval for the use of sex selection technology, both when questions were framed for personal use, and whether such technology should be generally available or made legal. In accordance with the findings of the current study, the review found stronger disapproval for personal use compared to general availability, and variation by proposed method, such that disapproval was higher for sex-selective abortion than for sex-selective IVF and for a hypothetical blue/pink pill. More recent studies have similar findings [12–14, 20–22], including one for Australia [23].

Our research adds to this international literature through investigating, for Australia, attitudes to sex selection for different reasons—medical, family balancing, any reason—changes in attitudes over time, and the demographic characteristics of those more likely to be opposed to sex selection.

What are the implications for Australian law of opposition to social sex selection? Currently, the blue/pink pill scenario for sex selection is still a hypothesis. It may be decades, if ever, before a sex-selective pill becomes a reality. And, in practice, early-term abortion is available on request in Australia, although what constitutes 'early-term' varies geographically as abortion law is state-based. Early maternal blood tests are now available that can determine fetal sex [24], and there is some evidence that sex-selective abortion is occurring in Australia, albeit on a very limited basis [25].

Any legal implications are most relevant for the use of IVF for sex selection. As noted in the Introduction, Australia's *Ethical Guidelines on the Use of Assisted Reproductive Technology in Clinical Practice and Research*, which have the force of law, prohibit the use of social sex selection "by whatever means". In practice, this prohibition had the effect of shutting down the use of IVF for social sex selection in Australian fertility clinics.

One school of thought is that legislation should be guided by community attitudes. This seems to be the position of the NHMRC, which in its 2017 revision of the *Ethical Guidelines* stated that "With any controversial practice, society's readiness to accept a practice is a relevant and important consideration." Our study finds that Australians are opposed to the use of sex selection, including via IVF, except where its use is recommended for medical reasons. Although the NHMRC has previously suggested that social sex selection for family balancing may be more acceptable than for other reasons [8, 9], our research shows that opposition by Australians to social sex selection is fairly consistent whether it is for family balancing for the second child, or third child, or for any reason.

A second school of thought is the legality of social sex selection should be guided by its potential for harm. However there is no consensus among ethicists and others about whether allowing social sex selection would result in harm or not. Possible harms that have been discussed include: distortions in the sex ratio of births, particularly if sons are preferred, as currently happens in some countries [1, 26, 27]; distortions in the sex ratio of first births, if boys and girls are equally desired, but there is a preference for first-born sons [7, 28, 29]; sex selection as expressed discrimination against females [1, 26, 27]; sex selection as a manifestation of normative gender stereotypes both within individual families and within society at large [26, 30, 31]; and sex selection as a "slippery slope" to designer babies [26, 27, 32].

The arguments for and against harm are equally vehement, and we are not in a position to judge most of them here. However, as demographers, we can comment on the first two possible harms mentioned: distortions in the overall sex ratio at birth, and in the sex ratio of first births. Previous research on parental behaviour and attitudes indicates that a change in the sex ratio of all births is unlikely in the Australian context, as sons and daughters are equally desired, with parents overall wishing for a mix of boys and girls [29, 33–35].

However, a previous study has found that a significant minority of Australians (40%) intending to have a first child in the future express a preference for the sex of that child, with first-born sons chosen over first-born daughters by more than two to one [34]. If social sex selection was permitted for any reason in Australia, it may lead to a distortion in the sex ratio of first-born children, with many more first-born boys than first-born girls. This is of concern, since research has found that first-borns are more likely to have attributes such as higher levels of intelligence, education and general achievements [29].

Conclusions

Assisted reproductive technology for social sex selection is banned in Australia. The prohibiting body noted in 2017 that community acceptance of the practice of social sex selection would be an important consideration in future regulatory change, but, currently, "there is limited research into the question of whether Australians support the use of sex selection for non-medical purposes" [6].

This study addresses this question, finding from analysis of a recent large national representative survey that around three-quarters of Australians believe the use of IVF for non-medical sex selection should not be legal, whether it be for family balancing or for any reason. In contrast, most Australians (58%) believe that sex selection through IVF should be legal for medical reasons.

Opposition to sex selection via IVF has strengthened over the past decade (as has opposition to sex selection via abortion). Clearly, the Australian community does not accept the practice of social sex selection. If regulatory change is to be guided by societal attitudes, then the prohibition against sex selection for non-medical reasons should remain in place.

If, instead, potential harms are paramount, then social sex selection should remain prohibited if there is a demonstrable harm from its use. Many potential harms have been raised, with a focus in this paper's discussion on possible distortions in the sex ratio at birth, if widespread social sex selection is used to choose many more sons than daughters, as happens in some other countries [1, 7]. Is such concern valid? Previous research finds that Australian parents have an overall equal preference for sons and daughters [29, 33–35], but that a large minority of intending parents have a preference for a first-born boy [34].

Thus, the legalisation of social sex selection is unlikely to lead to a surfeit of sons in Australia, but could result in a preponderance of first-born boys. Only allowing sex selection for family balancing after the first child would obviate any possible sex ratio distortions for first-borns. However such a recommendation depends on how much weight should be given to community attitudes, which in Australia are clearly against the use of social sex selection—even for the second or third child—with disapproval strengthening over the past decade.

Strengths and limitations of the study

A major strength of this study is that it is based on analysis of a large, nationally representative random survey of adult Australian citizens—the Australian Survey of Social Attitudes (AuSSA). The sample size was 2781 in 2007 and 1267 in 2016. Response rates fell over this period from 42% in 2007 to 25% in 2016. The collection of demographic characteristics of respondents means the data can be weighted to national population counts by age, sex and education, decreasing non-response bias. However, non-response bias due to other characteristics such as ethnicity or religion may remain. Because AuSSA is a broad survey of social attitudes, non-response is unlikely to be related to a reluctance to answer questions around the study topic [36]. Another limitation of this study is that we are unable to directly ascertain the reasoning behind the stated attitudes.

Acknowledgements
We thank three anonymous reviewers for their careful reading of our paper and their constructive comments and suggestions which significantly improved this work.

Funding
No funding was received for this research.

Authors' contributions
RK, EG and AE conceived and designed the study. RK analysed the data. RK, EG and AE interpreted the data, drafted and revised the manuscript, and give final approval of the version to be published. Each author has participated sufficiently in the work to take public responsibility for appropriate portions of the content, and has agreed to be accountable for all aspects of the work.

Competing interests
The authors declare that they have no competing interests.

Author details
[1]School of Rural Health, Monash University, 26 Mercy St, Bendigo, VIC 3552, Australia. [2]School of Demography, The Australian National University, Building 9, Acton, ACT 2601, Australia.

References

1. National Health and Medical Research Council. Ethical guidelines on the use of assisted reproductive technology in clinical practice and research. 2004. https://www.nhmrc.gov.au/guidelines-publications/e56. Accessed 19 Apr 2018.
2. Petersen K, Baker HWG, Pitts M, Thorpe R. Assisted reproductive technologies: professional and legal restrictions in Australian clinics. J Law Med. 2005;12(3):373–85.
3. Waters A-M, Dean JH, Sullivan EA. Supplement to Assisted reproduction technology in Australia and New Zealand 2003. Sydney: Australian Institute of Health and Welfare National Perinatal Statistics Unit; 2006.
4. Wang YA, Dean JH, Grayson N, Sullivan EA. Assisted reproduction technology in Australia and New Zealand 2004. Sydney: Australian Institute of Health and Welfare National Perinatal Statistics Unit; 2006.
5. National Health and Medical Research Council. Ethical guidelines on the use of assisted reproductive technology in clinical practice and research. 2007. https://www.nhmrc.gov.au/guidelines-publications/e78. Accessed 19 Apr 2018.
6. National Health and Medical Research Council. Ethical guidelines on the use of assisted reproductive technology in clinical practice and research. 2017. https://www.nhmrc.gov.au/guidelines-publications/e79. Accessed 19 Apr 2018.
7. Kippen R, Evans A, Gray E. Australian attitudes toward sex-selection technology. Fertil Steril. 2011;95(5):1824–6.
8. National Health and Medical Research Council. Question and answer: Ethical guidelines on the use of assisted reproductive technology in clinical practice and research. 2017. https://www.nhmrc.gov.au/_files_nhmrc/file/health_ethics/art_questions_and_answers.pdf. Accessed 16 July 2018.
9. National Health and Medical Research Council. Draft: Ethical guidelines on the use of assisted reproductive technology in clinical practice and research. Public consultation. 2015. https://consultations.nhmrc.gov.au/files/consultations/drafts/artdraftethicalguidelines150722.pdf. Accessed 16 July 2018.
10. Dickens BM, Serour GI, Cook RJ, Qiu R-Z. Sex selection: treating different cases differently. Int J Gynecol Obstet. 2005;90:171–7.
11. AuSSA. The Australian Survey of Social Attitudes. 2017. https://www.acspri.org.au/aussa. Accessed 21 Aug 2017.
12. Dahl E, Beutel M, Brosig B, Hinsch K. D. Preconception sex selection for non-medical reasons: a representative survey from Germany. Hum Reprod. 2003; 18(10):2231–4.
13. Dahl E, Gupta RS, Beutel M, Stoebel-Richter Y, Brosig B, Tinneberg H-R, et al. Preconception sex selection demand and preferences in the United States. Fertil Steril. 2006;85(2):468–73.
14. Himmel W, Dahl E, Michelmann H. Preconception sex selection: a survey of visitors to an internet-based health forum. Reprod BioMed Online. 2008; 16(1):18–26.
15. AuSSA. AuSSA Questionnaires. 2015. http://aussa.anu.edu.au/questionnaires.php. Accessed 21 Aug 2017.
16. Schenker JG. Assisted reproductive practice: religious perspectives. Reprod BioMed Online. 2005;10(3):310–9.
17. Betts K. Attitudes to abortion: Australia and Queensland in the twenty-first century. People and Place. 2009;17(3):25–39.
18. Dempsey D, Critchley C. Comfort with use of assisted reproductive technologies (ART) for family formation by same-sex and heterosexual couples: a survey of Australian social attitudes. Gay and Lesbian Issues and Psychol Rev. 2010;6(2):90–102.
19. Hall S, Reid E, Marteau T. Attitudes towards sex selection for non-medical reasons: a review. Prenat Diagn. 2006;26:619–26.
20. Woodward BJ, Sohan K, Dahl E. Gender preference and demand for preconception sex selection: a survey among pregnant women in the Caribbean. Hum Reprod. 2010;25(Suppl 1):i154–61.
21. Wilhelm M, Dahl E, Alexander H, Brähler E, Stöbel-Richter Y. Ethical attitudes of German specialists in reproductive medicine and legal regulation of preimplantation sex selection in Germany. PLoS One. 2013;8(2):e56390.
22. Winkelman WD, Missmer SA, Myers D, Ginsburg ES. Public perspectives on the use of preimplantation genetic diagnosis. J Assist Reprod Genet. 2015; 32(5):665–75.
23. Kovacs G, McCrann J, Levine M, Morgan G. The Australian community does not support gender selection by IVF for social reasons. Int J Reprod Med. 2013;242174:1–3.
24. Allyse M, Minear M, Rote M, Hung A, Chandrasekharan S, Berson E, et al. Non-invasive prenatal testing: a review of international implementation and challenges. Int J Women's Health. 2015;7:113–26.
25. Jain P, Liu N, Roberts B. Could gender-selective abortions be happening in Australia? SBS news. 2015. https://www.sbs.com.au/news/could-gender-selective-abortions-be-happening-in-australia. Accessed 19 Apr 2018.
26. Dahl E. Procreative liberty: the case for preconception sex selection. Reprod BioMed Online. 2003;7(4):380–4.
27. Savulescu J, Dahl E. Sex selection and preimplantation diagnosis. Hum Reprod. 2000;15(9):1879–80.
28. Pebley AR, Westoff CF. Women's sex preferences in the United States: 1970 to 1975. Demography. 1982;19(2):177–89.
29. Kippen R, Evans A, Gray E. Parental preference for sons and daughters in a western industrial setting: evidence and implications. J Biosoc Sci. 2007; 39(4):583–97.
30. Bhatia R. Constructing gender from the inside out: sex-selection practices in the United States. Fem Stud. 2010;36(2):260–91.
31. Browne TK. How sex selection undermines reproductive autonomy. J Bioeth Inq. 2017;14(2):195–204.
32. Rollins A. Sex selection a 'slippery slope' to designer babies: Gannon. Aust Med. 2016;28(7a):8.
33. Evans A, Barbato C, Bettini E, Gray E, Kippen R. Taking stock: parents' reasons for and against having a third child. Community, Work Fam. 2009;12(4):437–54.
34. Gray E, Kippen R, Evans A. A boy for you and a girl for me: do men want sons and women want daughters? People and Place. 2007;15(4):1–8.
35. Kippen R, Gray E, Evans A. The impact on Australian fertility of wanting one of each. People and Place. 2005;13(2):12–21.
36. Schofield TP, Butterworth P. Patterns of welfare attitudes in the Australian population. PLoS One. 2015;10(11):142792.

Sexual health of very young adolescents in South Western Uganda: a cross-sectional assessment of sexual knowledge and behavior

Elizabeth Kemigisha[1,2*], Katharine Bruce[1], Viola N. Nyakato[1], Gad Ndaruhutse Ruzaaza[1], Anna B. Ninsiima[3], Wendo Mlahagwa[1], Els Leye[2], Gily Coene[3] and Kristien Michielsen[2]

Abstract

Background: In most Sub-Saharan African countries, little is known about young adolescents' sexual and reproductive health (SRH). Though some efforts have been made to understand and improve SRH of older adolescents, very young adolescents (VYAs) are often overlooked, and little is known about their sexual knowledge and behaviors. The goal of this study was to describe SRH knowledge, information-seeking, and sexual behavior of VYAs in Uganda.

Methods: A cross-sectional survey was administered in 33 primary schools in June and July of 2016. Trained interviewers administered surveys to adolescents ages 10–14 regarding SRH knowledge, information-seeking, sexual behavior, and relevant covariates. Continuous variables were summarized as means (SD) or medians (IQR) whereas categorical variables were summarized as proportions (percentages).

Results: A total of 1096 adolescents were included in this analysis, 81.8% of which were from rural areas, with a median age of 12. Regarding sexually transmitted infections (STIs) knowledge; 95% knew HIV while 37% knew other STIs apart from HIV. Although 47% knew at least one way in which HIV is acquired only 8% knew at least four ways. Regarding contraceptive knowledge, 56% mentioned at least one modern method of preventing pregnancy (condoms, pills, intrauterine devices, implants, or injections). The majority (85%) of VYAs reported accessing SRH information in the media with 35% reporting accessing media with sexual content while 10% vs 22% consulted their father or mother respectively and 31% a school source. At least 7.6% of VYAs had ever had sexual intercourse, 90% of which were not using any protection.

Conclusion: Comprehensive SRH knowledge was low among VYAs in this study. Media remains an important source of information for SRH for this age group though it may be misused as some adolescents reported accessing sexual content that may be inappropriate. A large proportion of sexually active VYAs reported sexual risky behaviors. This study highlights the need for an accurate and more comprehensive SRH education approach for VYAs in Uganda at an opportune age before the majority engage in sexual behavior.

Keywords: Young adolescents, Sexuality, Uganda

* Correspondence: ekemigisha@must.ac.ug
[1]Mbarara University of Science and Technology, P.O. Box 1410, Mbarara, Uganda
[2]International Centre for Reproductive Health, Faculty of Medicine and Health Sciences, Ghent University, Ghent, Belgium
Full list of author information is available at the end of the article

Plain English summary

Uganda has the second youngest population in the world, with high rates of sexually transmitted diseases and adolescent pregnancy. Access to sexual and reproductive health (SRH) information and resources is a challenge, especially for very young adolescents (VYAs) aged 10–14. The goal of this study is to assess levels of SRH knowledge, SRH information seeking and sexual behavior among VYAs. We found that most students are aware of HIV, but few have detailed knowledge of how HIV is acquired, what other STIs exist, and what methods of pregnancy prevention are available. Seven percent of VYAs were already sexually active with most of them not using any form of protection such as condoms. The majority of VYAs had been exposed to SRH information in the media (television, radio or newspapers) with at least one third of them accessing media with sexual content, while far fewer had received such information in schools or from their parents. This study highlights the importance of implementing school-based SRH education at a young age. Because the majority of VYAs are not yet sexually active, SRH interventions in this age group may be more effective than those in older adolescents in delaying sexual onset and decreasing risky sexual behavior. Furthermore, because these students are already being exposed to sexual information in the media, it is important for schools and parents to provide accurate information that helps students to reflect more critically on SRH information in media sources.

Background

With a median age of just 15, Uganda has the second youngest population in the world [1]. Over half of the population is the under age of 18 years [2]. This youthful population presents unique challenges, especially with regard to sexual and reproductive health (SRH). Uganda's 2016 Demographic and Health Survey (DHS) found that 24.8% of girls ages 15–19 had already begun childbearing, which was as high as 53.9% among girls age 19 [3]. Uganda has one of the ten highest HIV prevalence rates in the world at 6.2% (4.7% among males and 7.6% among females) [4, 5]. Despite great initial success in decreasing HIV prevalence and incidence throughout the 1990s and early 2000s [6], HIV/AIDS remains the leading cause of death in Uganda [7], and the majority of new infections occur among adolescent women [3]. In this young population, comprehensive access to sexual and reproductive health knowledge and services is of upmost importance.

Access to SRH information and prevention services remains a challenge in most developing countries, including Uganda. The 2016 DHS found that only 40% of Ugandan adolescents ages 15–19 years have comprehensive HIV prevention knowledge [3]. A study among girls in Ugandan primary schools found low knowledge of menstruation and menstrual hygiene [8]. Inadequate SRH knowledge creates anxiety and shame, especially at the beginning of puberty [9]. While there is little data available on SRH outcomes among VYAs in Uganda, poor reproductive health outcomes become especially evident in late adolescence. A study among university students found high non-use of contraception, inconsistent condom use and low knowledge of proper condom use, especially among females and those who had early sexual debut [10, 11]. It is possible that intervening in early adolescence could mitigate adverse outcomes in older adolescence.

Despite these challenges, there has been a lot of pushback on SRH education in Uganda from parents, teachers, and even Members of Parliament (MPs), who feel that teaching these topics in schools will erode Uganda's culture and morality [12]. In 2016, the Ministry of Gender, Labor and Social Development banned sexuality education in schools [13]. The Ministry of Education and Sports recently released new national guidelines on sexuality education, but these guidelines are not comprehensive, they emphasize abstinence, and the future of their implementation is still unclear [14]. With no standardized SRH curriculum in schools and ongoing religious and political pushback on its relevance and appropriateness, adolescents in Uganda are left with few options to seek SRH information.

Following evidence on the proven benefits of comprehensive sexuality education in diverse settings [15], UNESCO recently released guidelines outlining recommendations for comprehensive sexuality education [16]. However, most of the existing SRH interventions in low and middle income countries, as well as most of the existing research, focus on older adolescents [15]. SRH needs of very young adolescents (VYAs), those aged 10–14 years, are often neglected in research and action [17–19] and there are many gaps in understanding SRH of young adolescents, especially in Sub-Saharan Africa (SSA) [20, 21]. This younger age group may be the ideal target for SRH interventions, as their behaviors and norms are less rigid [22]. Due to the fact that the majority of VYAs in Uganda are not yet sexually active [23], they are more susceptible to behavioral interventions than their older peers who have already started engaging in risky sexual behaviors. Bankole et al., 2007 found that 11% of Ugandan adolescents ages 12–14 are already sexually active [23], showing that SRH information is indeed relevant for this young age group, who are beginning to be exposed to SRH risks. Furthermore, research by Kemigisha et al., 2018 on Ugandan VYAs found that inequitable norms around gender and sexuality increase with age [24]. Harmful gender norms surrounding sexuality, consent and decision-making exacerbate SRH risks for boys as well as girls [25]. Interventions should target adolescents at a young age, before they have already developed harmful norms about gender and sex.

The goal of this study is to investigate the current status of sexual behavior, SRH knowledge, and information-seeking behaviors of adolescents ages 10–14 in Uganda. It aims to fill the gap in the literature regarding the SRH of VYAs in Uganda. This information should guide the development and implementation of educational SRH interventions across the country.

Methods

Study design and setting

This paper presents the results of a cross-sectional survey of very young adolescents in primary schools in Mbarara district of South Western Uganda. This data was collected as the baseline of a cluster randomized trial to evaluate the implementation and effectiveness of a comprehensive sexuality education program in primary schools. According to the 2015 District Education reports, Mbarara has a total of 248 primary schools with an estimated primary school enrolment of 80,924 [26].

Study population and selection of participants

Participant eligibility criteria included being 10–14 years old and in primary level 5 or 6 of education from rural and urban schools within Mbarara district. The final sample size included 1096 adolescents from 33 schools in both urban and rural settings. A list of primary schools in Mbarara was available in district records. We eliminated schools that had no upper classes (primary 5 to 7), and schools that offer unique services, including one school for children with hearing impairments and one school for children with visual impairments. The remaining schools were entered into an Excel spreadsheet and a formula was developed to randomly select the required 33 schools for the study. A second Excel formula was used to randomly assign each of the 33 schools to the treatment or control arm. Research assistants (RAs) selected the final sample of students in each school from class registration lists using systematic sampling methods and substituting pupils who were absent on the day that data was collected.

Data collection

The data were collected between June and July 2016. Standardized closed surveys were administered by trained RAs and were crosschecked by the onsite investigator and research monitors and cleaned for any errors. All RAs were fluent in both English and Runyankole (the local language) and surveys were administered based on each students' preference. Responses to all questions were recorded and coded either using scales or binary yes/no questions, with the option to refrain from responding. Additionally, questions that assessed pupils' knowledge included the option to respond with "I do not know". Anonymity was maintained throughout the study and participants' responses were deidentified.

Definitions for outcome variables

Sexual behavior was measured starting from a screening question: "have you ever been to a secret place alone with a friend of the opposite sex?" If the answer to this question was yes, further questions were asked regarding sexual experiences. These included "Did you ever kiss on the lips?", "Did you or your friend ever touch your private parts?", "Have you ever had sex?" "How old were you when you first had sex?", "What method did you use to prevent HIV/AIDS or STIs?" and "Were you willing to have sex the first time you did?"

Sexual and reproductive health knowledge was measured based on knowledge of puberty, HIV/STIs and pregnancy prevention. This included knowledge on how HIV/AIDS can be acquired, types of common Sexually Transmitted Infections, knowledge of pubertal changes in boys (such as having beards, deep voice etc.) and in girls (such as increase in breast size, having pubic or axillary hair etc.), and knowledge about ways to prevent pregnancy (such as abstinence, condom use or any other type of contraceptive).

Sources of Information on SRH were assessed. We asked students if they had sought SRH information from their mother, father, a school source, a community health facility and/or mass media sources. Media was further categorized into seeking information on SRH topics or sexual content.

Data was collected on socio-demographic variables such as age in years, pubertal stage, gender, religion, socio-economic status (assessed as a sum of the score for best water source, housing possessions and pupil possessions such as shoes or school uniform pairs), whether the school was located in rural or urban area and whether one, both or neither parents were alive.

Statistical analyses

Data was double entered into Epi-data 3.1 (EpiData, Odense, Denmark). The data utilized in this analysis represent the baseline data of a cluster randomized control trial evaluating the effectiveness of a Comprehensive Sexuality Education intervention. Based on an intra-class correlation calculated in a pilot test among 105 VYAs and an estimated drop-out rate of 20%, we determined that a minimum sample size of 1100 students was needed to measure a 10% score difference in outcomes between baseline and endline among the intervention vs control groups with a power of 90%. Data analysis was done using Stata® (College Station, Texas, USA). Continuous variables were summarized as means (SD) or medians (IQR) whereas categorical variables were summarized as proportions (percentages). In addition, a bivariate analysis among categorical variables was made using chi square. All analyses were stratified by gender. A p-value of less than 0.05 was considered a significant association.

Results

Description of participants

A total of 1096 pupils were interviewed between June and July 2016. The median age was 12 (IQR 11, 13) years and 58% were female. Over 80% of the study population were from rural areas and over 80% of the pupils had both parents alive. Twenty-nine percent were ranked as having a high socio-economic score, 47% ranked medium and 24% ranked low (Table 1). The majority of pupils had achieved some form of puberty, with 90% beyond (self-assessed) tanner stage 1 (i.e. beyond normal size of penis of 3 cm/testicular volume of 1.5 ml in boys or lack of glandular tissue or no areola enlargement in girls and no pubic hair in both) and about half were at tanner stage 2 (i.e. showing early signs of breast, bud development or testicular enlargement with pubic hair). About 26% of the girls had started menstruation and 23% of the boys mentioned they had experienced wet dreams.

Sexual health knowledge

Regarding knowledge about puberty, 27.9% vs 12.3% of the respondents knew at least 3 of 6 physical changes in

Table 1 Socio-demographic characteristics of the participants by gender

	Overall, n (%)	Male n (%)	Female n (%)	p-value
Gender				
Boys	460 (42.0)			
Girls	636 (58.0)			
Age in years, median (IQR)	12 (11,13)			
Pubertal age (Tanner 1–5)				
Tanner 1	130 (11.9)	49 (10.6)	81 (12.7)	1
Tanner 2	379 (34.6)	168 (36.5)	211 (33.2)	
Tanner 3	487 (44.4)	216 (47.1)	271 (42.6)	
Tanner 4 or 5	100 (9.1)	27 (5.8)	73 (11.5)	0.007
Ever experienced menstruation (female only)	155 (25.9)	–	155 (25.9)	NA
Ever experience wet dreams (male only)	101 (22.5)	101 (22.5)	–	NA
Education level				
= Primary 5 only	563 (51.4)	240 (52.2)	323 (50.8)	
= Primary 6 only	533 (48.6)	220 (47.8)	313 (49.2)	0.650
Socio economic status[a]				
Low	315 (29.0)	128 (28.2)	187 (29.6)	
Medium	511 (47.1)	215 (47.4)	296 (46.8)	
High	260 (23.9)	111 (24.4)	149 (23.6)	0.871
Religion				
Catholic	405 (37.1)	165 (36.0)	240 (37.8)	
Anglican	507 (46.4)	215 (46.9)	292 (46.0)	
Moslem	101 (9.2)	48 (10.5)	53 (8.4)	
Other	80 (7.3)	30 (6.6)	50 (7.8)	0.527
Location of school				
Rural	896 (81.8)	368 (80)	529 (83.2)	
Urban	199 (18.2)	92 (20)	107 (16.8)	0.178
Number of parents alive				
Both alive	905 (82.6)	378 (82.2)	527 (82.9)	
None/Single parent	124 (17.4)	82 (17.8)	109 (17.1)	0.767

[a]Social economic status assessed as a sum of the score for best water source, housing possessions and pupil possessions such as shoes or school uniform pairs with a possible score range of 1–25, median of 8.1. Was categorized as Low if scores were 1–5, medium for scores 6–10 and high if scores 11 till maximum score

puberty in boys vs 4 of 7 changes in girls respectively. A majority of respondents (95%) knew HIV is an STI and 37% knew other STIs apart from HIV. Although 47% knew at least one way in which HIV may be acquired, only 8% knew at least 4 methods by which HIV is acquired. Regarding contraceptive knowledge, 59% mentioned abstinence, 56% mentioned any of the more effective methods of preventing pregnancy (condoms, hormonal or surgical methods), and 3% knew natural methods for contraception. More boys than girls knew of any effective ways to prevent pregnancy and the difference was significant (Table 2).

Sources of SRH information

A total of 85% of VYAs reported accessing SRH information through radio or television media. In addition 35.5% had access to media with sexual content via mobile device/television, and 44.5% accessed sexual content in print media (newspapers and magazines). More boys than girls watched visual media with sexual content. A total of 31.7% reported seeking SRH information from a source at school. Only 22.3% and 9.9% had discussions about love or sex with their mother or father respectively. Pupils were more likely to communicate with a parent of their same gender, meaning more boys communicated with fathers and more girls communicated with mothers (Table 3).

Sexual behaviors

A total of 15.1% respondents had ever been in a secluded place with a girlfriend or boyfriend; 3.1% had kissed, 10.5% had either touched or been touched by a boyfriend or girlfriend in the genital area, and 7.6% had had sexual intercourse. Overall, more boys than girls reported having experienced any of these forms of sexual behavior. Of those who were sexually active, only 9.6% used condoms the first time they had sex. Of those who were not sexually active, 11.3% reported they felt pressured to have sex, of which 6.1% were boys and 3.9% were girls (Table 4).

Discussion

This study describes the sexual behavior, sexual health knowledge, and information seeking behavior of VYAs in Uganda, in an effort to inform interventions related to adolescent SRH. We found that 7% of adolescents were sexually active, and that a majority of these were not using condoms. Detailed SRH knowledge on HIV transmission, types of STIs and contraception was low. Furthermore, media was the most utilized source for SRH information, while school and parental sources were underutilized.

In Uganda, there is a lot of pushback against SRH education from many key stakeholders, including political, religious and cultural leaders, who feel that these topics are inappropriate for children and should not be taught in schools [12]. There are no clear guidelines on what, when, and in what setting SRH information should be disseminated to students [27]. However, this study shows that regardless of whether these topics are taught in schools, adolescents receive information on sex and relationships at a young age. We found that the majority (85.2%) of VYAs had been exposed to media on SRH topics with over one third accessing media with sexual content. More boys than girls had seen a movie or show

Table 2 Level of knowledge on Sexual and Reproductive Health by gender among Very Young Adolescents in South Western Uganda

Characteristic	Total	Male	Female	Chi	*p* value
Knowledge on pubertal signs					
Pubertal signs in boys (at least 3/6)	305 (27.9)	158 (34.4)	147(23.2)	16.58	< 0.001
Pubertal signs in girls (at least 4/7)	134 (12.3)	56 (12.2)	78 (12.4)	0.09	< 0.926
Knowledge on STIS					
Knows HIV as an STI	1037 (95.1)	441 (96.5)	596 (94.2)	3.15	0.076
Knows any STI apart from HIV	402 (36.7)	183 (39.8)	219 (34.4)	3.29	0.07
Knowledge of HIV transmission					
Knows at least 1 way of HIV acquisition	516 (47.1)	218 (47.4)	298 (46.9)	0.03	0.861
Knows 4 ways of HIV acquisition	86 (7.9)	42 (9.1)	44 (6.9)	1.81	0.179
Knows a person who looks healthy can still have HIV	710 (65.3)	350 (76.8)	360 (57.1)	54.05	< 0.001
Knowledge on pregnancy prevention					
Knows abstinence	627 (59.0%)	264 (58.9)	363 (59.1)	0.004	0.95
Knows natural methods	33 (3.1%)	21 (4.7)	12 (2.0)	6.43	0.01
Knows more effective methods	592 (55.8%)	297 (66.4)	295 (48.0)	35.50	< 0.001

Table 3 Sources of information on Sexual and Reproductive Health for Very Young Adolescents in SW Uganda

Characteristic	Total	Male	Female	Chi	*p* value
Ever sought information on SRH					
Father	82 (9.9)	44 (11.5)	38 (7.2)	4.97	0.03
Mother	222 (22.3)	58 (13.9)	164 (28.4)	29.39	< 0.001
School source (of 791 who were aware of services)	251 (31.7)	57 (19.9)	194 (38.7)	28.80	< 0.001
Community health facility	61 (5.6)	29 (6.3)	32 (5.0)	1.09	0.58
Any mass media with educative SRH topics	923 (85.2)	396 (87.2)	527 (83.7)	2.66	0.10
Ever watched a movie or show with sexual content	389 (35.5)	191 (41.5)	198 (31.2)	12.45	< 0.001
Ever read a newspaper or magazine describing sexual content	487 (44.5)	220 (47.9)	267 (42.1)	3.73	0.05

with sexual content. However, far fewer adolescents received this information in school or from their parents.

Much of the SRH information in the media that adolescents are exposed to may be inaccurate or misleading [28, 29]. Although some public health institutions in Uganda use media to provide adolescents with accurate and relevant SRH information [30, 31], it is hard for adolescents to determine which sources are accurate and which are not [28, 29]. Moreover, media with sexual content has been associated with early sexual debut among adolescents in Africa [32]. Findings from a qualitative study in Uganda indicate use of media with sexual content is perceived to contribute to persistence of inequitable norms, especially in depicting women as submissive and men being sex driven [33]. In another study in a subset of these VYAs, we found inequitable sexual socialization tendencies beginning to emerge in early adolescence [25]. Both of these studies highlighted the role that media can play in shaping VYAs ideas about sex and relationships including norms that can be harmful to both boys and girls.

Schools and parents could serve as valuable resources for adolescents in mitigating potential harm of misleading media sources. One study in Uganda found that parents were in fact effective in mediating the effects of inappropriate media use among their adolescent children [34]. Furthermore, the National Sexuality Education Framework released by the Ugandan Ministry of Education and Sports includes modules on analyzing SRH information in the media [14]. Though this framework has not yet been implemented, it may enable schools to help students identify which information sources are accurate and credible, and which sources are not.

While the majority (95.1%) of VYAs were aware of HIV, few were aware of the four most common ways that HIV is transmitted and over a third said that it is not possible for a person who looks healthy to have HIV. Similar findings about SRH knowledge were earlier described by Bankole et al., 2007 [23]. This shows that despite the extremely high level of HIV awareness, adolescents had inadequate in-depth knowledge on HIV transmission. Furthermore, only one third knew any STI other than HIV. This implies that they may not be equipped with sufficient information to protect themselves from acquiring HIV and other STIs. Knowledge of contraceptive methods was moderate, with just over half mentioning abstinence or modern methods. Inadequate contraceptive knowledge may lead to poor utilization of these methods. This is supported by a previous study among sexually active adolescents that found that contraceptive knowledge and uptake has been significantly lower in younger women compared to older women [35, 36]. Clearly there are significant gaps in the information that young people are receiving about SRH. It is important that VYAs are aware of the health risks involved in sexual activity beyond HIV.

In this study, 7.6% of VYAs were sexually active, which is lower than previous findings among the same age group in Sub-Saharan Africa of 11–15% [23, 37]. More boys than girls reported being sexually active, which may relate to underreporting among Ugandan girls, who are often less comfortable and more stigmatized for being

Table 4 Description of sexual behavior of Very Young Adolescents by gender

Characteristic	Total	Male	Female	chi	*p* value
Ever went in seclusion with friend of opposite sex	165 (15.1)	101 (22.0)	64 (10.1)	29.29	< 0.001
Have (been) kissed	34 (3.1)	26 (5.7)	8 (1.3)	4.20	0.04
Have (been) fondled	115 (10.5)	80 (17.4)	35 (5.5)	11.15	< 0.001
Had penetrative sex	83 (7.6)	67 (14.6)	16 (2.5)	26.78	< 0.001
Used condoms on the last sexual experience (among sexually active only)	8 (9.6)	7 (10.4)	1 (6.7)	0.26	0.61
Have no sexual experience but are under pressure to have it	114 (10.4)	69 (15.0)	45 (7.1)	26.00	< 0.001

sexually active before marriage [25] . However, it was noted in this study that the majority of sexually active young adolescents did not use condoms, which puts young adolescents at risk of STIs, HIV and early pregnancy. These findings are supported with an established association that early sexual debut is a risk factor for risky sexual practices in Uganda [38, 39]. Furthermore, recent evidence shows that adolescents especially those of better social economic background globally experience puberty at a younger age [10, 40, 41]. Simultaneously, they are choosing to get married later than previous generations [9]. Attainment of biological maturity much earlier than socioeconomic independence and marriage imposes a wider biosocial gap among adolescents that may expose them to sexual and reproductive health risks prior marriage [42].

Furthermore, because the majority of these students are still not sexually active, this is an opportune age to implement behavioral SRH interventions. A plethora of studies in low and middle income countries have shown that comprehensive SRH education is associated with delayed sexual onset [15, 43], but these programs can only delay sexual onset if they are implemented before target students are sexually active. Additionally, about 96% of Ugandan children attend some primary school, while only 34% go on to secondary education [44]. If SRH interventions only target secondary school students, the majority of Ugandan adolescents will miss out on this vital information. By targeting VYAs in primary school, SRH interventions can reach the majority of Ugandan adolescents with accurate information before they become sexually active. This study highlights the vital need for comprehensive, school-based SRH education for VYAs that will enable young people make informed decisions about their sexual health.

Study limitations

Sexual behavior was self-reported and this being a sensitive subject, under reporting could have occurred among some participants. During data collection, we ensured privacy and tried as much as possible to have interviewers of the same sex as respondents conduct the interviews in an effort to limit reporting bias, a form of information bias. While dichotomizing certain variables was helpful in demonstrating statistical results, this may have led to a loss of relevant data. Furthermore, because this was a cross sectional survey, we could not determine the direction of causality. Finally, due to cultural and legal restrictions around homosexuality in Uganda, we were only able to ask students about heterosexual behavior, and did not ask about homosexual activity.

Conclusion

Very young adolescents in Uganda face great challenges in SRH, having low SRH knowledge, early sexual debut and risky sexual practices. SRH education should start during early adolescence, before the majority of these students are sexually active and while most of them are still in school. Comprehensive, accurate, school-based SRH education is crucial. Further research should be conducted and used by policy makers in the development of nation-wide policies regarding SRH education for VYAs.

Acknowledgements
We would like to thank the study participants and all the research assistants and data management team for their contribution to the study.

Funding
Funding was obtained from VLIR-OUS for implementation of a team project between universities in Uganda and Belgium Mbarara (reference ZEIN2015PR411). The funders had no role in the study design, data collection, analysis or interpretation of data. The funders had no role in writing of the manuscript.

Authors' contributions
EK participated in design, data analysis and writing of the initial manuscript. KB participated in the data analysis, writing and editing of the initial manuscript. KM and VNN participated in data analysis and manuscript editing. GNR, WM, ABN, GC and EL participated in editing of the manuscript. All authors read and approved the final manuscript.

Competing interests
The authors declare that they have no competing interests.

Author details
[1]Mbarara University of Science and Technology, P.O. Box 1410, Mbarara, Uganda. [2]International Centre for Reproductive Health, Faculty of Medicine and Health Sciences, Ghent University, Ghent, Belgium. [3]RHEA, Centre of Expertise on Gender, Diversity and Intersectionality, Vrije Universiteit Brussel, Brussels, Belgium.

References
1. CIA. The World Fact Book 2017 [21 Mar 2018]. Available from: https://www.cia.gov/library/publications/the-world-factbook/fields/2177.html. Accessed 21 Mar 2018.

2. Uganda Bureau of Statistics [UBOS]. National Population and Housing Census 2014, Provisional Results. Kampala, Uganda: UBOS. 2014. Retrieved from http://library.health.go.ug/publications/leadership-andgovernance-monitoring-and-evaluation/population/national-population-an-0. Accessed 10 June 2018.

3. Uganda Bureau of Statistics [UBOS], & ICF International. (2017). Uganda Demographic Health Survey 2016: Key Indicators Report. Kampala, Uganda: UBOS, and Rockville, Maryland,USA: UBOS and ICF International. Retrieved from https://www.ubos.org/onlinefiles/uploads/ubos/pdf%20documents/Uganda_DHS_2016_KIR.pdf. Accessed 20 Feb 2018.
4. CIA. The World Fact Book, Country Comparison HIV/AIDS Adult prevalence rate 2016 [27th February 2018]. Available from: https://www.cia.gov/library/publications/resources/the-world-factbook/rankorder/2155rank.html. Accessed 27 Feb 2018.
5. UPHIA(2016–2017). Uganda Population Based HIV Impact Assessment 2017 [21 June 2018]. Available from: http://www.afro.who.int/sites/default/files/2017-08/UPHIA%20Uganda%20factsheet.pdf. Accessed 21 June 2018.
6. Green EC, Halperin DT, Nantulya V, Hogle JA. Uganda's HIV prevention success: the role of sexual behavior change and the national response. AIDS Behav. 2006;10(4):335–46.
7. Institute for health metrics and evaluation; [27th February 2018]. Available from: http://www.healthdata.org/uganda. Accessed 27 Feb 2018.
8. Boosey R, Prestwich G, Deave T. Menstrual hygiene management amongst schoolgirls in the Rukungiri district of Uganda and the impact on their education: a cross-sectional study. Pan Afr Med J. 2014;19:253.
9. Bello BM, Fatusi AO, Adepoju OE, Maina BW, Kabiru CW, Sommer M, et al. Adolescent and parental reactions to puberty in Nigeria and Kenya: a cross-cultural and intergenerational comparison. J Adolesc Health. 2017;61(4):S35–41.
10. Mehra D, Agardh A, Odberg Petterson K, Östergren P-O. Non-use of contraception: determinants among Ugandan university students. Glob Health Action. 2012;5(1):18599.
11. Mehra D, Östergren P-O, Ekman B, Agardh A. Inconsistent condom use among Ugandan university students from a gender perspective: a cross-sectional study. Glob Health Action. 2014;7(1):22942.
12. Annah N. The sex education debate has been blown out of proportion – UNFPA 2016 [20 June 2018]. Available from: http://capitalradio.co.ug/sex-education-debate-blown-proportion-unfpa/. Accessed 20 June 2016.
13. Time to lift the ban on se education in schools [press release]. Kampala, Uganda 2017. http://www.monitor.co.ug/News/Education/Time-to-lift-ban-on-sex-education-in-schools/688336-4007894-mm27t8z/index.html. Accessed 20 June 2018.
14. Ministry-of-Education-and-Sports-Uganda. National Sexuality Education Framework https://www.education.go.ug/files/downloads/UNFPA_68_090518.pdf: 2018. Accessed 20 June 2016.
15. Fonner VA, Armstrong KS, Kennedy CE, O'Reilly KR, Sweat MD. School based sex education and HIV prevention in low-and middle-income countries: a systematic review and meta-analysis. PLoS One. 2014;9(3):e89692.
16. UNESCO, UNAIDS, UNFPA, UN Women and WHO, (2018). International Technical Guidance on Sexuality Education, an evidence-informed approach, revised edition. Retrieved from http://unesdoc.unesco.org/images/0026/002607/260770e.pdf. Accessed 20 June 2018.
17. WHO/RHR/11.11. The sexual and reproductive health of young adolescents in developing countries. Geneva: research DoRHa; 2010. http://apps.who.int/iris/bitstream/10665/70569/1/WHO_RHR_11.11_eng.pdf
18. Igras SM, Macieira M, Murphy E, Lundgren R. Investing in very young adolescents' sexual and reproductive health. Global Public Health. 2014;9(5):555–69.
19. Blum RW, Astone NM, Decker MR, Mouli VC. A conceptual framework for early adolescence: a platform for research. Int J Adolesc Med Health. 2014;26(3):321–31.
20. Fearon E, Wiggins RD, Pettifor AE, Hargreaves JR. Is the sexual behaviour of young people in sub-Saharan Africa influenced by their peers? A systematic review. Soc Sci Med. 2015;146:62–74.
21. Albert B, Brown S, Flanigan CM. 14 years and younger: The sexual behavior of young adolescents. Washington: National Campaign to Prevent Teen Pregnancy; 2003.
22. Ministry of Education and Sports, (2018). National Sexuality Education Framework 2018. Kampala, Uganda: Ministry of Education and Sports. Retrieved from https://www.education.go.ug/files/downloads/NATIONAL%20SEXUALITY%20EDUCATION%20FRAMEWORK.pdf. Accessed 21 June 2018.
23. Bankole A, Biddlecom A, Guiella G, Singh S, Zulu E. Sexual behavior, knowledge and information sources of very young adolescents in four sub-Saharan African countries. Afr J Reprod Health. 2007;11(3):28.
24. Kemigisha E, Nyakato VN, Bruce K, Ndaruhutse Ruzaaza G, Mlahagwa W, Ninsiima AB, et al. Adolescents' sexual wellbeing in southwestern Uganda: a cross-sectional assessment of body image, self-esteem and gender equitable norms. Int J Environ Res Public Health. 2018;15(2):372.
25. Ninsiima AB, Leye E, Michielsen K, Kemigisha E, Nyakato VN, Coene G. "Girls have more challenges; they need to be locked up": a qualitative study of gender norms and the sexuality of young adolescents in Uganda. Int J Environ Res Public Health. 2018;15(2):193.
26. Mbarara District Education Office. Report on Schools and enrollment in Mbarara District, (2015). Unpublished data.
27. Darabi L, Bankole A, Serumaga S, Neema S, Kibombo R, Banoba P et al. Protecting the next generation in Uganda: new evidence on adolescent sexual and reproductive health needs (2008). Retrieved from https://www.guttmacher.org/sites/default/files/report_pdf/png_uganda_mono.pdf. Accessed 20 June 2018.
28. Bar-on ME, Broughton DD, Buttross S, Corrigan S, Gedissman A, de Rivas MG, et al. Sexuality, contraception, and the media. Pediatrics. 2001;107(1):191–4.
29. Hust SJ, Brown JD, L'Engle KL. Boys will be boys and girls better be prepared: an analysis of the rare sexual health messages in young adolescents' media. Mass Commun Soc. 2008;11(1):3–23.
30. Bull SS, Levine DK, Black SR, Schmiege SJ, Santelli J. Social media–delivered sexual health intervention: a cluster randomized controlled trial. Am J Prev Med. 2012;43(5):467–74.
31. Straight Talk Foundation, (2017). Straight Talk Annual report 2017. Retrieved from http://straighttalkfoundation.org/index.php/resources/annual-reports/55-annual-report-2017/file. Accessed 21 June 2018.
32. Mulugeta Y, Berhane Y. Factors associated with pre-marital sexual debut among unmarried high school female students in bahir Dar town, Ethiopia: cross-sectional study. Reprod Health. 2014;11(1):40.
33. Miller AN, Nalugya E, Gabolya C, Lagot S, Mulwanya R, Kiva J, et al. Ugandan adolescents' sources, interpretation and evaluation of sexual content in entertainment media programming. Sex Educ. 2016;16(6):707–20.
34. Miller AN, Gabolya C, Mulwanya R, Nabaseke G, Kiva J, Nalugya E, et al. The relationship between parental mediation of adolescent media use and Ugandan Adolescents' sexual attitudes and behavior. Howard J Commun. 2017:1–14.
35. Dennis ML, Radovich E, Wong KL, Owolabi O, Cavallaro FL, Mbizvo MT, et al. Pathways to increased coverage: an analysis of time trends in contraceptive need and use among adolescents and young women in Kenya, Rwanda, Tanzania, and Uganda. Reprod Health. 2017;14(1):130.
36. Wolf HT, Teich HG, Halpern-Felsher BL, Murphy RJ, Anandaraja N, Stone J, et al. The effectiveness of an adolescent reproductive health education intervention in Uganda. Int J Adolesc Med Health. 2017;29(2)
37. Wellings K, Collumbien M, Slaymaker E, Singh S, Hodges Z, Patel D, et al. Sexual behaviour in context: a global perspective. Lancet. 2006;368(9548):1706–28.
38. Mbalinda SN, Kiwanuka N, Eriksson LE, Wanyenze RK, Kaye DK. Correlates of ever had sex among perinatally HIV-infected adolescents in Uganda. Reprod Health. 2015;12:96.
39. Mmari KN, Kaggwa E, Wagman J, Gray R, Wawer M, Nalugoda F. Risk and protective correlates of young women's first sexual experiences in Rakai, Uganda. Int Perspect Sex Reprod Health. 2013;39(3):153–62.
40. Sidze EM, Elungata'a P, Maina BW, Mutua MM. Does the quality of parent–child connectedness matter for adolescents' sexual behaviors in Nairobi informal settlements? Arch Sex Behav. 2015;44(3):631–8.
41. Kabiru CW, Mumah JN, Maina BW, Abuya BA. Violence victimisation and aspirations–expectations disjunction among adolescent girls in urban Kenya. Int J Adolesc Youth. 2017:1–10.
42. Fathalla MF. Global trends in women's health. International Journal of Gynecology & Obstetrics. 1997;58(1):5–11.
43. Kirby DB. The impact of abstinence and comprehensive sex and STD/HIV education programs on adolescent sexual behavior. Sex Res Soc Policy. 2008;5(3):18–27.
44. Uganda Bureau of Statistics [UBOS], & ICF International. (2012). Uganda Demographic and Health Survey 2011. Kampala, Uganda: UBOS and ICF International. Retrieved fromhttps://www.ubos.org/onlinefiles/uploads/ubos/UDHS/UDHS2011.pdf. Accessed 20 Feb 2018.

10

mHealth intervention to improve the continuum of maternal and perinatal care in rural Guatemala

Boris Martinez[1,8], Enma Coyote Ixen[1], Rachel Hall-Clifford[2], Michel Juarez[1], Ann C. Miller[3], Aaron Francis[4], Camilo E. Valderrama[4], Lisa Stroux[5], Gari D. Clifford[4,6] and Peter Rohloff[1,7*]

Abstract

Background/objective: Guatemala's indigenous Maya population has one of the highest perinatal and maternal mortality rates in Latin America. In this population most births are delivered at home by traditional birth attendants (TBAs), who have limited support and linkages to public hospitals. The goal of this study was to characterize the detection of maternal and perinatal complications and rates of facility-level referral by TBAs, and to evaluate the impact of a mHealth decision support system on these rates.

Methods: A pragmatic one-year feasibility trial of an mHealth decisions support system was conducted in rural Maya communities in collaboration with TBAs. TBAs were individually randomized in an unblinded fashion to either early-access or later-access to the mHealth system. TBAs in the early-access arm used the mHealth system throughout the study. TBAs in the later-access arm provided usual care until crossing over uni-directionally to the mHealth system at the study midpoint. The primary study outcome was the monthly rate of referral to facility-level care, adjusted for birth volume.

Results: Forty-four TBAs were randomized, 23 to the early-access arm and 21 to the later-access arm. Outcomes were analyzed for 799 pregnancies (early-access 425, later-access 374). Monthly referral rates to facility-level care were significantly higher among the early-access arm (median 33 referrals per 100 births, IQR 22–58) compared to the later-access arm (median 20 per 100, IQR 0–30) ($p = 0.03$). At the study midpoint, the later-access arm began using the mHealth platform and its referral rates increased (median 34 referrals per 100 births, IQR 5–50) with no significant difference from the early-access arm ($p = 0.58$). Rates of complications were similar in both arms, except for hypertensive disorders of pregnancy, which were significantly higher among TBAs in the early-access arm (RR 3.3, 95% CI 1.10–9.86).

Conclusions: Referral rates were higher when TBAs had access to the mHealth platform. The introduction of mHealth supportive technologies for TBAs is feasible and can improve detection of complications and timely referral to facility-care within challenging healthcare delivery contexts.

Keywords: Barriers to care, Lay midwives, mHealth, Perinatal monitoring, Referral system, Guatemala, Indigenous, Resource-constrained healthcare, Traditional birth attendants

* Correspondence: peter@wuqukawoq.org
[1]Wuqu' Kawoq | Maya Health Alliance, 2a. Calle 5-43 Zona 1, Santiago Sacatepéquez, Guatemala
[7]Division of Global Health Equity, Brigham and Women's Hospital, Boston, MA, USA
Full list of author information is available at the end of the article

Plain English Summary

The indigenous Maya population in Guatemala has one of the highest rates of dying from complications during pregnancy and childbirth in Latin America. Due to many contributing factors, most Maya women opt for home deliveries attended by traditional birth attendants (TBAs). TBAs are required to arrange referrals when complications arise, however they usually lack support from and linkages to public hospitals. We have designed a smartphone application that provides support and guidance to TBAs while they evaluate patients. In this study, we evaluated the impact of this smartphone application on utilization of higher-level medical care for rural patients in Guatemala.

Collaborating TBAs were randomly assigned to either have early-access or later-access to the smartphone application. TBAs in the early-access group used the application for the whole study period. TBAs in the later-access group initially provided standard care to patients and then, half-way through the study, they began using the smartphone application. An emergency on-call team was available for TBAs in both groups to provide support during the referral process.

We found that referral rates for pregnancy and childbirth complications were higher when TBAs had access to the smartphone application. Our findings show that the introduction of such technology in the practice of TBAs is feasible and can lead to improvements in the detection of pregnancy and childbirth complications and timely referral of patients to hospital care.

Background

Improving maternal and neonatal health in resource-limited settings is a key priority in global health [1]. Around 300,000 women die each year from pregnancy or labor-related complications, most of these in Low- and Middle-Income Countries (LMICs) [2]. Perinatal deaths (stillbirths and early neonatal death) are similarly concentrated in LMICs, at an overall rate of 5.4 million per year [3]. Guatemala, the most populous country in Central America, has one of the highest perinatal and maternal mortality rates in Latin America [4, 5]. These poor outcomes particularly impact Guatemala's rural indigenous Maya population, where both perinatal and maternal mortality rates are markedly higher than for Guatemala's non-indigenous population [6, 7].

Contributing factors to these disparities include lack of rural infrastructure for early detection and referral of maternal and neonatal complications and systemic discrimination against Maya women in healthcare facilities, leading to a strong cultural preference for home births [8–10]. Indeed, at least 50% of births in rural Maya communities in Guatemala occur in the home under the care of Traditional Birth Attendants (TBAs) [7, 11].

Therefore, addressing the continuum of maternal and perinatal care in Guatemala requires not only increasing access to facility-level births, but also improving the early detection of complications in community-based care and the formal linkages of TBAs to higher levels of care [9–12]. A few studies have demonstrated the promise of mHealth systems for improving maternal and neonatal outcomes in LMICs [13]. However, with a few exceptions, most of these have focused on community health workers with a higher level of literacy and formal healthcare system engagement than is typical for TBAs [14, 15].

We have recently designed a low-cost, real-time decision support smartphone application for use by non-literate Maya TBAs, which is augmented by input from commercially-available sensors, including 1-D Doppler ultrasound, pulse oximetry, and oscillometric blood pressure [16, 17]. In this study, we report results from a pragmatic feasibility trial of this system by 44 TBAs in rural Guatemala. The goals of the trial were to characterize, for the first time, baseline rates of complication detection and facility-level referral by TBAs in rural Guatemala, and to evaluate the impact of the mHealth system on these rates. We hypothesized that the system would improve maternal and perinatal complication detection and referral rates to facility-level care.

Methods

Study design

This was a pragmatic, randomized controlled trial assessing the effectiveness of a mHealth decision support system to improve maternal and perinatal complication detection and referral rates to facility-level care by TBAs. Forty-four indigenous Maya TBAs from one rural municipality (Tecpán, Chimaltenango, pop. 95,000) in rural Guatemala participated. TBAs were randomized to have either early- or later-access to the mHealth platform. TBAs in the early-access arm used the mHealth platform through the whole study duration. Initially, TBAs in the later access-arm provided usual care and subsequently transitioned to use of the mHealth platform in a unidirectional cross-over. The study was conducted in collaboration with Maya Health Alliance (MHA), a Guatemalan primary health care organization with a clinical center in Tecpán. The study was approved by the Institutional Review Boards of MHA (Protocol number WK-2015-001) and Emory University (Protocol number IRB00076231). The study protocol and replication data set are available online at: https://doi.org/10.7910/DVN/VCJKH7. The trial was registered at ClinicalTrials.gov, NCT02348840.

Participants

All TBAs aged 18–65 years who were independently practicing in the Tecpán municipality, who had attended at least 5 deliveries per year in the previous 5 years, and who held a valid license to practice issued by local health authorities were eligible to participate in the study. A list of 150 TBAs from the study area was produced in collaboration with local health officials. Eighty-six TBAs did not met eligibility criteria. All TBAs meeting eligibility criteria ($n = 64$) were invited to attend an informational session led by research staff, 49 TBAs attended this meeting. Subsequently, 44 of them (29% of total TBAs, 69% of eligible TBAs) agreed to participate, and written informed consent was obtained by study staff bilingual in Spanish and Kaqchikel Maya, the language spoken by most of the TBAs.

During the study, all TBAs continued to provide usual home-based care to their patients. TBAs alerted study staff to new pregnant patients in their practice. A study staff member bilingual in Kaqchikel and Spanish subsequently visited patients (and the biological father, when available) in the home to explain the study and obtained written informed consent for collection of individual-level health information and pregnancy perinatal outcomes data. All pregnant patients over 18 years of age and under the care of a TBA were eligible to participate.

Randomization and masking

Stratified randomization of TBAs to two study arms (early-access or later-access to the mHealth technology) was performed using a computer-based randomization process. A Montecarlo statistical analysis using a rank sum test was used to ensure median ages, community origin, and distance to municipality were not significantly different between study arms. The allocation and assignment procedures were performed by a study author (GC) prior to meeting participants and not otherwise involved in the recruitment of participants or daily conduct of field work. Due to the pragmatic nature of a trial involving access to mHealth technology, neither TBAs, pregnant subjects, nor study personnel could be blinded to allocation. However, many TBAs resided/practiced in a single isolated rural settlement within the municipal catchment area, with minimal overlap with other TBAs. In addition, when more than one TBA resided/practiced within the same settlement, they were allocated to the same study arm. This resulted in 23 TBAs from 13 villages being assigned to the early-access arm, and 21 TBAs from 15 mutually exclusive villages being assigned to the later-access arm.

Intervention

A perinatal monitoring mHealth platform was introduced in the daily practice of participating TBAs in a unidirectional cross-over study design. We hypothesized that such a system would improve timely and accurate TBA-initiated referrals to higher levels of care, measured as referral rates per number of births and as the proportion of successful referrals respectively, by improving the diagnostic capabilities of participating TBAs and connecting them with an existing referral network. Use of the mHealth platform by TBAs was supported by an existing referral support structure at MHA outlined in Fig. 1, consisting of an on-call clinical team who provided triage support and coordinated transportation to hospital if referral was needed. This wrap-around support structure at MHA existed prior to the mHealth intervention, helping with emergency care for MHA patients and patients referred from collaborating health districts. However, prior to this study, attempts had not been made to integrate TBAs into this network.

The mHealth platform used in this study was developed for the Android operating system (4.2.2; Google Inc.) and installed on Samsung S3 mini smartphone devices (costing about $100). This smartphone platform also provided integrated use of peripheral sensor devices, including a pulse oximeter (Onyx II, Model 9560, Nonin Medical, Inc.), a hand-held 1-dimensional Doppler ultrasound device (AngelSounds Fetal Doppler JPD-100 s, Jumper Medical Co., Ltd.), and—via a customized camera application—a self-inflating oscillometric blood pressure cuff (Omron M7, OMRON Healthcare). We have previously described in more detail the technical aspects of the design and end-user testing by TBAs for this platform [16, 17].

In terms of decision support, the smartphone application allowed collection of simple demographics, maternal and perinatal symptoms and clinical signs, maternal vital signs (pulse, oxygen saturation, systolic and diastolic blood pressure), and the fetal heart rate. While using the application, TBAs are guided through a pictographic list of common maternal and perinatal complications grouped by visit type, as outlined in Table 1 and depicted in Fig. 2a. Checking complications triggered automatic communications with the on-call clinical team by voice call or text message, as outlined in Table 1. Vital sign abnormalities also triggered alert text messages to the on-call team (maternal: heart rate ≤ 60 or ≥ 100 bpm, oxygen saturation $\leq 90\%$, systolic blood pressure ≤ 70 or ≥ 140 mmHg, diastolic blood pressure ≥ 90 mmHg; fetal heart rate ≤ 120 or ≥ 160 bpm).

TBAs randomized to the early-access arm ($n = 23$) participated in a four-day training led by study nurses, where they first refreshed key medical concepts related to perinatal complications, including risk factors for maternal and neonatal morbidity and mortality, indications for referral to higher levels of medical care, importance of timely assessment, and use of the smartphone decision support platform (Fig. 2a, Table 1). This and subsequent training described below were similar in design to other courses previously conducted by MHA, relying on adult-learning and low-literacy strategies such as interactive narrative stories and pictorial informational and

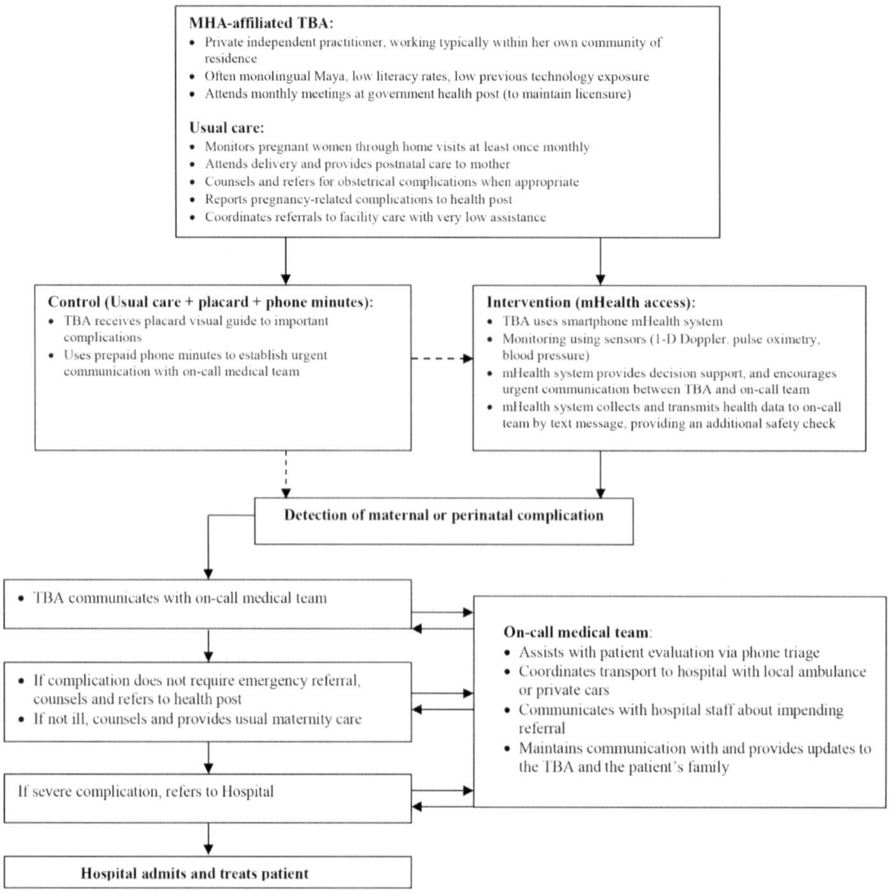

Fig. 1 A schematic view of the traditional birth attendant obstetric referral strategy. Figure outlines the emergency referral workflow between TBAs and supporting medical team and details the integration of the mHealth system into this workflow

Table 1 Guided list of complications included in the mHealth platform by visit type

Prenatal	Perinatal	Postnatal
Seizures[a]	Seizures[a]	Maternal:
Hemorrhage[a]	Rupture of membranes without labor[a]	Seizures[a]
Premature rupture of membranes[a]	Prolonged labor[a]	Hemorrhage[a]
Difficulty breathing[a]	Multiple pregnancy[a]	Difficulty breathing[a]
Abdominal pain	Fetal malpresentation or malposition[a]	Abdominal pain
Blurred vision	Placenta previa[a]	Fever
Fever	Nuchal cord[a]	Blurred vision
Edema	Hemorrhage[a]	Headache
Severe headache	Placental retention[a]	Neonatal:
	Previous C-section[a]	Difficulty breathing[a]
	Difficulty breathing[a]	Fever[a]
	Severe abdominal pain[a]	Hypothermia[a]
	Blurred vision[a]	Low-birth weight[a]
	Fever[a]	Very small baby[a]
	Edema[a]	Jaundice
	Severe headache[a]	Breastfeeding difficulties
		Umbilical infection

Complications marked with an superscripted ([a]) triggered an automatic emergency call to the on-call clinical team (interrupting the work-flow of the visit). Remaining complications triggered an alert screen upon conclusion of the visit requesting a call to the team. All complications data were also automatically conveyed to the on-call team by a text message at the end of the visit encounter. Adapted from Stroux L et al [16]

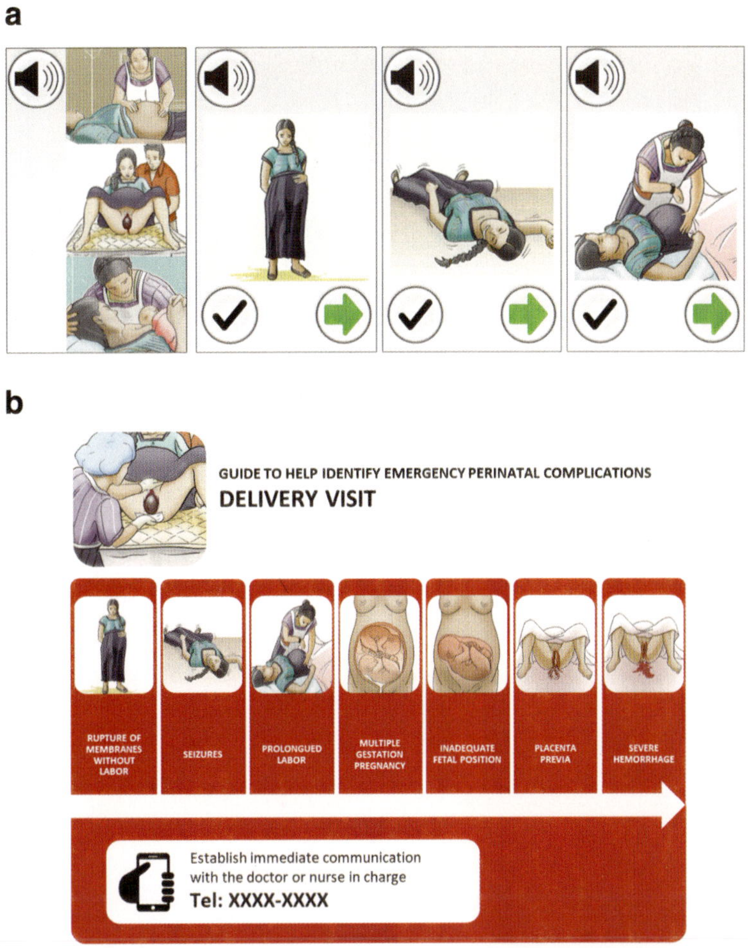

Fig. 2 Example of decision support workflows for facilitating obstetric emergency referral. **a** Shows an example of workflow on the mHealth platform. In the left-most illustration, the TBA selects the appropriate visit type (prenatal, perinatal, postnatal). The TBA is then guided through a series of pictorial warning signs, with audio prompts as necessary. Checking a warning sign generates an emergency call and text-message to on-call team. **b** Shows the same pictorial partial workflow through warning signs for a typical perinatal visit for TBAs using the visit placard in the later-access arm (during the non-intervention period), where an emergency telephone number is provided. All images were adapted from existing public sector resources in Guatemala [33]

instructional material. After completion of this study training, three standardized patient encounters were used to evaluate each participant's use of the mHealth platform when facing common maternal and perinatal complications. Each standardized encounter was observed by a study staff member, using an observation checklist with 60 discrete tasks (minimum passing score of 90%), who assessed the TBA's ability to detect the complication, use the mHealth platform, and establish communication with the emergency on-call team. Six of 23 TBAs (26%) failed the first evaluation, received a two-day retraining session, and subsequently passed.

TBAs randomized to the later-access arm ($n = 21$) received a separate, two-day training containing the same medical content as the early-access arm, less the mHealth content. Instead of training on the mHealth system, they received a laminated placard containing the same images of the maternal and perinatal complications used in the smartphone system, as well as emergency contact numbers and instructions for initiating referrals (Fig. 2b). Similar standardized patient encounters and an evaluation checklist were also used to evaluate each participant's use of the placard-based complication guide. All TBAs passed the evaluation and subsequently received a copy of the placard. After month 7 of the study, TBAs in the later-access arm received training on the smartphone platform, as described above, and began to use the mHealth platform (Fig. 3). Two of 21 TBAs (10%) failed the first evaluation, but were subsequently retrained and passed.

Outcomes

The primary outcome was the number of monthly referrals to facility-level care from TBAs for maternal and

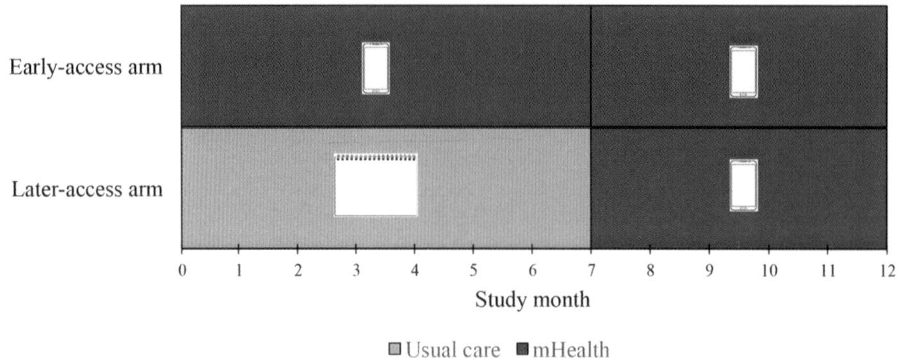

Fig. 3 Intervention design. TBAs in the early-access arm used the mHealth platform (intervention) through the whole study duration, depicted as a cell phone device in this and related figures. TBAs in the later-access arm provided usual care during the first 7 months of the study (non-intervention period), assisted with a placard-based complication guide (depicted as a notebook sheet in this and related figures), and subsequently crossed into use of the mHealth platform (intervention period)

perinatal complications, adjusted by the monthly birth volume. A secondary outcome was the proportion of referrals which were completed, defined as successfully receiving facility-based care after a TBA-initiated referral. A computer-based list of births attended was updated every two weeks by the study team with direct input from each TBA. Referrals outcomes were adjudicated by the study team with input from the TBA, and were considered successful if the subject received facility-level medical care. Outcomes data collection was overseen by study staff (physician and nurse), and monthly monitored for missing data, correct data entry errors, and to ensure consistency in collection and reporting over time.

The mHealth intervention involved the use of standard smartphones and CE-approved peripheral sensors (1-D Doppler ultrasound, pulse oximeter, and oscillometric blood pressure cuff). Therefore, no adverse study-related outcomes were anticipated. Nevertheless, study staff maintained a spreadsheet of all clinical outcomes from referrals, as well as morbidity and mortality data reported by TBAs, updated daily. A study physician not otherwise involved in the intervention reviewed these data, determining whether an adverse clinical outcome was possibly study-related. None of the reported adverse events were adjudicated as study related.

Statistical analysis

This was an exploratory, pragmatic pilot trial designed to explore baseline maternal and perinatal referral rates by practicing TBAs in rural Guatemala to facility-level care, and to explore the feasibility of and impact from use of a smartphone decision support application by these TBAs. As such, no formal sample size calculations were conducted [18]. Rather, the study was conducted within a single municipal catchment area, defined as a high-priority target by the implementing partner given locally high rates of maternal and perinatal complications, and could be used to inform future sample size calculations. Within this target area, initial estimates from the partner were that 50 practicing TBAs would meet eligibility criteria and, with an average of 10 births per year per TBA, we anticipated evaluating referral outcomes for 500 pregnancies over the course of the 12 month study.

We generated descriptive statistics describing sociodemographic and practice for TBAs in both study arms. We also generated descriptive statistics for key baseline sociodemographic indicators and prior maternal and perinatal outcomes for patients cared for by the TBAs in both study arms. Only patients for whom written informed consent was obtained were included in this descriptive baseline analysis. Categorical data were reported as absolute numbers and percentages, and compared using the chi-square or Fisher's exact test, as appropriate. Non-normally distributed continuous variables were reported as medians with interquartile ranges (IQR), and compared using the Wilcoxon-Mann-Whitney test.

For the primary outcome, in unadjusted intention-to-treat analysis, we compared the volume of monthly referrals for maternal and perinatal complications adjusted for monthly birth volume, using the Wilcoxon-Mann-Whitney test. Subsequently, to assess the effect of accessing the mHealth technology adjusting for seasonal variation and repeated-measures clustering by TBA, we also conducted an exploratory analysis using a generalized estimating equations (GEE) model (Poisson family distribution, log link function). For secondary outcomes, risk ratios (RR) with 95% confidence intervals (CI) were calculated. For all outcomes, a nominal p value of less than 0.05, without adjustment for multiple comparisons, was considered to indicate statistical significance. For patient-level outcomes, p-values were adjusted for clustering by TBA. All statistical analyses were conducted using Stata 13 (StataCorp, College Station, Texas).

Results

Participants

Forty-four TBAs consented participation in the study and underwent randomization (early-access arm: 23; later-access arm: 21; Fig. 4). Baseline demographic characteristics of participating TBAs in the two study arms were well balanced (Table 2). Eligible participant patients were recruited from April 2016 to March 2017. Throughout the study, TBAs reported 799 completed pregnancies (early-access arm: 241 completed pregnancies reported during the first study period, 184 completed pregnancies during the second study period; later-access arm: 222 and 152 respectively) (Fig. 4). Baseline demographic and clinical data were available for 335 patients in the early-access arm and 327 in the later-access arm. There were no statistically significant differences in baseline characteristics between patients in the two study arms (Table 3), except for proportion of women who experienced scarce economic resources as a barrier to obstetric care in the previous pregnancy ($p = 0.009$). Two TBAs in the early-access arm (9%) and one in the later-access arm (5%) discontinued their participation in the study but continued to report outcomes data, allowing for inclusion in the intention-to-treat analysis. Outcome and referral data was available for all completed pregnancies (Fig. 4).

Outcomes

For primary outcomes, the rate of monthly emergency referrals over birth volume during the first study period (Fig. 3) was significantly higher ($p = 0.03$) for the early-access arm (median 33 referrals per 100 births, IQR 22 to 58; Table 4)

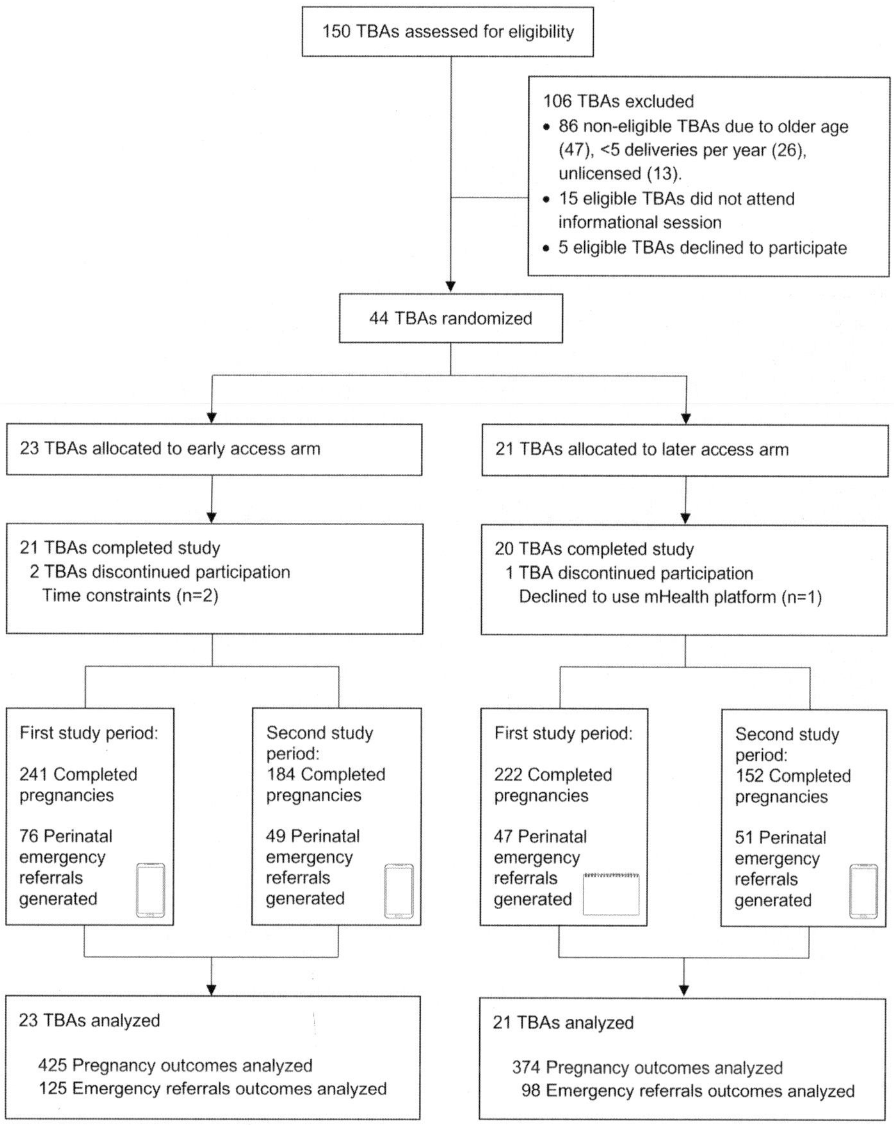

Fig. 4 Study flow diagram. Enrollment, randomization, and follow-up

Table 2 Baseline characteristics of study participants (traditional birth attendants)

Characteristic[a]	Early-Access Arm ($N = 23$)	Later-Access Arm ($N = 21$)
Age (years)	47 [40–55]	51 [43–55]
Education (years)	0 [0–2]	1 [0–4]
Spanish Literacy[b]	5 (22)	4 (19)
Monolingual Maya	13 (57)	9 (43)
Years in practice (years)	12 [10–20]	16 [10–24]
Distance from town (Km)	15 [5–21]	11 [7–18]
Travel time from town (min)	45 [15–60]	40 [15–60]

[a]Data are median [IQR], or n (%)
[b]Defined as able to read and write a simple sentence in Spanish

in comparison to the later-access arm (median 20 referrals per 100 births, IQR 0 to 30; Table 4). During the second study period (Fig. 3) after the later-access arm transitioned to the mHealth platform, referral rates were not significantly different between the study arms ($p = 0.58$), with referral rate increasing as expected in the later-access arm after crossover into the mHealth intervention (Table 4). For secondary outcomes, the proportions of successful referrals were high (> 90%) for both study arms during both study periods (Table 4), without statistically significant differences. Non-successful referrals were due to refusal to referral (lack of permission to complete the referral from another family member ($n = 5$), patient's fear to hospital due to cultural or language barriers ($n = 4$), or the patient not recognizing the complication as an emergency (n = 4)) or due to logistical difficulties during emergency communication or transportation ($n = 3$). To adjust for seasonal variation and repeated-measures clustering by midwife, we conducted an exploratory analysis using a generalized estimating equations (GEE) model; results from the GEE analysis similarly showed an increase in referral rates in the early-access arm, although this did not reach statistical significance (coefficient 1.24, 95% CI -0.93 – 3.40).

Pregnancy outcomes and adverse events were monitored for both arms throughout the study. The study arms did not differ significantly with respect to mode of delivery (home, hospital, or caesarian delivery) (Table 5). There were no significant differences between study arms in the proportion of reported maternal and perinatal complications, with one exception: the rate of reported hypertensive disorders in pregnancy was higher among TBAs in the early-access arm than among TBAs in the later-access arm (3.53% vs 1.07%; $P = 0.03$). All complications reported in Table 5 are final diagnoses as determined at the time of emergency referral by the treating healthcare provider. Three maternal deaths due to preeclampsia or eclampsia were reported, with no difference in occurrence between the study arms (Table 5). Ten neonatal deaths were reported, with two thirds occurring in the first two days of life (6/10), and with no significant difference in occurrence between the study arms.

Discussion

This pragmatic, randomized-controlled feasibility trial showed that the introduction of a mHealth decision support technology into the routine community-based practice of a group of TBAs in rural Guatemala resulted in a significant increase in the rate of emergency referrals to facility-care for maternal and perinatal complications. We designed this study with the goal of conducting foundational implementation research on the utility of

Table 3 Baseline demographic and clinical characteristics of patients treated by participating traditional birth attendants

Characteristic[a]	Early-Access Arm ($N = 335$)[b]	Later-Access Arm ($N = 327$)[b]	p value
Age (years)	26 [22–31]	26 [22–31]	0.59
Nulliparous	71 (21)	61 (19)	0.43
Number of pregnancies	3 [2–5]	3 [2–5]	0.73
Previous caesarian section[c]	27/263 (10)	33/263 (13)	0.41
Previous facility birth[c]	88/261 (34)	91/261 (35)	0.78
Previous perinatal complication[c]	84/265 (32)	83/263 (32)	0.97
Referral to hospital in last pregnancy[c]	60/262 (23)	59/262 (23)	0.92
Obstetric care barriers in last pregnancy	20/60 (33)	17/59 (29)	0.59
Lack of transportation	14 (70)	12 (71)	0.97
Scarce economic resources	8 (40)	14 (82)	0.009
Distance to hospital	4 (20)	5 (29)	0.51
Hospital mistreatment	5 (25)	2 (12)	0.31

[a]Data are median [IQR], or n (%)
[b]Where individual data was missing or not applicable for the entire sample, the denominator used to calculate each characteristic is given
[c]Calculated after excluding nulliparous individuals

Table 4 Effect of intervention on emergency referral volume and successful referral completion by study arms

Outcome[1]	Early Access Arm ($N = 23$)	Later Access Arm ($N = 21$)	p value[2]
Adjusted monthly emergency referral rate (referrals/births) per 100 births			
First study period	33 [22–58]	20 [0–30]	0.03
Second study period	31 [10–42]	34 [5–50]	0.58
Referral success proportion (successful/referrals)			
First study period	69/76 (90.79)	44/47 (93.61)	0.74
Second study period	48/49 (97.95)	47/51 (92.16)	0.36

[1]Rates reported as median [IQR], and proportions as no./total no. (%)
[2]Wilcoxon-Mann-Whitney test for rates, Fisher's exact test for proportions

smart phone technology to improve health decision-making and linkages to higher-level obstetrical care by TBAs, the de facto front line health workers for rural, indigenous women in much of Guatemala. Using a pragmatic, randomized controlled design, we demonstrated that TBAs who received early access to a smartphone-based decision support technology, integrated into their routine community-based practice, had increased monthly referral rates compared to those who provided usual care, even when given manual access to referral processes via training and a laminate reminder card. Furthermore, when TBAs in the usual care arm subsequently received access to the technology, their referral rates also increased similarly to the early-access arm. Interestingly, referral success rates were very high for both arms throughout the study. This suggests that, at least within the MHA institution context which provides meaningful wrap-around support to coordinate emergency referral, the most important impact of the mHealth intervention is on increasing detection of complications.

Rates of most maternal and neonatal complications were similar in both study arms. Although one might expect that increased detection of early warning signs and referral to higher-level care might decrease complication rates, this was an exploratory feasibility study. Baseline complication rates were unknown for the study population, and the study was not powered to detect a difference in the rate of any complication. However, we did find an increase in the proportion of hypertensive disorders detected in the early-access arm. This finding is

Table 5 Mode of delivery, reported complications, and adverse outcomes for completed pregnancies during the study

Outcome[1]	Early-Access Arm ($N = 425$)[2]	Later- Access Arm ($N = 374$)[2]	Risk Ratio (95% CI)	p value[3]
Mode of delivery				
Home delivery	345 (81.18)	318 (85.03)	0.95 (0.90–1.02)	0.35
Hospital delivery	42 (9.88)	29 (7.75)	1.27 (0.81–2.00)	0.43
Caesarian section	38 (8.94)	27 (7.22)	1.24 (0.77–1.99)	0.50
Emergency Referrals				
Maternal Complications				
• Labor progression abnormality	51 (12.00)	36 (9.63)	1.25 (0.83–1.87)	0.51
• Hypertensive disorders of pregnancy	15 (3.53)	4 (1.07)	3.3 (1.10–9.86)	0.03
• Hemorrhage	9 (2.12)	10 (2.67)	0.79 (0.33–1.93)	0.52
• Premature labor	5 (1.18)	6 (1.60)	0.73 (0.23–2.38)	0.64
• Fetal cardiac rate abnormality	4 (0.94)	4 (1.07)	0.88 (0.22–3.49)	0.84
Neonatal Complications				
• Suspected sepsis	4 (0.94)	5 (1.34)	0.70 (0.19–2.60)	0.62
• Respiratory compromise	5 (1.18)	2 (0.53)	2.2 (0.43–11.27)	0.46
• Preterm newborn	4 (0.94)	0	–	0.06
Death				
Maternal deaths	2 (0.47)	1 (0.27)	1.76 (0.16–19.33)	0.65
Neonatal deaths	7 (1.65)	3 (0.80)	2.05 (0.53–7.88)	0.23

[1]Outcomes reported as no. (%)
[2]N = reported births. All births were singleton
[3]p values are adjusted for clustering by TBA using logistic regression

remarkable, because use of the mHealth technology here included an automated oscillometric blood pressure monitoring (Fig. 1). This suggests that the mHealth technology improved detection of hypertensive disorders of pregnancy, which are a leading cause of maternal and perinatal deaths [19–21]. In fact, in an analysis of data from the international Global Network for Women's and Children's Health Research Maternal and Neonatal Health Registry—which includes data from the same region of Guatemala where this study occurred—hypertensive disorders were the strongest predictor of maternal death [22]. In-home blood pressure monitoring is not routinely available or utilized by TBAs in rural Guatemala, and integrating this technique into their skillset as our intervention does here has the potential to directly impact the high rates of maternal and perinatal mortality [23, 24].

Our study has several strengths. To our knowledge, it is the first attempt to quantify baseline TBA-initiated referral rates for maternal and neonatal complications in the region. These data will be important both for policy and public health initiatives as well as for planning large-scale clinical trials. Secondly, pragmatic incorporation of the mHealth intervention into an existing primary care collaboration linking TBAs to the formal healthcare system allowed for more direct evaluation of the hypothesis that mHealth decision support could increase referral rates. The overall high proportion of successful referrals before and after access to the mHealth technology suggests that the quality of the wrap-around support environment for TBAs was similar for both study arms while using or not the mHealth platform and that, therefore, the increase in rate of referral was due to use of the platform. Finally, TBAs attrition was low and the use of the mHealth platform was high, despite the low literacy and lack of previous exposure to technology. This suggests that the research team's use of agile design with early end-user feedback [16, 17] helped produce a functional system which integrated easily into the usual daily practice of participating TBAs. Potential limitations of our study should be considered. This was a pragmatic feasibility trial designed to explore the use of mHealth to improve referral volume. Given this context and the fact that the intervention involved introduction of sophisticated technology, it was not possible to blind study staff and TBAs to study arm allocation. Additionally, the study was not powered to detect differences in clinical outcomes. Finally, due to the unidirectional cross-over study design, there was no complete control arm without any access to the intervention. Furthermore, TBAs in the study self-reported pregnancy and referrals outcomes, which may have led to underreporting of patients and pregnancies with certain characteristics or unfavorable outcomes. Effects of possible confounders, particularly temporality, on secondary patient-level endpoints were not addressed, given the small overall sample size and small number of observed complications. Our study took place in rural Guatemala in collaboration with indigenous Maya TBAs and patients and, therefore, our technology intervention and findings may not be generalizable to different settings or populations. Finally, in exploratory analysis, referral rates (although encouraging) were not significantly different when adjusted for repeated-measures clustering. This may be a simple statistical power issue which will be addressed in a future study powered to detect these adjusted differences. However, it also illustrates the need, in future work, to better define and address variation in TBAs' practice parameters and ability to optimize use of the mHealth technology.

This study is, to our knowledge, the first report of supportive mHealth technology for low-literate TBAs with little previous exposure to technology in a challenging rural healthcare delivery context, as well as the first report of referral rates by TBAs in indigenous populations, and it adds to the evidence of community-based intervention packages for improving maternal and perinatal outcomes [25, 26] and of mHealth interventions integrated within existing healthcare systems as potential solutions for addressing maternal health in LMICs [13, 27–29]. For example, in a study conducted in rural Pakistan by Jokhio et al. [30], training TBAs to recognize maternal and perinatal complications, alongside efforts made to better integrate them into the formal health system, resulted in increased referral rates to facility-care for emergency obstetrical care. Similarly, a recent study in rural Guatemala connecting community health workers – with higher levels of clinical training and literacy than the TBAs in our study – to medical specialists via cell-phones [31], showed a promising trend toward reductions in maternal mortality.

In future research, we plan to validate incorporation of mHealth decision support into TBA workflows in a larger scale study adequately powered to detect differences in important maternal and perinatal clinical outcomes and to include a cost analysis of our intervention. By providing estimates of baseline referral and complication rates, as well as observations on variations in individual TBA practice, this pilot feasibility study will assist in planning that study. We are also in the process of collecting and analyzing qualitative feedback from TBAs, patients, and staff at health facilities on the systems' impact, in terms of improving the quality of healthcare for women and the integrations of TBAs into the healthcare system. Our overall goal remains improving linkages of TBAs in rural Guatemala to the formal healthcare system and respectful maternity care for indigenous mothers [32].

Conclusion

Our trial showed an increase in the rate of referrals to higher-level obstetrical care among TBAs utilizing a mHealth decision support platform. Our results show that the introduction of mHealth technologies for TBAs is feasible and may improve referral to facility-care within a challenging healthcare delivery context such as rural Guatemala. As an early-stage pragmatic trial, our findings are subject to many limitations. Therefore, further research needs to be conducted to explore the effects of mHealth systems on perinatal and maternal morbidity and mortality and to rigorously examine the impact of temporal trends and individual TBA practice variation on obstetrical referral. Nevertheless, despite these limitations, our promising results help make a strong case for continued investments in TBA training and technologies to improve linkages of TBAs to the formal healthcare system.

Abbreviations

LMIC: Low- and middle-income country; MHA: Maya Health Alliance; mHealth: Mobile Health; TBA: Traditional birth attendant

Acknowledgements

We thank the traditional birth attendants, their patients, families, and communities for participating in the study. We are grateful to the staff from local public health posts, ambulance and car drivers, and staff from Hospital Nacional de Chimaltenango for their collaboration in the referral process for the patients involved in the study.

Funding

This work was funded by the Eunice Kennedy Shriver National Institute of Child Health & Human Development and The Fogarty International Center at the National Institute of Health (1R21HD084114–01). The funder had no role in the design of the study and collection, analysis, and interpretation of data, or writing and reporting of the manuscript.

Authors' contributions

BM supervised the study, analyzed and interpreted data, and produced the first manuscript draft. EC and MJ collected and analyzed data. GDC and LS designed the hardware configuration. LS and AF programmed the app for data collection and user interaction. AF and CEV worked on data curation. ACM analyzed and interpreted study data. RHC, GDC, and PR designed and supervised the study. All authors critically revised the manuscript and made substantial contributions to the final draft. All authors read and approved the final manuscript.

Competing interests

BM, ECI, MJ, and PR are current staff members at Maya Health Alliance, the partnering healthcare organization for this study in Guatemala; the authors declare that they have no competing interests.

Author details

[1]Wuqu' Kawoq | Maya Health Alliance, 2a. Calle 5-43 Zona 1, Santiago Sacatepéquez, Guatemala. [2]Departments of Sociology and Anthropology and Public Health, Agnes Scott College, Decatur, GA, USA. [3]Department of Global Health and Social Medicine, Harvard Medical School, Boston, MA, USA. [4]Department of Biomedical Informatics, Emory University, Atlanta, GA, USA. [5]Institute of Biomedical Engineering, Department of Engineering Science, University of Oxford, Oxford, UK. [6]Department of Biomedical Engineering, Georgia Institute of Technology and Emory University, Atlanta, GA, USA. [7]Division of Global Health Equity, Brigham and Women's Hospital, Boston, MA, USA. [8]Department of Medicine, Saint Peter's University Hospital, New Brunswick, NJ, USA.

References

1. United Nations. Sustainable Development Goals. http://www.un.org/sustainabledevelopment/health/ (2015). Accessed 10 Oct 2017.
2. World Health Organization. Maternal mortality. In: Fact sheet #348. Geneva: World Health Organization; 2015. Accessed 10 Oct 2017. http://www.who.int/mediacentre/factsheets/fs348/en/.
3. World Health Organization. Maternal and perinatal health. Geneva: World Health Organization; 2016. Accessed 10 Oct 2017. http://www.who.int/maternal_child_adolescent/topics/maternal/maternal_perinatal/en/
4. The World Bank. Indicator: Maternal mortality ratio. http://data.worldbank.org/indicator/SH.STA.MMRT (2015). Accessed 10 Oct 2017.
5. The World Bank. Indicator: Mortality rate, under-5 (per 1,000 live births). http://data.worldbank.org/indicator/SH.DYN.MORT (2016). Accessed 11 Oct 2017.
6. Stollak I, Valdez M, Rivas K, Perry H. Casas Maternas in the rural highlands of Guatemala: a mixed-methods case study of the introduction and utilization of birthing facilities by an indigenous population. Glob Health Sci Pract. 2016;4:114–31.
7. Ministerio de Salud Pública y Asistencia Social. VI Encuesta Nacional de Salud Materno Infantil. Guatemala City: Ministerio de Salud Pública y Asistencia Social; 2015.
8. Walsh LV. Beliefs and rituals in traditional birth attendant practice in Guatemala. J Transcult Nurs. 2006;17:148–54.
9. Goldman N, Glei DA. Evaluation of midwifery care: results from a survey in rural Guatemala. Soc Sci Med. 2003;56:685–700.
10. Chary A, Díaz AK, Henderson B, Rohloff P. The changing role of indigenous lay midwives in Guatemala: new frameworks for analysis. Midwifery. 2013;29:852–8.
11. Garces A, Mcclure EM, Hambidge KM, Krebs NF, Figueroa L, Aguilar ML, et al. Trends in perinatal deaths from 2010 to 2013 in the Guatemalan western highlands. Reprod Health. 2015;12(Suppl 2):S14.
12. Homer CS, Friberg IK, Dias MA, ten Hoope-Bender P, Sandall J, Speciale AM, et al. The projected effect of scaling up midwifery. Lancet. 2014;384:1146–57.
13. Colaci D, Chaudhri S, Vasan A. mHealth interventions in low-income countries to address maternal health: a systematic review. Ann Glob Health. 2016;82:922–35.
14. Munro ML, Lori JR, Boyd CJ, Andreatta P. Knowledge and skill retention of a mobile phone data collection protocol in rural Liberia. J Midwifery Womens Health. 2014;59:176–83.
15. Lori JR, Munro ML, Boyd CJ, Andreatta P. Cell phones to collect pregnancy data from remote areas in Liberia. J Nurs Scholarsh. 2012;44:294–301.
16. Stroux L, Martinez B, Coyote Ixen E, King N, Hall-Clifford R, Rohloff P, et al. An mHealth monitoring system for traditional birth attendant-led antenatal risk assessment in rural Guatemala. J Med Eng Technol. 2016;40:356–71.
17. Martinez B, Hall-Clifford R, Coyote E, Stroux L, Valderrama CE, Aaron C, et al. Agile development of a smartphone app for perinatal monitoring in a resource-constrained setting. J Health Inform Dev Ctries. 2017;11:e1–19.
18. Leon AC, Davis LL, Kraemer HC. The role and interpretation of pilot studies in clinical research. J Psychiatr Res. 2011;45:626–9.
19. Say L, Chou D, Gemmill A, Tunçalp Ö, Moller AB, Daniels J, et al. Global causes of maternal death: a WHO systematic analysis. Lancet Glob Health. 2014;2:e323–33. https://doi.org/10.1016/S2214-109X(14)70227-X.

20. Kassebaum NJ, Bertozzi-Villa A, Coggeshall MS, Shackelford KA, Steiner C, Heuton KR, et al. Global, regional, and national levels and causes of maternal mortality during 1990–2013: a systematic analysis for the global burden of disease study 2013. Lancet. 2014;384:980–1004.
21. World Health Organization. WHO recommendations for prevention and treatment of pre-eclampsia and eclampsia. Geneva: World Health Organization; 2011.
22. Bauserman M, Lokangaka A, Thorsten V, Tshefu A, Goudar SS, Esamai F, et al. Risk factors for maternal death and trends in maternal mortality in low-and middle-income countries: a prospective longitudinal cohort analysis. Reprod Health. 2015;12(Suppl 2):S5.
23. Garces A, McClure EM, Chomba E, Patel A, Pasha O, Tshefu A, et al. Home birth attendants in low income countries: who are they and what do they do? BMC Pregnancy Childbirth. 2012;12:34.
24. Milne F, Redman C, Walker J, Baker P, Bradley J, Cooper C, et al. The pre-eclampsia community guideline (PRECOG): how to screen for and detect onset of pre-eclampsia in the community. BMJ. 2005;330:576–80.
25. Lassi ZS, Bhutta ZA. Community-based intervention packages for reducing maternal and neonatal morbidity and mortality and improving neonatal outcomes. Cochrane Database Syst Rev 2015; Issue 3. Art. No.: CD007754. https://doi.org/10.1002/14651858.CD007754.pub3.
26. ten Hoope-Bender P, de Bernis L, Campbell J, Downe S, Fauveau V, Fogstad H, et al. Improvement of maternal and newborn health through midwifery. Lancet. 2014;384:1226–35.
27. Tamrat T, Kachnowski S. Special delivery: an analysis of mHealth in maternal and newborn health programs and their outcomes around the world. Matern Child Health J. 2012;16:1092–101.
28. Mechael P, Batavia H, Kaonga N, Searle S, Kwan A, Goldberger A, et al. Barriers and gaps affecting mHealth in low and middle income countries: Policy white paper. 2010. http://www.globalproblems-globalsolutions-files.org/pdfs/mHealth_Barriers_White_Paper.pdf. Accessed 18 Jan 2018.
29. Clifford GD. E-health in low to middle income countries. J Med Eng Technol. 2016;40:336–41.
30. Jokhio AH, Winter HR, Cheng KK. An intervention involving traditional birth attendants and perinatal and maternal mortality in Pakistan. N Engl J Med. 2005;352:2091–9.
31. Martínez-Fernández A, Lobos-Medina I, Díaz-Molina CA, Chen-Cruz MF, Prieto-Egido I. TulaSalud: an m-health system for maternal and infant mortality reduction in Guatemala. J Telemed Telecare. 2015;21:283–91.
32. Austad K, Chary A, Martinez B, Juarez M, Juarez Martin Y, Coyote Ixen E, et al. Obstetric care navigation: a new approach to promote respectful maternity care and overcome barriers to safe motherhood. Reprod Health. 2017;14:148.
33. FARMAMUNDI, ASECSA, MSPAS, KOICA, UNFPA y OSAR. Más que una sanadora, Manual práctico de comadronas tradicionales para una maternidad sana. Guatemala. 2014.

11

Quality of care during childbirth in Tanzania: identification of areas that need improvement

Andrea Solnes Miltenburg[1*], Richard Forget Kiritta[2], Tarek Meguid[3] and Johanne Sundby[1]

Abstract

Background: Making use of good, evidence based routines, for management of normal childbirth is essential to ensure quality of care and prevent, identify and manage complications if they occur. Two essential routine care interventions as defined by the World Health Organization are the use of the Partograph and Active Management of the Third Stage of Labour. Both interventions have been evaluated for their ability to assist health providers to detect and deal with complications. There is however little research about the quality of such interventions for routine care. Qualitative studies can help to understand how such complex interventions are implemented. This paper reports on findings from an observation study on maternity wards in Tanzania.

Methods: The study took place in the Lake Zone in Tanzania. Between 2014 and 2016 the first author observed and participated in the care for women on maternity wards in four rural and semi-urban health facilities. The data is a result of approximately 1300 hours of observations, systematically recorded primarily in observation notes and notes of informal conversations with health providers, women and their families. Detailed description of care processes were analysed using an ethnographic analysis approach focused on the sequential relationship of the 'stages of labour'. Themes were identified through identification of recurrent patterns.

Results: Three themes were identified: 1) Women's movement between rooms during birth, 2) health providers' assumptions and hope for a 'normal' birth, 3) fear of poor outcomes that stimulates intervention during birth. Women move between different rooms during childbirth which influences the care they receive. Few women were monitored during their first stage of labour. Routine birth monitoring appeared absent due to health providers 'assumptions and hope for good outcomes. This was rooted in a general belief that most women eventually give birth without problems and the partograph did not correspond with health providers' experience of the birth process. Contextual circumstances also limited health worker ability to act in case of complications. At the same time, fear for being held personally responsible for outcomes triggered active intervention in second stage of labour, even if there was no indication to intervene.

Conclusions: Insufficient monitoring leads to poor preparedness of health providers both for normal birth and in case of complications. As a result both underuse and overuse of interventions contribute to poor quality of care. Risk and complication management have for many years been prioritized at the expense of routine care for all women. Complex evaluations are needed to understand the current implementation gaps and find ways for improving quality of care for all women.

Keywords: Maternal Health, Quality of Care, Participant Observation, Partograph, Active Management of Third Stage of Labour

* Correspondence: a.solnesmiltenburg@gmail.com
[1]Institute of Health and Society, Department of Community Medicine and Global Health, Faculty of Medicine, University of Oslo, Oslo, Norway
Full list of author information is available at the end of the article

Plain English summary

Good routines for management of normal childbirth are essential to ensure quality of care and timely actions in case of complications. There is however little research about the quality of routine care. This paper reports on findings from the maternity ward, from an observation study in Tanzania. The study took place in the Lake Zone in Tanzania. Between 2014 and 2016 the first author observed and participated in the care for women on maternity wards in four rural and semi-urban health facilities. The data is a result of approximately 1300 hours of observations. Our findings show that facility infrastructure requires women to move between different rooms during active childbirth. This influences the care they receive. We observed few women were monitored during birth. This is partly because health workers have an assumptions and hope for good outcomes. At the same time health workers fear for being held personally responsible for outcomes. This triggers the use of interventions to speed up birth even if there was no indication to intervene. Insufficient monitoring leads to poor preparedness of health providers both for normal birth and in case of complications. Risk and complication management have for many years been prioritized at the expense of routine care for all women. To understand the current gaps between what care is desired and what happens in reality complex evaluations are needed to find ways for improving quality of care for all women.

Background

During the past two decades the global maternal mortality ratio (MMR) has nearly halved. Although this is reason for optimism, many countries in sub Sahara Africa did not achieve the Millennium Development Goal 5 target of 75% MMR reduction [1]. Nevertheless, in many of these countries there was substantial increase in coverage of facility births [2]. Persisting high mortality and morbidity figures despite increase in service utilization, is thought to be due to a gap in the quality of care [2, 3]. Quality of care is insufficient due to poor facility capacity to provide timely emergency obstetric care (EmOC) and limited health provider knowledge to prevent, identify and manage complications [4]. Additionally, the push for increased numbers of facility births in countries with weak health systems also threatens the quality of routine care for uncomplicated births.

High quality of childbirth care includes provision of both routine care and emergency care. The majority of women giving birth in the health facility only require routine care. One reason for coming to a facility is to be near interventions provided by competent personnel if a complication occurs. Lack of good quality routine care may lead to more complications or late detection of these. However limited systematic research is available on the quality of routine care in low-middle income countries [4]. Quality of care assessments for management of complications are guided by the EmOC signal functions but similar signal functions for routine care are not well defined [4–6]. The WHO quality standard for childbirth care [7] suggests a selected number of process measures for quality assessment of routine monitoring during childbirth covering two essential interventions: 1) initiation and use of the partograph for monitoring and management of first and second stage of labour and 2) active management of the third stage of labour (AMTSL). Both interventions are intended to allow for controlled monitoring of the natural processes of birth, early identification of complications and preparedness of potential interventions when things deviate [8].

Use of the partograph and AMTSL are complex interventions because they contain a variety of interacting components and rely on good clinical skills [9]. Both interventions have been evaluated for their ability to help health providers detect and deal with complications. Little attention however has been paid to such intervention as part of routine care [4] beyond assessment of coverage of selected elements (e.g administration of oxytocin). It is increasingly acknowledged that there is a gap between global strategies, coverage of services and what actually happens when women reach health facilities to give birth [10]. Measurement of coverage of services and outcomes of care, although relevant, do not inform us on how care is provided and under which circumstances. Nor does it inform us about the health workers evaluation of clinical findings and decision making process. Qualitative studies are therefore important to increase our understanding of how such care processes take place and what this tells us about the quality of interventions such as the partograph and AMTSL for routine care [11]. This paper reports on findings from an observation study in Tanzania. Through description and holistic analysis of partograph use and AMTSL we intend to provide an understanding of the quality of routine care for uncomplicated childbirth in an African setting.

Methods

Setting

The study took place in the Lake Zone in Tanzania. Although Tanzania has made significant progress between 1999 and 2015 in increasing facility births (from 47% to 63%) the maternal mortality ratio has remained the same (from 578 in 2000 with CI 466-690 to 556 in 2015 with CI 446-666) [12]. Other sources suggest there has been substantial progress (MMR of 398 in 2015, CI 281-570) [13] but current reduction rates and wide confidence intervals suggest it remains unlikely Tanzania will reach the 2030 target MMR of 140 maternal deaths per 100.000 live births [14]. Maternity care in Tanzania is organized along a referral pyramid with dispensaries being the first formal health unit at primary level, followed by health centres and district hospitals [15]. All facility levels are expected to provide routine care for pregnant women and basic EmOC. District hospitals are expected to provide Comprehensive EmOC including availability of blood transfusion and caesarean sections [16].

Observer and Observations

Over the course of 25 months between 2014 and 2016 the first author [ASM], a medical doctor, observed and participated in the care for women on maternity wards in four health facilities. ASM speaks Kiswahili and lived in Tanzania for the past three years engaging with peoples lives in both urban and rural settings. For 6 months, ASM taught nursing and medical students on a weekly basis while volunteering alongside midwives and doctors on the maternity ward in one urban district hospital. This was followed by 8 months of volunteering full time as a medical doctor at a semi-urban faith-based health centre, before entering a systematic PhD program. As the research role evolved the final 11 months more focused observations were performed in a second rural district hospital and rural government health centre where the researcher had no clinical responsibilities. During these final months a research assistant (a nurse) also provided observations at the district hospital. As she was less able to intervene and participate this helped to increase understanding of routine care processes. For practical reasons observations only took place during the daytime and evenings. The research role of observing versus participating often fluctuated and shifted depending on the situation.

Being a medical doctor, ASM was naturally engaged in the defences of best practices in obstetric care from a technological point of view, following essential guidelines as promoted by the WHO. As a result of this, beyond participating in care provision, there were situations where ASM would intervene in normal care. For example if the situation was interpreted to potentially endanger the woman (either physically or psychologically) or cause unnecessary harm. Intervening in normal care included active discussion with providers about the course of action, give solicited or unsolicited advice or take action.

Taking action would always be in agreement with the women, the health providers or their seniors and only if the researcher felt capable to do so. For the final 11 month of observations the researcher had no authority to intervene independently. This was clear to the staff because observations were not on a daily basis and the researcher never established a formal role in these institutions. On some occasions the researcher faced difficult decision whether to intervene in the process of care or not. Situations occurred where women were prepared for a caesarean section without proper indication or where women received harmful treatment or practices, which went against most standards of care. When the researcher intervened this sometimes resulted in clashes or arguments with some of the staff. When the researcher did not intervene, and remained in the observer role, feelings of guilt for allowing things to evolve gave internal conflict. If the researcher intervened this was documented in the observation reports and taken into account for analysis.

Data collection

The data is a result of approximately 1300 hours of participant observation and consist of systematically recorded observation notes, notes of informal conversations with health providers, women and their families. In addition we reviewed clinical notes, handover books, staff schedules, reporting books and clinic cards while being present at the facilities. Observations mainly focused on the perspective of the health provider. During observations, activities and timing of care provision for individual women were documented using key words if the situation allowed for it. This usually started with description of the situation on the maternity wards after arrival. Researchers selected women that arrived at the nursing station or that were already admitted with what was expected to be an uncomplicated birth. Where possible individual women were followed until they had given birth. In additional other remarkable situations were noted, this could include situations where women developed complications. Although focus for our observations was uncomplicated births, it was important to document other happenings as they influenced and determined health worker's other activities. Full observation reports were written after each observation day. To the best of the researchers ability details of the day were documented. In addition personal reflections including feelings and interpretation of the activities were written down in the same reports.

Data analysis

Preliminary analysis of findings took place throughout the observation period. As a reference to standards of care we made use of a modification of the Maternal and Newborn Quality of Care Survey Labor and Delivery Observation Checklist developed by the Maternal and Child Health Integrated Program (MCHIP) [17]. The modified checklist is provided as Additional file 1. Detailed analysis was done after completion of the data collection using an ethnographic analysis approach comprising of four subsequent techniques: domain-, taxonomic-, componential- and theme analyses [18]. Domain analysis helped to meaningfully describe observations. For example one domain that we identified was 'the admission process' and all activities that these include (e.g. review of antenatal record, history taking, physical examination). For this paper domain analysis focused on identifying the 'stages of labour'[1] (see Table 1). Our reference point and terms used included the three stages of labour, around which standards of care have been organized in both international and local protocols with focus on normal, uncomplicated, childbirth.

Taxonomy analysis resulted in identification of subdomains within the different stages of labour (e.g movements between stages, locations of service provision, actions performed, consequences of clinical findings etc). This helped to identify how procedures and actions were organized and understand behaviour of women and health providers in the different stages and how they related to each other. Subsequently compound analysis helped to identify contrasting dimensions and its attributes (e.g. characteristics of woman and health providers, expectations of services, actual observed practices for monitoring and actions taken in case of deviations across the stages of labour). Themes were identified through identification of recurrent patterns in the previous steps.

Results

During analysis the following themes were identified: 1) Women's movement between rooms during birth, 2) health providers' assumptions and hope for a 'normal' birth, 3) fear of poor outcomes that stimulates intervention during birth.

Moving between rooms

Women accessed at least two rooms during childbirth at the health facility: the waiting room and/or the birth room (see Table 2).

> *In the maternity ward, women who are in latent phase or early stages of childbirth are admitted to the waiting room or antenatal room. In practice, this includes all women who are in the first stage of labour. There are 8 beds in the waiting room and women often have to share a bed when it is crowded.*

Table 1 Stages of Labour [8]

Latent phase
Presence of contraction which can both be regular and irregular, cervical dilatation < 4 cm
Active phase
First stage: Presence of frequent and regular contractions, cervical dilatation > 4 cm
Second stage: Full cervical dilatation and urge to push, birth of the baby
Third stage: After birth of the baby, placental separation and expulsion

> *[...] When approaching the second stage of labour, women need to shift to the birth room. Women need to walk approximately 15-20 meters to get to this room, carrying their own belonging and supplies. On their way to this room women pass the nursing station, which is located adjacent to the birth room. The birth room has six delivery beds, three on each side, although one of the beds is mainly used for supplies and materials. Rarely all beds are occupied. (Observation note district hospital)*

The admission process at the nursing station was the start of the care process. Examination was part of this process and took place in the birth room. Most of the time, it included assessments of the fundal height, fetal heart rate and vaginal examination to determine the cervical dilatation. Women arriving before the second stage of labour were considered not to be 'in labour' and they were placed in the waiting area together with women who were not in active phase of labour (for stages of labour see Table 1). When the beds in the birth room were not occupied, nurses would say 'it is not busy' or 'we don't have anyone in labour' while several women could be in active stage of labour in the waiting room. Women were required to walk from the waiting area to the birth room for physical examinations, complete certain stadia of birth within an expected timeframe (e.g cervical dilatation of 1 cm per hour) and adhere to the rules of the health facility (e.g. ensure availability of necessary supplies, wear appropriate clothing) for each step in the process. Although most births fit well into this local flow of care provision, some women had a faster birth than expected. For example Mrs P (18 years, primigravida).

> *Mrs P came to the hospital at 10.40am. At 11 am the nurse examines her abdomen and checks how far her cervix has dilated. She then informs Mrs P that she has to try and walk around, drink tea and can come back later: 'After four hours we measure you again'. Mrs P goes to the waiting area and the nurse documents that she has a cervical dilatation of 7cm on the admission form and the partograph. An hour later, another nurse brings Mrs P back to the nursing station, saying: 'This mama was pushing above her basin'. The nurse informs Mrs P it is not yet time. She should drink her tea and come back when she feels strong pushing urge. Mrs P quietly walks back to the waiting area. After 5 minutes, another pregnant woman comes to inform the nurses someone is pushing in the waiting area. Not long after cries of a baby can be heard and Mrs P has given birth to her daughter in the waiting area, assisted by her own mother. (Observation notes District Hospital)*

Table 2 Matrix of stages of labour in waiting area and birth room

Stage	Latent	Early first	Late first	Early second		Late second	Third
Location	Waiting area			Birth room			
Birth expected	Birth not imminent			Birth imminent			NA
Labour	Not in labour	Beginning in labour		In labour			After birth
Cervix	Tip of finger, closed,<4 cm	3-7cm	7or 8cm	8or9cm	Fully dilated head high/far	Fully dilated head close	NA
Time allowed	Days	Up to 1 day	Up to 6 hours	Up to 4 hours	1-2 hours	1 hour	5-15min
Nursing proximity	Far			Hearing distance		Close by	
Monitoring frequency	None	4hourly, upon shift change, doctors round, upon request		Frequent		None	
Monitoring activity	None	Cervical dilatation, foetal heart rate		Cervical dilatation		None	
Care seeking	Woman needs to approach the nurse by walking to the nursing station			Nurse will approach the woman, woman can ask for help when nurses are in hearing distance or on the labour ward			
Visitors/birth companion	Allowed on set times inside but women are able to go outside as they please			Not Allowed, only when instructed by nursing staff to bring supplies and materials			
Mobility	Women are able to walk around freely, urinate at the toilet, can position herself in any way but has to lie flat on her back during examination			Women are confined to the labour bed, urinate in a basin next to the labour bed which is brought by the woman herself, has to position herself lying flat on her back for pushing or other nursing activities			
Food and drink	Is allowed to eat and drink as she pleases			Is only allowed tea when this is instructed by the staff			

'Whatever will be, will be'

After admission women's antenatal card and files including a partograph remained at the nursing station. The type of partograph used at the health facilities was the composite partograph and was integrated in the admission form used at the maternity ward. Partographs were often not filled in immediately after admission, even though women where in active phase of labour. There was usually no organized filing system and from the admission files it was not clear which women required monitoring or were expected to give birth the coming hours. Sometimes women were admitted for days without any notes of observations until they eventually presented themselves at the nursing station in second stage of labour. The following case of Mrs S (32 years, gravida 6, para 5) illustrates poor monitoring and insufficient use of the partograph:

> *At 11am, the nurse says they are having a prolonged labour case, which they are thinking of referring. When we go to review the case of Mrs S, it becomes clear no partograph was filled in so the nurse decides to fill in her findings of this morning. Mrs S, who has given birth 5 times before with only two living children, informs us she was checked twice, upon arrival at 10pm yesterday evening and early morning at 6am. Some scattered notes show us her cervix was 5 cm dilated on arrival. There is no documentation of the examination of 6am, but the nurse checked Mrs S at 9.30am after the ward rounds and found her cervix was 6 cm dilated. (Observation notes Health Centre)*

Routine 'checks' and monitoring of women in the active stage occurred primarily during nurses' shifts changes (around 7am, 1pm and 7pm) and if there was a doctors ward round (between 9 and 10am). Nurses would collect all admission papers and pass by the different rooms on the maternity wards. If vaginal examination was needed women were asked to come to the nursing station one by one after the ward round. The time intervals between such routines during daytime were relatively short which allowed for somewhat regular monitoring. However, during the evening and night shifts many women like Mrs S were often left unattended and unnoticed until morning hours. Sometimes women presented themselves at the nursing station requesting to be examined

If the partograph was used, nurses appeared to prioritize some parts of the partograph, while leaving out others. If examination took place for the purpose of monitoring, this primarily included routine assessment of cervical dilatation. Less invasive assessments such as blood pressure measurement, assessment of fetal heart rate, number of contractions per 10 minute, pulse rate or temperature were rarely measured nor discussed in relation to the birth progress or well-being of the mother. Blood pressures were sometimes documented based on the findings during the last clinic visit, because the blood pressure machine was not readily available and a temperature of 37.5 C was often written assuming the woman had no fever. Assessment findings were not always recorded on the partograph, but rather in separate notes. Some assessments were filled in through 'guessing' rather than actual measuring.

While assisting the nurse with documentation on the partograph, I asked her how much the fetal heart rate was. She listened for a few seconds with the fetoscope and said '136'. I wondered how she calculated this so quickly. [Observation notes district hospital]

Usually nurses expressed an expectation that, even though based on the partograph the firsts stage appeared to take too long, most women would eventually give birth without problems and with mostly positive outcomes. If women seemed to approach the action line on the partograph nurses would sometimes dismiss previous documented cervical dilatation or make changes to what was filled in on the partograph before and rather allow women more time to progress without intervention. Sometimes nurses preferred to avoid documentation on the partograph or did not actively monitor women unless women themselves called the nurses for assistance. This lack of monitoring could result in staff being unprepared for in-facility 'sudden events'. Women who had been admitted for days could appear with 'sudden' onset of complications, give birth 'suddenly' on their own in the waiting area or 'suddenly' appear in second stage at the birth room with staff being unprepared, for example Mrs D (19 years, primigravida).

After finishing at the ANC clinic, at 1pm, a nurse rushes to the birth room where she quickly puts on some gloves. A young girl, Mrs D, is lying on the bed in second stage of labour. The nurse says: 'This girl was admitted to the ward since yesterday, now suddenly she comes in second stage'.[...] Her file states that Mrs D was examined this morning and that her cervix was 2 cm dilated. [...] Shortly after, she gives birth to a 3kg baby girl. (Observation notes Health Center)

Nurses were also hesitant to start the partograph at early first stage of labour, saying this would result in 'too many women reaching the action line'. The action line would indicate 'poor progress' requiring immediate action, which was not always easy to manage in their setting. The decision that birth was not progressing resulted in a range of consequences for both families and health providers in the example of Mrs. S:

When we examined Mrs. S at 11am she had mild contractions but a cervical dilatation of 8 cm with the head high and membranes intact. The fetal heart rate was fine. There was hesitation to rupture the membranes because of the long distance to the district hospital in case of problems after rupturing. [...] The doctor- in charge, who was on his way to the hospital, instructed the nurse to rupture the membranes and to give Mrs. S 500ml IV fluids. [...] There was slight meconium stained fluid but a good fetal heart rate of 140 beats per minute [bpm]. At 12.30 Mrs S was still 8 cm and not showing signs of progress and the nurse suggested to refer her for further management. But lack of available ambulance would require the family to make their own arrangements.[...] The doctor in-charge was still on his way and informed us he would come to perform a caesarean section. [...] The family was instructed to buy a catheter and the nurse asked the laboratory technician to perform hemoglobin measurement. The doctor arrived at 2pm. Meanwhile the contractions of Mrs S had increased, although she had progressed, there were signs of obstruction. Family members were asked to bring supplies and water for cleaning the operating theatre at 3pm. Finally at 4pm Mrs S delivered a baby boy by caesarean section. (Observation notes Health Center)

In the example of Mrs S several delays occurred after poor progress was diagnosed. The nurses, and the researcher, experienced they had little influence on these delays. The researcher had suggested to drive Mrs S to the district hospital in her private car. Although both the nurses and Mrs S where happy with this option the medical doctor refused this saying he would arrive soon to assess the situation. When he finally arrived, family members where instructed to make necessary arrangements before the caesarean section was possible, resulting in more delay. Similar delays were also observed at the district hospital. One afternoon nurses adequately and timely called for supervision for a case of obstructed labour. It took an entire night before the woman was taken to the operating theatre the next morning.

Active management out of fear of poor outcomes

After women arrived in the birth room we observed nurses appeared to have a sense of urgency to intervene and make sure women gave birth as quickly as possible. Failure to complete a stadium, for example poor descend of the head within the expected time, or failure according to expected social norms, such as screaming out of pain and being perceived demanding, was considered a deviation of 'normal' and required intervention and active management. If women did not give birth soon enough after arriving to the birth room nurses would fear poor progress would lead to poor fetal outcome and therefore required active management. For example Mrs A (21 years, gravida 3, para 0), who was lying in the birth room with what was perceived to be poor progress because she had been in the birth room since early morning. The following events occurred:

Funding
ASM was supported by the Research Council of Norway through the Global Health and Vaccination Programme (GLOBVAC) for her PhD, project number 244674. The funding body had no role in the design of the study and collection, analysis, and interpretation of data, nor in writing of the manuscript.

Authors' contributions
ASM performed the observations. RFK provided local expert advice and feedback on observations. JS spent a few days in the field, and JS and TK provided supervision and helped ASM to reflect on findings. All authors analysed and interpreted the data. ASM drafted the manuscript. All authors read and approved the final manuscript.

Ethics approval and consent to participate
Ethical approval was granted by the National Institute of Medical Research in Tanzania (MR/53/100/103-349-399) and a research permit was granted by the Tanzanian Commission for Science and Technology (No.2015-255-ER-2013-32). The Regional Committee for Medical and Health Research Ethics, Section A, South East Norway (2015/1827), and the Norwegian Social Science Data Service (44482/3/MHM) both reviewed the study and found the study in accordance with the Norwegian Personal Data Act. The first author was also registered at the Medical Council of Tanganyika as a medical practitioner (Reg.no 5533) during the time of the research. As soon as the research role became more explicit in 2015 we requested permission from relevant local health authorities for the research. Health workers were informed of the study and were asked for written informed consent. Women were asked for verbal consent where possible. Because of the sensitivity of the subject we ensured anonymity in note taking and for this reason hospital and clinic names are also not included in this paper.

Competing interests
The authors declare that they have no competing interests.

Author details
[1]Institute of Health and Society, Department of Community Medicine and Global Health, Faculty of Medicine, University of Oslo, Oslo, Norway. [2]Department of Obstetrics and Gynaecology, Sekotoure Regional Referral Hospital, Mwanza, Mwanza Region, Tanzania. [3]Department of Obstetrics & Gynaecology, Mnazi Mmoja Hospital, Zanzibar, Tanzania.

References

1. Victora CG, Requejo JH, Barros AJD, Berman P, Bhutta Z, Boerma T, et al. Countdown to 2015: a decade of tracking progress for maternal, newborn, and child survival. Geneva: UNICEF and WHO; 2015. Available from: http://www.ncbi.nlm.nih.gov/pubmed/26477328.
2. Montagu D, Sudhinaraset M, Diamond-smith N, Campbell O, Gabrysch S, Freedman L, et al. Where women go to deliver: understanding the changing landscape of childbirth in Africa and Asia. Health Policy Plan. 2017;32:1146–52.
3. Koblinsky M, Moyer CA, Calvert C, Campbell J, Campbell OMR, Feigl AB, et al. Quality maternity care for every woman, everywhere: A call to action. Lancet. 2016;388(10057):2307–20.
4. Campbell OMR, Calvert C, Testa A, Strehlow M, Benova L, Keyes E, et al. The scale, scope, coverage, and capability of childbirth care. Lancet. 2016; 388(10056):2193–208.
5. Gabrysch S, Civitelli G, Edmond KM, Mathai M, Ali M, Bhutta ZA, et al. New Signal Functions to Measure the Ability of Health Facilities to Provide Routine and Emergency Newborn Care. PloS Med. 2012;9(11):e1001340.
6. Brenner S, De Allegri M, Gabrysch S, Chinkhumba J, Sarker M, Muula AS. The quality of clinical maternal and neonatal healthcare a strategy for identifying routine care signal functions. PLoS One. 2015;10(4):1–19.
7. WHO. Standards for improving quality of maternal and newborn care in health facilities. Geneva: WHO; 2016.
8. WHO. United Nations Population Fund, UNICEF. Pregnancy, childbirth, postpartum and newborn care: a guide for essential practice (3rd edition). Geneva: WHO; 2015.
9. Bedwell C, Levin K, Pett C, Lavender DT. A realist review of the partograph: when and how does it work for labour monitoring? BMC Pregnancy Childbirth. 2017;17(1):31.
10. Freedman LP. Implementation and Aspiration gaps: Who's view counts? Lancet. 2016;388(10056):2068–9.
11. Pope C, Campbell R. Qualitative research in obstetrics and gynaecology. Br J Obstet Gynaecol. 2001;108(3):233–7.
12. Ministry of Health, Community Development, Gender, Elderly and Children (MoHCDGEC) [Tanzania Mainland], Ministry of Health (MoH) [Zanzibar], National Bureau of Statistics (NBS), Office of the Chief Government Statistician (OCGS), and ICF. Tanzania Demographic and Health Survey and Malaria Indicator Survey (TDHS-MIS) 2015-16. Dar es Salaam: MoHCDGEC, MoH, NBS, OCGS, and ICF; 2016.
13. World Health Organization. World health statistics 2017: monitoring health for the SDGs, Sustainable Development Goals. Geneva: WHO; 2017.
14. Afnan-holmes H, Magoma M, John T, Levira F, Msemo G, Armstrong CE, et al. Tanzania ' s Countdown to 2015 : an analysis of two decades of progress and gaps for reproductive , maternal, newborn, and child health, to inform priorities for post-2015. Lancet Glob Health. 2015;3(7): e396–409.
15. Pembe AB, Carlstedt A, Urassa DP, Lindmark G, Nyström L, Darj E. Effectiveness of maternal referral system in a rural setting: a case study from Rufiji district, Tanzania. BMC Health Serv Res. 2010;10:326.
16. Ministry of Health, Community Development, Gender, Elderly and Children (MoHCDGEC). The national road map stratecic plan to improve reproductive, maternal, newborn, child and adolescent health in Tanzania (2016 - 2020). Dar es Salaam: MoHCDGEC. p. 2016.
17. MCHIP. Maternal and Newborn Quality of Care Surveys: labour and delivery observtion checklist. Wachington: MCHIP; 2014. Available at: http://www.qualityofcarenetwork.org/resources/assessments/maternal-and-newborn-quality-caresurvey-ld-observation-checklist#.
18. Spradley J. Participant Observation. copyright 1980. 2016th ed. Long Grove: Waveland Press; 2016.
19. Davis-Floyd R. The technocratic, humanistic, and holistic paradigms of childbirth. Int J Gynaecol Obstet. 2001;75Suppl1:S5–S23.
20. Friedman EA. Primigravid labor: a graphicostatistical analysis. Obstet Gynecol. 1955;6(6):567–89.
21. WHO. Preventing prolonged labour: a practical guide. The partograph Part I: Principles and strategy. Geneva; WHO, 1994.
22. Zhang J, Troendle JF, Yancey MK. Reassessing the labor curve in nulliparous women. Am jouranal. Obstet Gynecol. 2002:824–8.
23. Zhang J, Landy HJ, Branch DW, Burkman R, Haberman S, Gregory KD, et al. Contemporary Patterns of Spontaneous Labor With Normal Neonatal Outcomes. Obs Gynecol. 2010;116(6):1281–7.
24. Lavender T, Hart A, Smyth R. Effect of partogram use on outcomes for women in spontaneous labour at term. CochDatabase Syst Rev. 2013;10(7): CD005461.
25. Fistula Care and Maternal Health Task Force. Fistula care revitalizing the partograph: does the evidence support a global call to action? New York; Fistula Care and Maternal Health Task Force, 2012.
26. WHO. Care in Normal Birth: a practical guide. Geneva: WHO; 1996.
27. Duysburgh E, Zhang WH, Ye M, Williams A, Massawe S, Sié A, et al. Quality of antenatal and childbirth care in selected rural health facilities in Burkina Faso, Ghana and Tanzania: Similar finding. Trop Med Int Heal. 2013;18(5):534–47.
28. Delvaux T, Aké-Tano O, Gohou-Kouassi V Alérie, Bosso P, Collin S, Ronsmans C. Quality of normal delivery care in Côte d'Ivoire. Afr J Reprod Health 2007;11:22–32.
29. Maimbolwa MC, Ransjo-Arvidson AB, Ng'andu N, Sikazwe N, Diwan VK. Routine care of women experiencing normal deliveries in Zambian maternity wards: a pilot study. Midwifery. 1997;13(3):125–31.

30. Ollerhead E, Osrin D. Barriers to and incentives for achieving partograph use in obstetric practice in low-and middle-income countries: a systematic review. BMC Pregnancy Childbirth. 2014;14:281.
31. Nyamtema AS, Urassa DP, Massawe S, Massawe A, Lindmark G, van Roosmalen J. Partogram use in the Dar es Salaam perinatal care study. Int J Gynecol Obstet. 2008;100(1):37–40.
32. Mathibe-Neke J, Lebeko F, Motupa B. The partograph: A labour management tool or a midwifery record? Int J Nurs Midwifery. 2013;5(8):145–53.
33. Scamell M, Alaszewski A. Fateful moments and the categorisation of risk: Midwifery practice and the ever-narrowing window of normality during childbirth. Health, Risk and Society. 2017;14(2):207–21.
34. WHO. Every Woman, Every Child, Every Adolescent: Achievements and prospects: the final report of the independent Expert Review Group on Information and Accountability for Women's and Children's health. Geneva: WHO; 2015.
35. Campbell J, Dussault G, Buchan J, Pozo-Martin F, Guerra Arias M, Leone C, Siyam A, Cometto G. A universal truth: no health without a workforce. Forum Report, Third Global Forum on Human Resources for Health, Recife, Brazil. Geneva: Global Health Workforce Alliance and World Health Organization; 2013.
36. Shimoda K, Leshabari S, Horiuchi S, Shimpuku Y, Tashiro J. Midwives' intrapartum monitoring process and management resulting in emergency referrals in Tanzania: a qualitative study. BMC Pregnancy Childbirth. 2015;15(1):248.
37. Mc Court C. Chapter 2: Cosmologies, concept, and theories: Tme and Childbirth in cross-cultural perspective. In: Mc Court C. Childbirth, Midwifery and the concept of time. Parkin D, Tremayne S, Inhorn M, editors. eBook edition 2013. New York: Berghahn Books; 2013
38. Litorp H, Mgaya A, Mbekenga CK, Kidanto HL, Johnsdotter S, Ess B. Fear, blame and transparency : Obstetric caregivers' rationales for high caesarean section rates in a low-resource setting. Soc Sci Med. 2015;143:232–40.
39. Chuma C, Kihunrwa A, Matovelo D, Mahendeka M. Labour management and Obstetric outcomes among pregnant women admitted in latent phase compared to active phase of labour at Bugando Medical Centre in Tanzania. BMC Pregnancy Childbirth. 2014;14(1):68.
40. Miller S, Abalos E, Chamillar M, Ciapponi A, Colaci D, Comande D, et al. Beyond Too Little, Too Late and Too Much, Too Soon': A pathway towards evidence-based, respectful maternaity care worldwide. Lancet. 2016; 6736(16):1–17.
41. Brownlee S, Chalkidou K, Doust J, Elshaug AG, Glasziou P, Heath I, Nagpal S, et al. Evidence for overuse and underuse of medical services around the world. Lancet. 2017;390(10090):156–68.
42. Maaløe N, Sorensen BL, Onesmo R, Secher NJ, Bygbjerg IC. Prolonged labour as indication for emergency caesarean section: A quality assurance analysis by criterion-based audit at two Tanzanian rural hospitals. BJOG. 2012;119(5):605–13.
43. Heemelaar S, Nelissen E, Mdoe P, Kidanto H, van Roosmalen J, Stekelenburg J. Criteria-based audit of caesarean section in a referral hospital in rural Tanzania. Trop Med Int Heal. 2016;21(4):525–34.
44. Litorp H, Kidanto HL, Nystrom L, Darj E, Essén B. Increasing caesarean section rates among low-risk groups: a panel study classifying deliveries according to Robson at a university hospital in Tanzania. BMC Pregnancy Childbirth. 2013;13:107.
45. Wagner M. Fish can't see water: the need to humanize birth. Int J Gynaecol Obstet. 2001;75:S25–37.
46. Saini V, Garcia-armesto S, Klemperer D, Paris V, Elshaug AG, Brownlee S, et al. Drivers of poor medical care. Lancet. 2017;90(10090):178–90.
47. Stanton C, Armbruster D, Knight R, Ariawan I, Gbangbade S, Getachew A, et al. Use of active management of the third stage of labour in seven developing countries. Bull World Health Organ. 2009;87(3):207–15.
48. Oladapo OT, Akinola OI, Fawole AO, Adeyemi AS, Adegbola O, Loto OM, et al. Active management of third stage of labor: evidence versus practice. Acta Obstet Gynecol Scand. 2009;88(11):1252–60.
49. Roth AD. Managing motherhood, managing risk: fertility and danger in west central Tanzania. Ann Arbor: University of Michigan; 2004.
50. WHO. WHO Recommendations for the Prevention and Treatment of Postpartum Haemorrhage. Geneva: WHO; 2012.
51. Ten Hoope-Bender P, De Bernis L, Campbell J, Downe S, Fauveau V, Fogstad H, et al. Improvement of maternal and newborn health through midwifery. Lancet. 2014;384(9949):1226–35.
52. Maaløe N, Housseine N, Van RJ, Bygbjerg IC, Tersbøl BP, Khamis RS, et al. Labour management guidelines for a Tanzanian referral hospital: The participatory development process and birth attendants ' perceptions. BMC Pregnancy Childbirth. 2017:1–11.
53. Maaløe N, Housseine N, Meguid T, Nielsen BB, Jensen AKG, Khamis RS. Effect of locally tailored labour management guidelines on intrahospital stillbirths and birth asphyxia at the referral hospital of Zanzibar : a quasi-experimental pre-post study (The PartoMa study); 2017. p. 1–11.
54. Sakala C, Newburn M. Meeting needs of childbearing women and newborn infants through strengthened midwifery. Lancet. 2014;384(9948):e39–40.
55. Renfrew MJ, McFadden A, Bastos MH, Campbell J, Channon AA, Cheung NF, et al. Midwifery and quality care: Findings from a new evidence-informed framework for maternal and newborn care. Lancet. 2014;384(9948):1129–45.
56. Bohren MA, Vogel JP, Hunter EC, et al. The Mistreatment of Women during Childbirth in Health Facilities Globally: A Mixed-Methods Systematic Review. Plos Medicine. 2015;12(6):1–32.
57. Fathalla MF. Human Rights Aspects of Safe Motherhood. Best Pract Res Clin Obstet Gynaecol. 2006;20(3):409–19.
58. Cook RJ, Dickens BM, Wilson OAF, Scarrow SE. Advancing safe motherhood through human rights. Geneva: WHO; 2001.
59. Meguid T. Re Humanising Health Care – Placing Dignity and Agency of the Patient at the Centre. Nordic J Hum Rights. 2016;34(1):60–4.
60. Hodnett E, Gates S, Gj H, Sakala C, Weston J. Continuous support for women during childbirth. CochDatabase Syst Rev. 2011;2:CD003766.
61. Lawrence A, Lewis L, Gj H, Styles C. Maternal positions and mobility during first stage labour. CochDatabase Syst Rev. 2013;10:CD003934.

12

"It's something that marks you": Abortion stigma after decriminalization in Uruguay

Roosbelinda Cárdenas[1,2*], Ana Labandera[3], Sarah E. Baum[4], Fernanda Chiribao[3], Ivana Leus[3], Silvia Avondet[3] and Jennifer Friedman[1]

Abstract

Background: Abortion stigma is experienced by women seeking abortion services and by abortion providers in a range of legal contexts, including Uruguay, where abortion was decriminalized up to 12 weeks gestation in 2012. This paper analyzes opinions and attitudes of both abortion clients and health professionals approximately two years following decriminalization and assesses how abortion stigma manifests among these individuals and in institutions that provide care.

Methods: In 2014, we conducted twenty in-depth, semi-structured interviews with abortion clients ($n = 10$) and health care professionals ($n = 10$) in public and private facilities across Uruguay's health system. Interviews were recorded, transcribed, and then coded for thematic analysis.

Results: We find that both clients and health professionals express widespread satisfaction with the implementation of the new law. However, there exist critical points in the service where stigmatizing ideas and attitudes continue to be reproduced, such as the required five-day waiting period and in interactions with hospital staff who do not support access to the service. We also document the prevalence of stigmatizing ideas around abortion that continue to circulate outside the clinical setting.

Conclusion: Despite the benefits of decriminalization, abortion clients and health professionals still experience abortion stigma.

Keywords: Uruguay, Latin America, Abortion stigma, Decriminalization, Abortion

Plain English summary

Abortion stigma is experienced by women seeking legal induced abortion services and by abortion providers in a range of legal contexts. This paper analyzes abortion stigma in Uruguay, where abortion was decriminalized up to 12 weeks gestation in 2012. In it, we explore the opinions and attitudes of both abortion clients and health professionals approximately two years after decriminalization in order to assess if and how stigma manifests within institutions that provide abortion services.

Respondents were interviewed after participating in a survey at the clinical setting where they provide or receive reproductive health services. Our qualitative analysis found that both clients and health professionals express widespread satisfaction with the implementation of the new law. However, despite clear improvements in quality of care, there exist critical points in the service where stigmatizing ideas and attitudes continue to be reproduced. Overall, we conclude that despite the benefits of decriminalization, abortion clients and health professionals still experience abortion stigma both inside and outside the clinical setting.

Background

Abortion stigma

Stigma has been found to be an obstacle in delivery of some health services due to negative consequences for those who are, or who fear being, stigmatized [1, 2]. Erving Goffman, a key figure in the sociological definition of stigma, conceptualizes it as "an attribute that is deeply discrediting" that "reduces an individual from a

* Correspondence: rooscardenas@gmail.com
[1]International Planned Parenthood/Western Hemisphere Region, New York, USA
[2]Hampshire College, Amherst, USA
Full list of author information is available at the end of the article

whole and usual person to a tainted, discounted one" [3]. Goffman presents three types of stigma: blemishes of character, deformations of the body, and group identity [3]. Link and Phelan, in response to the assertion that stigma was "vaguely defined" and "individually focused," explain it as a social process in which individuals are marked as different, associated with negative attributes, conceived of as "others," separated from society, and subject to loss of status and discrimination. This process places them in a framework of economic, political, and social power relations that perpetuate stigma in order to maintain the status quo [4].

Every year over 40 million women in the world have an abortion [5], making it one of the most common and safe medical procedures [6]. Yet it is still loaded with strong social stigma expressed in negative attitudes and secrecy by both women who get abortions and clinicians involved in the process. Thus, abortion stigma is one of the main barriers to women seeking termination of an unwanted pregnancy and a challenge to abortion service providers. This stigma translates into shame and silence for women and into marginalization for providers, and creates or perpetuates myths and misunderstandings about abortion [2, 7]. Stigma manifests differently depending on legal frameworks, religious beliefs, and social and cultural contexts [8].

Kumar, Hessini, and Mitchell define abortion stigma as "a negative attribute ascribed to women who seek to terminate a pregnancy that marks them, internally or externally, as inferior to ideals of womanhood" [9]. They explain that when a woman has an abortion, she transgresses socially-accepted concepts, such as that sexual relations are only for reproductive purposes; that maternity is inherent in the condition of being a woman, and therefore inevitable; and that the role established for women is motherhood and the nurturing of children [9].

At the individual level, stigma can be classified into three main manifestations: 1) perceived stigma, which are ideas about what others may think about abortion and about what could happen if their own experience is made public (rejection by the family or partner, impaired social relationships, loss of friendships, criticism, abuse, and isolation); 2) experienced stigma, which are actual acts of discrimination, harassment, and aggression by others; and 3) internalized stigma, which refers to the materialization of the two previous forms in feelings of guilt, shame, anxiety, or other negative ideas [9, 10].

Shellenberg et al. [10] and Sorhaindo et al. [11] focus on how internalized stigma was experienced by women who had abortions in Mexico and Peru. Feelings of guilt, sadness, and shame were common, as well as widespread silence and secrecy around abortion, especially in small communities. Some of the women interviewed by Shellenberg et al. [10] initially said that their abortions were spontaneous, a strategy to distance themselves from stigma, although they later explained that they had induced abortions. Some women in the study by Sorhaindo et al. [11], said that they had changed their perception about abortion based on their own experience. Yet despite changing their prejudiced views of women who terminate their pregnancies, they were unable to approve of abortion even after having one. The accounts in these studies reflect experiences of isolation among women who choose to not share their experiences or seek support [9, 10].

Health care providers who counsel women and dispense abortion medication, as well as pharmacists and other personnel who work in facilities that provide abortion services are also affected by stigma [10–12]. This stigma often discredits them and excludes them from full participation in their professional community. For example, abortion providers have been called "dirty workers" in the social psychology literature. "Dirty work" refers to professions stigmatized by their associations with contamination that is physical (grime, dirt), social (interaction with stigmatized individuals), or moral (primarily sin) [12]. Studies conducted with abortion providers where abortion is illegal reveal that they frequently feel isolated from the general medical community and that they are afraid to speak openly about their work [8, 12]. Under these conditions, many choose not to get involved in abortion provision, or if they do, they do not speak openly about it in their social and professional circles [13].

Even though research that specifically explores how abortion stigma operates among Latin American women and health professionals is incipient, there is a growing body of work that provides solid bases with which to develop theoretical frameworks that are grounded on empirical evidence [10, 11, 16–19].

Although an increasing number of countries Latin America have achieved partial decriminalization of abortion in recent years, it is still estimated that the region has the highest percentage of unsafe abortions in the world [5, 14]. Furthermore, research shows that in settings where abortion is legal, risks to the lives of women and abortion-related stigma are lower than in those where it is criminalized [14, 15]. Thus, this paper emerges from the broad idea that perceptions and attitudes toward abortion vary depending on legal contexts, and that these tend to be more favorable when a woman's legal right to terminate her pregnancy is recognized. The study's overall objective was to uncover and analyze these patients' and health professionals' perceptions and attitudes towards abortion. Specifically, to explore if and how stigma continues to operate in decriminalized clinical abortion settings.[1]

Legal framework

In 2012 (Law 18,987), Uruguay decriminalized medicated and surgical abortion, without specifying grounds but under strict compliance with two requirements: to not exceed twelve weeks of pregnancy and that the woman meet with a multidisciplinary team of three health professionals (gynecologist, psychologist, and social worker), which must ensure that she has all necessary information available to make an informed and responsible decision. The law and its regulations (Decree No. 375/012) state that a woman must attend four visits and during the process, the woman must think over her decision for five days except in cases where the pregnancy represents a risk to the woman's life, is a result of rape, or when there is fetal malformation. In addition, the IVE[2] manual published by the Ministry of Health following decriminalization privileges medicated abortion over surgical procedures. For this reason, women who go through a regular abortion process will routinely receive a medicated abortion and will not be asked for their preference of method. All public facilities in Uruguay's Integrated Health System are required to follow the law and conscientious objection is permitted among physicians as long as the facilities where objectors work inform women on how and where to access services.[3]

In the Uruguayan model of care, teams of health professionals in abortion services are organized in first level clinics and in hospitals, and they include physicians, nurses, midwives, psychologists, social workers, and sonographers. Under the law, abortion clients must follow the following steps: a first appointment where the woman expresses her intent to terminate a pregnancy (Visit 1), a second appointment with the interdisciplinary team where she receives counseling and is informed about the required reflection period (Visit 2), a five-day waiting period, a third appointment where the woman expresses her final decision and the procedure is initiated (Visit 3), and a fourth appointment to confirm whether the abortion has been completed (Visit 4).

Methods

Recruitment and data collection

In order to test whether the legal recognition of the right to terminate a pregnancy has an impact on stigma, we collected data from a group of abortion clients and a group of health professionals who provide abortion care in Uruguay in 2014, two years following decriminalization.[4] In Uruguay, women were recruited at the Sexual and Reproductive Health Service of the Complejo Hospitalario Pereira Rossell, a major public hospital in the capital city, Montevideo.[5] At the end of the second appointment (Visit 2), following counseling by the interdisciplinary team, women were invited by a nurse to participate in the study. Women received necessary information about the research and, if they were interested in participating, provided their verbal consent and contact information to be contacted later. Interviews were conducted in person or by telephone following the fourth appointment (Visit 4). The interviews analyzed in this paper are a subsample of a larger group of abortion clients who completed a survey for a quantitative analysis. Of a total of 203 abortion clients recruited for the quantitative study, ten were chosen by convenience sampling to be interviewed in person. Semi-structured in-depth interviews (from 30 to 90 min long) were conducted with participants aged 22 to 38 years. Although most lived in Montevideo, some respondents lived outside Uruguay's capital city. Health professionals were also invited to participate in an interview following participation in a quantitative study. Among a sample of 72 health professionals in facilities around the country who completed the quantitative survey, ten completed an in-depth interview including seven women and three men. These included physicians, midwives, social workers, and a psychiatrist. Interviews lasted from 20 to 60 min. Most interviews were conducted in person by trained study coordinators; some were conducted by telephone due to long travel distances. This study was approved by the Allendale Investigational Review Board (Old Lyme, CT, USA).

All interviews were recorded, transcribed, and coded for analysis using Dedoose software. The research team jointly developed two codebooks, one for interviews with health professionals and one for interviews with women. The codebooks were created independently to capture unique topics in the semi-structured interview guides and in vivo codes that emerged directly from the participants; however the codebooks reflected similar overarching themes such as attitudes towards the abortion law, disclosure and interactions with people in their community, and experiences in different phases of the abortion process, among others. Analysis was led by a team of two researchers and two coders who jointly developed a codebook and carried out thematic analysis of the data. Each of the codes was individually scrutinized first and subsequently the team identified key themes and patterns in responses.

Results

Opinions and attitudes among abortion clients

Attitudes towards abortion and women who have abortions

While some women believe that Uruguay continues to be a conservative country where abortion is still taboo, others said they saw major progress in social attitudes, including the fact that decriminalization had been achieved. Almost all interviewees felt that abortion is their right and that they have the prerogative to decide what to do with their bodies and their lives. In general, abortion is seen as an individual experience that is only incumbent on the person who has to get one. Although most spoke with their partner, family members, or friends, a few did not share the experience with anyone other than the legal abortion team that provided care during the process.

> "I have nothing to say; what needed to be said got said and that's that. I did it, I'm fine, and ciao." (Age 23).

> "I didn't talk about it with my husband, or my sister, or my friends, or with anybody. The topic is now closed, that's that." (Age 34).

Religious ideas were almost nonexistent in interviewees' discourse. However, they all reported some level of guilt, describing "pangs of conscience," and other feelings, such as "a non-physical pain," shame, sadness, anger, depression, and loneliness, and some referred to themselves as selfish. All interviewees shared the idea that the abortion was an experience that marked them for life:

> "[...] I think I'm going to carry this until I die." (Age 23).

> "I think it is a trauma that one does not get over, even though one learns to live with it [...] this guilt is going to be lifelong." (Age 22).

> "When I think about going to the gynecologist and they are going to ask me about my medical history, I'm ashamed to have to tell them that I just had an abortion." (Age 38).

Still, one abortion client expressed positive feelings about having access to a legal abortion as compared to an unsafe option:

> "It was strange because it was a new experience, but it was a lifesaver. You avoid the trauma of doing it in a clandestine place where they can do anything to you and where no one is going to take responsibility for anything." (Age 29).

Despite recurring feelings of guilt, none of the participants said they regretted their abortion. However, these clients experienced their process as something that they do not want to have to go through again. In fact, all of them said that, until discovering an unwanted pregnancy, they saw abortion as a very remote possibility, something that they would not have to go through or that they would not be capable of doing.

> "[...] I had sworn to myself that I would never have an abortion and I ended up doing it. It was kind of ironic and I was surprised to find myself contradicting myself about something that I said I wouldn't do." (Age 23).

> "[...] I said it would never happen to me and it happened." (Age 34).

Several of them said they were against abortion even after having terminated a pregnancy, while others expressed a change of opinion prompted by the experience.

> "I'm against abortion, so it was a very difficult decision to make and to this day it still weighs on me." (Age 31).

> "[..] I was against abortion until it was my turn." (Age 22).

> "In line with my upbringing, I had always been against it; I imagined it to be pretty cruel because of what they say and they tell you." (Age 27).

They all confirmed that it was the best decision they could make, given that it was not the right time to have a child because of various reasons: poor economic or health situations, instability with a partner, or because they already had several children.

Interestingly, with the exception of one interviewee, participants harshly judged other women who have abortions, and even more severely those who have more than one. Although they fully justified their own abortion saying things like "I didn't want to do it, but of course my situation wasn't easy" (Age 27), they saw other women's abortions as acts of irresponsibility, selfishness, and immaturity.

> "If you already did it once, why are you going to do the same thing again? Once is fine, but those who do it two, three, four times, [it's] like they kind of do it just for fun." (Age 22).

> "I see many women who do it like just for fun [...] people who say: 'well, I got pregnant and I can do it one, two, and even three times.'" (Age 31).

> "[...] others get pregnant real easy and have abortions [as easily/often as] they change their jeans." (Age 23).

> "[...] there are other cases of women where it's like they don't care if they get pregnant and abort and go

back and repeat the story [...] it's different for those who want to come every year to do it, but for women whose case is like mine, it's okay." (Age 38).

"I think there should be limits because they're going to get pregnant ten times and they're going to take the life of an innocent being [...] Names and record numbers should be recorded and tell them 'look, there's a limit, you can't get pregnant five times and get rid of it every time you feel like it.'" (Age 22).

Attitudes towards abortion health professionals and services

For the women interviewed, the most common feelings before visiting facilities to request an IVE or legal abortion service were shame, fear of rejection, or fear of undergoing a procedure that could endanger their health.

"At first, I was a little afraid of the whole procedure. After the counseling, I felt safe and calm. I felt confident." (Age 29).

Overall, women had positive experiences with the health care teams at the facility where they received their service. Almost all said that they did not feel judged by the interdisciplinary team. Rather, they said they were surprised by the thorough information they received and that they felt welcomed and well-understood.

"I thought they would be a little more hostile, because of the fact that one is killing a person, but no, everything [was] just fine." (Age 22).

"You arrive afraid that you're going to be judged by the same doctors whose job is to save lives, but it was nothing like that, everything super good, marvelous, in fact, they protect you." (Age 29).

Only one of the clients reported having felt rejected by one of the health professionals who treated her:

"When I came in for the ultrasound, the person who was doing it looked at me and said 'I don't do IVE and they looked me up and down. When I gave them the paper, they looked at it and said that the doctor didn't do IVE and the other went and told them: 'it doesn't matter, she's a patient and you have to take care of her'. She went and took her the paper and the woman came and told me to my face, 'I don't do IVE. There were a lot of people outside the examining room and even though not everyone knows what IVE is, it was like [...] they were judging me." (Age 38).

During the interview, women were asked about a hypothetical doctor refusing to provide abortion services. Even though they talked about how disappointing and upsetting it would be for a doctor to disapprove of their decision and said they might have changed their minds had they encountered something like this, they did agree that health professionals should be allowed to object to providing abortion services.

All abortion clients in our sample had a medicated abortion. Despite having expressed a high level of satisfaction with the overall service, many of the women said they would have liked to have been able to choose between a medicated and surgical procedure. Two women said they would have preferred a surgical abortion because they perceived the hospital to be a safer place to have the procedure.

"I thought they were going to do the procedure here, not that it had to be in my home. I was very scared. If I had been given a choice, I would have liked to be admitted because I would have felt calmer" (Age 22).

"When they sent me home to take the pill I thought it was risky and that it would be much better to be seen in a hospital" (Age 22).

Opinions on the Uruguay abortion law

Almost all the women interviewed knew about decriminalization of abortion from seeing it on television or in the press, which suggests that the issue had been present in the public discourse. Most found the facility where they obtained abortion services by searching online. All said they were relieved that they did not have to have an illegal or clandestine abortion and saw decriminalization as a major advance with regard to the rights of women in Uruguay. Further, they believed that decriminalization had contributed to changing Uruguayans' overall attitude towards abortion.

"Since there's the law, more [people] are in favor [of women's right to choose]." (Age 22).

"Hopefully no one stops this law, it saves us all, it's a choice so that one can live as one wants, as one likes. It makes no sense to have children to keep them deprived. It's a choice they give us to live well." (Age 29).

These abortion clients became aware of the details of the law and the service—such as the gestational age limit and the abortion method specified in the medical guides—during their first visit to the health care center. When asked about their opinion about the specific aspects of the law, almost all felt that the twelve-week limit was appropriate. Some even felt that it should be earlier due to preconceived—and sometimes inaccurate—views that they held regarding the risks involved and the state of development of the fetus.

> "Up to 12 weeks is okay and that is already a lot, because the baby [sic] is already formed and it's somewhat traumatic, it gives you quite a shock, it had everything: its fingers were formed, even the features on its face. I say that eight weeks would be okay." (Age 29).

However, the majority of those interviewed were in disagreement with the required five-day reflection period, calling it excessive, unnecessary, and torturous.

> "Those five days were endless for me, because when you are sure and you want to be done with it, you want it to be now." (Age 38).

> "If it is already a difficult decision and they make you wait, it becomes torture." (Age 22).

> "You want to be done with it. When they give you that requirement, they don't strictly consider it to be five days. In my case, it was fifteen days." (Age 29).

For these women, there was nothing to think over since they had made up their minds before setting foot in the facility for the first time.

Opinions and attitudes among health professionals who participate in abortion services

Attitudes towards abortion and women who have abortions

In general, health professionals who participate in abortion services in Uruguay had positive opinions about the right to choose and they supported women and their choices. Although each health professional has their own limits with regard to the different aspects of the process, all felt that their perspectives should not influence the care they give their patients. The health professionals interviewed said that they saw abortion as a woman's right and that the decision to terminate a pregnancy is her own business. They believe that each woman has her reasons, that these reasons are worthy, and that their role as medical professionals is not to judge.

> "The reasons are worthy; no one can decide what a woman should do or what is best for her." (Physician).

> "Every woman has the right to terminate a pregnancy for whatever reason. I don't think that it's right or wrong." (Physician).

> "One doesn't stop being a person, but my feelings don't matter when I'm supporting the women. If a woman comes in who is using contraceptives, lives alone, has four children, does not have a pension, and gets pregnant, of course we'll feel more empathy than for a woman who does not take care of herself, who doesn't care whether she gets pregnant; but regardless of my feelings and opinions, the decision is the woman's." (Physician).

All participants felt that their professional duty was strictly to provide information and services. One health professional expressed this recurrent feeling eloquently by explaining that their professional duty is defined in terms of how they can support the patient's needs:

> "What matters most to me is to support the patient; that's why I became a gynecologist." (Physician).

In general, health professionals saw abortions as difficult situations for women; as an experience that no woman wants to have to begin with, and certainly as one that none would want to repeat. Thus, they see abortion overall as a watershed experience in their lives.

> "The experience is an abortion in general, whether medicated or surgical. The experience marks a before and an after." (Physician).

In terms of their opinion of abortion itself, several health professionals saw it simply as one more sexual and reproductive health service; as a routine procedure in their daily professional life, the same as a gynecological exam or a pelvic exam on a pregnant woman. With regard to repeat abortions, most saw them as a result of errors of a medical system that is unable to provide effective training on contraception and the Uruguayan mentality that still sees sexuality as a taboo. But nonetheless, they did not believe that women use abortion as contraception.

> "It's mostly the system's fault, due to a lack of understanding, time, or information. It is not an ideal

situation; it's not that I like it, but I don't place the blame on the patient." (Physician).

We did not find a clear trend regarding health professionals' preference about whether or not to talk about providing abortion services outside the workplace. Some health professionals talk about it openly:

"I talk about my job with everyone. Family, friends, colleagues. At the family level, sometimes there are differences on the subject of principles or religious values." (Physician).

While others prefer discretion, noting that they only "talk about [their] job with few people." (Midwife).

In general, these health professionals expressed great satisfaction with the increase of legal abortion services in the country, without denying that abortion stigma still exists in Uruguayan society. When asked directly about its existence, the interviewed health professionals described this stigma in the following ways:

"[...] it shows in abortion clients' fear, and is manifested quietly, with rejection and with indifference." (Physician).

"[...] it exists. I don't know if it's to such an extent as to produce consequences. When the law was being defended, a segment of society demonstrated their opposition." (Physician).

"Many patients who do terminate [pregnancies] want to keep it a secret for fear of what others might say. Where I work, it's a small town; people gossip about this and are judgmental. These comments affect patients emotionally." (Physician).

"Uruguay is a stigmatizing society around abortion and a number of other issues." (Psychiatrist).

Attitudes towards health professionals who participate in abortion services

In general, health professionals said they were comfortable with their work teams and believe that their experiences since decriminalization have been positive. Only one health professional reported difficulties in the social context where they work, which is not in the city of Montevideo:

"Since it's a small town, people ask questions and try to judge, but we try to maintain confidentiality." (Physician).

One of the most common complaints was that there is great demand for abortion services and few service health professionals:

"[...] the greatest obstacle is patient demand where sometimes we feel a little overloaded; more human resources are needed and more time given to visits." (Physician).

High demand sometimes hinders the process:

"Delays in the process make [some] women still prefer clandestine abortions. The process is very long; so they prefer to do it outside." (Midwife).

Although all of those interviewed respected the right of other health professionals to object, they see objection as a significant obstacle, since it can affect women's decisions and hinder overall service. Some health professionals also mentioned health centers that have not been able to put together abortion teams because in some cases there is a scarcity of gynecologists who are willing to prescribe the abortion medication.

Health professionals felt that administrative staff within hospitals also needed further training, given that, together with the objectors, when they manifest stigmatizing views they too constitute a substantial barrier that negatively impacts the quality of abortion services.

"Improving access to the different services and the interaction among them, for example, with the administrative side, nursing, medical staff, laboratory, they should have periodic meetings to fine-tune issues. Administrators and doctors see voluntary termination of pregnancy in totally different ways." (Physician).

"Not a single administrator works with us [the IVE teams]; there is a lot of turnover in receptionists and they aren't trained." (Midwife).

"Very good work is done on logistics, on timing, coordination. The only detail is with the sonographers, because this needs special handling and technicians are not always trained and can intimidate patients." (Physician).

The majority of the health professionals who participate in legal abortion services reported having received training before the law went into effect. However, all participants expressed interest in receiving further training in abortion service delivery, including some who want to be trained in vacuum aspiration procedures or care for complications from incomplete abortions.

Health professionals mentioned the bias that exists in the type of abortion procedure they provide, which is almost always medicated abortion. They all confirmed that women are not given a choice between a surgical and medicated procedure. One reason they preferred to provide medicated abortion was because they perceived surgical abortion to have more complications and to cost more.

> "It is an option that suits all parties: the woman, because she can do it at home in a setting that is not unfamiliar and if we talk about it as a law, that abortion is medicated and not surgical, it serves the state itself and the different institutions, and health professionals. It's more economical than hospitalizing all those women." (Physician).

Others explain the preference for medicated abortion in terms of training, in other words, many health professionals have not been trained to provide aspiration abortions. But in general, most are quite pleased with the widespread use of medicated abortion. Some health professionals also described preference for providing the pills because they could avoid being present during expulsion. Some even said that if they had to perform aspiration abortions they would become objectors.

> "If the woman requests the surgical method, I withdraw. I wouldn't have my colleagues' support. The situation would get messy. I believe that the woman has to accept that she is the one who is terminating the pregnancy." (Physician).

> "I always say what I do, and that I don't have to actively participate in the termination. If I had to participate actively I would conscientiously object. I had a very bad experience with a fetus when I was a resident, and I said that I wouldn't do that again because it was very traumatic." (Physician).

However, several health professionals believe that patients should be able to choose their preferred abortion method and that health professionals should adhere to their role of providing complete and accurate information on the available options. For most, their primary concern was to not endanger the woman's life and to prevent complications in order to minimize the risk of empowering their opponents:

> "We take care of the woman and we take care of the law because if a complication occurs the opponents will take advantage of it." (Physician).

Opinions on the Uruguay abortion law

Some health professionals believed that following decriminalization in 2012, attitudes in the medical community changed and that the right to choose is increasingly being seen in a better light.

> "Yes, I have seen colleagues who were not very convinced that this is a right [...], and there are others who are conscientious objectors. But in general, the attitude [towards abortion] is more open now." (Physician).

> "Discussion about the issue is a little more fluid and open; even though you may or may not agree, the woman's decision is respected." (Physician).

> "Colleagues who were very negative seem calmer now." (Physician).

Almost everyone believes that implementation of legal abortion services has been very successful across the country. However, the health professionals interviewed outside the capital thought that this success is more obvious in Montevideo and that women outside the capital continued to experience much more difficulty in accessing services.

Opinion was divided on the five-day reflection period. Some think that rather than being a time for reflection, the five days are disrespectful to the patient and stigmatize her, because they challenge a decision that has already been made.

> "I don't think it's advisable, I think it's more a contradiction: we say that we respect the patient and then we tell her to go think about her decision." (Physician).

> "Most women have already thought about it and they come in to terminate; very few decide to continue with the pregnancy after counseling." (Physician).

> "There shouldn't be a set time period. For some it simply does more harm. The person already thought about it before coming to the clinic." (Midwife).

Some health professionals would prefer to have this requirement removed. Other health professionals believe that it is an adequate period, as long as the wait does not result in exceeding the legal gestational age limit. Others believed that the five days were critical because they enabled women to think without pressure and, in some cases, to continue their pregnancies.

There was consensus that the gestational age limit was appropriate although some believe the limit should be lowered to ten weeks. This is due to the overall view that "[t]he more weeks that go by, the greater the risk to the patient." (Physician).

Discussion

Qualitative studies in Uruguay before decriminalization of abortion discussed how the restrictive context was creating high levels of fear, uncertainty, and anxiety among women seeking to terminate a pregnancy. Not only was there a high risk to the health and lives of these women, but some were also exposed to painful emotional experiences and to stigma related to clandestine abortion [20, 21]. This paper sought to take the pulse of this abortion stigma after the legal context changed in Uruguay, following the decriminalization of abortion up to 12 weeks of pregnancy. Therefore, attitudes and perceptions were assessed not only from legal abortion clients, but also from health professionals who participated in abortion services.

It is likely that Uruguay is a unique country in the region in two ways: first, there is a deep commitment by the health professionals who have been advancing the sexual and reproductive rights agenda, in particular through the development and implementation of an innovative harm-reduction model, which helped increase access to safe abortion and usher in decriminalization. Second, in Uruguay there seems to be surprisingly little influence of religious sectors and of religious beliefs on sexual and reproductive health issues. For both abortion clients and health professionals, decriminalization in Uruguay followed logically from this unique history of experimentation with a harm-reduction model that significantly reduced maternal morbidity and mortality. Both health professionals and abortion clients in this study saw decriminalization as a key factor that contributed to mitigating negative social views surrounding abortion and to a substantial reduction of clandestine abortions. In this sense, it is undeniable that decriminalization has contributed towards reducing abortion stigma for both women and health professionals [22, 23].

That said, abortion stigma continues to exist for both women seeking an abortion and health professionals involved in abortion services. In particular, there are several key moments within the service where stigma is more likely to emerge. The first of these involves the mandated five-day reflection period, which almost all clients and some of the health professionals saw as onerous and unnecessary. This requirement has the potential to reproduce stigma because it carries within it an implicit distrust of women's decision and an assumption that women have not fully considered its consequences before arriving to seek care.

Secondly, the exclusive use of medicated abortion also has the potential to reproduce stigmatizing ideas about abortion as "dirty work." On the one hand, some health professionals see the preferential use of medicated abortion as a welcome means to avoid hands-on participation in a medicated procedure deemed undesirable. On the other hand, as evidenced by our data, the near-exclusive use of medicated abortion allows some providers to shift the moral and de facto onus of interrupting a pregnancy entirely to women. The implicit message in both of these cases is clear: these professionals prefer to separate themselves from "participating" in abortions, thereby emphasizing the idea that abortion is "dirty work." Finally, although there is strong scientific evidence to support the prevalent use of medicated abortions [3, 24, 25], the failure to provide women with a choice may negatively impact their experience with the service. In an ideal setting, as our informants corroborate, women would be given an opportunity to choose their preferred abortion method. Since the law permits both types of procedures, it is clear that in the Uruguayan case there is space for additional training that expands medical expertise in the epidemiology and technical aspects of various methods, in particular vacuum aspiration.

Finally, with respect to the operation of stigma within the clinical setting, both health professionals and clients identified clinical personnel who do not participate in abortion services as potential perpetuators of stigma. Clinical personnel who were not involved in abortion services can be divided into two types: broad administrative staff and objectors. The latter were identified as enhancers of stigma when their behavior chastised or otherwise "exposed" clients as wrongdoers. In the case of administrative personnel more broadly, both clients and health professionals identified some of them as de facto gatekeepers who actively obstruct access to abortion services or treat abortion clients differently than clients seeking other services. Health professionals in particular saw this as a shortcoming in the structure of service provision resulting from a lack of training and awareness-raising for hospitals' technical and administrative personnel with whom women are obliged to interact.

Health professionals were generally comfortable about their jobs in abortion teams and expressed overwhelmingly positive attitudes towards the law. Women also expressed that they felt supported by health professionals who through their compassionate and efficient care often dissipated many of the fears and preconceptions that women held before arriving at the clinic. Health care providers and women benefited from strong professional abortion teams, which provided emotional and technical support to all involved. This aspect of clinical care is reflected in other decriminalized contexts and is a component of the Uruguayan model that should be considered for replication. Both clients and health professionals felt that social attitudes were visibly changing as a result of decriminalization. Future research should continue to document the unfolding of long-term impact of decriminalization on women's access to safe abortion provision as well as perceived and experienced stigma.

It is clear from our interviews, however, that both women and health professionals believed that abortion is always and necessarily a traumatic experience for women; an experience that marks them for life. That is, although perceptions of the law, of safe abortion, and of the rights of women were generally positive, women and providers still looked down on women that had one or more abortions, saw abortion as a weight that women were to carry for the rest of their lives, and that necessarily marked a before and after. In many of these cases the persistence of guilt or judgment reveals the persistence of social stigma despite the legal change. Thus, it is recommended that interventions designed to reduce stigma should not be limited to clinical settings, but rather should include community-level interventions aimed at interrupting stigmatizing social views, and providing spaces for the reproduction of ideas and practices that normalize abortion and contribute towards further de-stigmatization.

Finally, we would like to point to some of the limitations of this study. In particular, the fact that women were interviewed immediately following their fourth visit meant that the data cannot track whether attitudes towards abortion changed substantially over longer periods of time. It is also important to note that we only interviewed women and providers involved in legal abortion services and therefore this study cannot speak towards the circulation of stigma in clandestine settings.

Conclusion

Overall, this study reveals that although decriminalization does contribute to mitigating abortion stigma, even in legal clinical settings, there can remain practices that perpetuate the notion that abortion is a dirty and morally questionable practice. For example, the refusal to carry out surgical procedure replicates the idea that direct involvement is "dirty work." Medicated abortion devolves the moral responsibility to women and since it is the only method available de facto, it limits opportunities for women to choose the way the termination will be carried out. Likewise, the five-day reflection period questions a woman's motives and would seem to implicitly suggest that the ideal decision would be to continue the pregnancy. Further, while abortion clients reported high levels of satisfaction with services, we have identified several key points where stigma is prone to reappearing in service delivery. For example, stigma affects services when women interact with personnel that do not participate in the abortion teams and who are not sensitive to the issue, or when women are unable to obtain care when encountering objectors. Among women and health professionals alike the idea prevails that abortion is something that leaves a mark, and in the case of women this is accompanied by a negative moral judgment toward other women who have abortions, in particular those who have more than one abortion, and those who do not show remorse. Yet, almost all women said that they themselves did not feel judged during the procedure and the health professionals stated that they did not feel rejected by their colleagues, including those are objectors. It is important to underscore that the legal framework has had a decisive impact on abortion stigma and greatly improves women's experience seeking abortion care.

Endnotes

[1]Hereon after, we will refer to abortion providers as health professionals who participate in abortion services, or simply as health professionals. We do this in order to highlight the broad spectrum of work that these professionals are involved in, rather than pigeonholing their work as simply abortion provision.

[2]IVE is the acronym for *Interrupción Voluntaria del Embarazo* (Voluntary Interruption of Pregnancy), which has become a term in its own right in Uruguay, and is often used instead of the word abortion. Accordingly, IVE1, IVE 2, IVE3 and IVE 4 are used to refer to each of the four mandatory clinical visits established by the clinical guides. In this piece, we primarily use the word abortion but have opted to keep IVE when its meaning is not fully captured by the term abortion. In addition, we have used Visit 1, 2, 3, and 4 to substitute for the IVE terminology described above.

[3]Note that in August 2015, a ruling by the Court of Administrative Disputes overturned 7 of the 11 articles in the decree, which were challenged by a group of gynecologists arguing that it restricted their right to conscientious objection. As a result of this ruling, the scope of objection was expanded to include not only gynecologists who prescribe the drug, but also other health providers (e.g., sonographers and nurses) who are involved in preparatory procedures and consultations prior to the termination where information and counseling are provided (Visits 1 and 2).

[4]It bears to note that in Uruguay abortion outside the health system continues to be penalized.

[5]Within the hospital, recruitment and analysis was done in partnership with *Iniciativas Sanitarias*, a leading coalition of sexual and reproductive health professionals whose work advances sexual and reproductive health and rights as a basic human right for women and men in Uruguay.

Acknowledgements
The authors would like to acknowledge the women who participated in the interviews and shared their experiences.

Funding
The funding for this research was made possible by anonymous private donors.

Authors' contributions
RC participated in the research design, data collection, analysis and write up of the article. AL participated in the research design and helped facilitate local data collection by identifying interviewers and streamlining recruitment of participants. SB participated in the research design, data collection, analysis and write up of the article. FC coordinated all local interviewers, oversaw participant recruitment and follow up, and revised preliminary drafts of the manuscript. IL recruited and interviewed research participants and revised preliminary drafts of the manuscript. SA recruited and interviewed research participants and revised preliminary drafts of the manuscript. JF secured funding for this research project, managed local and international research teams, participated in research design and revised preliminary drafts of the manuscript.

Competing interests
The authors declare that they have no competing interests.

Author details
[1]International Planned Parenthood/Western Hemisphere Region, New York, USA. [2]Hampshire College, Amherst, USA. [3]Iniciativas Sanitarias, Montevideo, Uruguay. [4]Ibis Reproductive Health, Oakland, USA.

References
1. Ellison MA. Authoritative knowledge and single women's unintentional pregnancies, abortions, adoption, and single motherhood: social stigma and structural violence. Med Anthropol Q September. 2003;17:322–47.
2. Major B, Gramzow RH. Abortion as stigma: cognitive and emotional implications of concealment. J Pers Soc Psychol October. 1999;77:735–45.
3. Goffman E. Stigma; notes on the management of spoiled identity. Englewood cliffs, NJ: Prentice-Hall; 1963.
4. Link BG, Phelan JC. Conceptualizing Stigma. Annu Rev Sociol. 2001;27:363–85.
5. Sedgh G, Henshaw S, Singh S, Åhman E, Shah IH. Induced abortion: estimated rates and trends worldwide. Lancet October. 2007;370:1338–45.
6. Finer LB, Zolna MR. Unintended pregnancy in the United States: incidence and disparities, 2006. Contraception November 2011;84:478–485.
7. Cockrill K, Nack A. 'I'm not that type of person': managing the stigma of having an abortion. Deviant Behav December. 2013;34:973–90.
8. Norris A, Bessett D, Steinberg JR, Kavanaugh ML, Zordo SD, Becker D. Abortion stigma: a reconceptualization of constituents, causes, and Consequences Womens Health Issues May 2011;21 Suppl 3: 49–54.
9. Kumar A, Hessini L, Mitchell EMH. Conceptualising abortion stigma. Cult Health Sex August. 2009;11:625–39.
10. Shellenberg KM, Moore AM, Bankole A, Juarez F, Omideyi AK, Palomino N, et al. Social stigma and disclosure about induced abortion: results from an exploratory study. Glob Public Health September 2011;6 Suppl 1:111–125.
11. Sorhaindo AM, Juárez-Ramírez C, Díaz Olavarrieta C, Aldaz E, Mejía Piñeros MC, Garcia S. Qualitative evidence on abortion stigma from Mexico City and five states in Mexico. Women Health. 2014;54:622–40.
12. Joffe CE. Doctors of conscience: the struggle to provide abortion before and after roe v. Wade. Boston: Beacon Press; 1995.
13. Harris LH, Debbink M, Martin L, Hassinger J. Dynamics of stigma in abortion work: findings from a pilot study of the providers share workshop. Soc Sci med 1982. October. 2011;73:1062–70.
14. World Health Organization: Trends in maternal mortality: 1990 to 2015. http://www.who.int/reproductivehealth/publications/monitoring/maternal-mortality-2015/en/ (2015). Accessed 23 Aug 2016.
15. Organización Mundial de la Salud: Estadísticas Sanitarias Mundiales 2012. http://www.who.int/gho/publications/world_health_statistics/2012/es/ (2012). Accessed 23 Aug 2016.
16. Lamas M. Entre el estigma y la ley: La interrupción legal del embarazo en el DF. Salud Públ Méx February 2014;56(1):56–62.
17. Galli B, Sydow E. Autonomia Reprodutiva EM Questão: Relatos De Mulheres sobre Aborto E Estigma EM Mato Grosso do Sul (reproductive autonomy at stake: Women's histories on abortion and stigma in Mato Grosso do Sul, Brazil). Social Science Research Network. 2010; http://papers.ssrn.com/abstract=2703948 Accessed 15 Jun 2016
18. Zordo SD. Representações e experiências sobre aborto legal e ilegal dos ginecologistas-obstetras trabalhando em dois hospitais maternidade de Salvador da Bahia. Ciênc Saúde Coletiva. 2012;17:1745–54.
19. Faúndes A, Duarte GA, Osis MJD. Conscientious objection or fear of social stigma and unawareness of ethical obligations. Int J Gynecol Obstet. 2013; 123 Suppl 3:57–9.
20. Lopez GA, Berro EC. Efectos del aborto clandestino en la subjetividad de las mujeres: resultados de una investigación cualitativa en Uruguay. BDDOC CSIC: Sumarios ISOC - Ciencias Sociales y Humanidades. 2010; http://revpubli.unileon.es/ojs/index.php/cuestionesdegenero/article/view/3784 Accessed 23 Aug 2016
21. Rostagnol S, Viera M, Grabino V, Mesa S. Transformaciones y continuidades de los sentidos del aborto voluntario en Uruguay: del AMEU al misoprostol. Bagoas. 2013;7:17–42. http://www.mec.gub.uy/innovaportal/file/48018/1/transformaciones-y-continuidades-de-los-sentidos-del-aborto-voluntario-en-uruguay.pdf . Accessed 15 Jun 2016
22. Briozzo, L. From risk and harm reduction to decriminalizing abortion: the Uruguayan model for women's rights. Int J Gynaecol Obstet 2016; 134 Suppl1: 3–6.
23. Labandera A, Gorgoroso M, Briozzo L. Implementation of the risk and harm reduction strategy against unsafe abortion in Uruguay: from a university hospital to the entire country. Int J Gynaecol Obstet. 2016;134(Suppl 1):7–11.
24. Zamberlin N, Romero M, Ramos S. Latin American women's experiences with medical abortion in settings where abortion is legally restricted. Reprod Health; December 2012;9:34.
25. Fiol V, Rieppi L, Aguirre R, Nozar M, Gorgoroso M, Coppola F, Briozzo L. The role of medical abortion in the implementation of the law on voluntary termination of pregnancy in Uruguay. Int J Gynaecol Obstet. 2016;134(Suppl 1):12–5.

Experiences of antenatal care among pregnant adolescents at Kanyama and Matero clinics in Lusaka district, Zambia

Bwalya C. Bwalya[1*], Doreen Sitali[2], Kumar Sridutt Baboo[2] and Joseph M. Zulu[2]

Abstract

Background: Adolescent pregnancy is among the many public health concerns not only in Zambia but also in other parts of the world. Exploring pregnant adolescents' experiences of antenatal care may help to identify specific problems and the contextual relevant strategies to improve the access to antenatal care. The purpose of this study was to explore and describe the lived experiences of antenatal care among pregnant adolescents aged between 12 to 19 years old at Kanyama and Matero Referral Clinics in Lusaka district of Zambia.

Methods: This was a qualitative study which used in-depth interviews to collect data. Maximum variation sampling technique was used to select 12 pregnant adolescents of 12 to 19 years age range that attended antenatal care. Data were analysed thematically with the help of Nvivo software version 10.

Results: The study revealed that the adolescents experienced positive and negative antenatal care. While there were some reported cases of caring and friendly health care providers and older pregnant women, there were also reported cases of poor attitudes and behaviours by the older pregnant women and health care providers towards the adolescents. In addition, other issues that were reported by the adolescents were the opening hours for the health facilities which was not favourable to all adolescents and the lack of specific spaces for adolescents as well as inadequate privacy and confidentiality. Some solutions were suggested to overcome some of the problems such as reducing the waiting hours or time for consultations at the clinic and to have specific rooms or spaces for pregnant adolescents at the clinic.

Conclusion: Appropriate interventions targeting pregnant adolescents with emphasis on making antenatal care services more adolescent friendly may improve the quality of and accessibility of antenatal services. The adolescent friendly antenatal services should integrate health promotion activities aimed at sensitising elderly women within the health facilities on the importance of supporting pregnant adolescents.

Keywords: Pregnant adolescents, Antenatal care, Experiences

Plain English summary

There are several adolescent pregnancies in Zambia and other low and middle income countries. These adolescent pregnancies pose a serious health risk to the adolescents. Meanwhile, many of these adolescents have difficulties to access antenatal care services and comprehensive strategies to address these challenges are lacking.

* Correspondence: bwalyasinyangwe@gmail.com; bwalyachisosobwalya@yahoo.com
[1]Ministry of Education, Matero Girls Secondary School, P.O Box 32979, Lusaka, Zambia
Full list of author information is available at the end of the article

Using interviews with 12 adolescent mothers, the study explored the challenges and positive issues that adolescents aged between 12 to 19 years experience when accessing antenatal care at Kanyama and Matero Referral Clinics in Lusaka district of Zambia. Also, strategies to address these challenges were documented.

Adolescents reported that the barriers to accessing health services included poor attitudes and behaviours of some older pregnant women and health care providers towards the adolescents, the opening hours for health facilities being unfavourable to most adolescents, lack of specific rooms or spaces for adolescents as well as inadequate privacy and confidentiality. In order to improve the access to the services, adolescents recommended that it was important to reduce the waiting time before consultations at the clinic and to have specific rooms or spaces for pregnant adolescents.

In conclusion, to effectively improve the access to antenatal services by pregnant adolescents, there is need for increased sensitisation of adult women and health workers on the importance of supporting adolescents during antenatal care.

Background

Adolescent pregnancy is one of the sexual and reproductive health (SRH) problems that several low and middle income countries (LMICs) [1] experience. It accounts for about 11% of all births worldwide (WHO, 2014) and 95% of these births occur in LMICs [1]. In Zambia, approximately 3 in every 10 adolescents aged between 15 to 19 years have either given birth or are pregnant [2]. However, adolescent pregnancy is associated with various maternal health-related complications and deaths. For instance, it has been documented worldwide that pregnancy and childbirth related complications are among the leading causes of death for adolescent girls aged between 15 to 19 years [1, 3]. In addition, research has also shown that girls who give birth before the age of 16 years are three to four times more likely to suffer maternal death than women in their twenties [2].

Additionally, adolescents are more likely to suffer from other pregnancy related complications [2, 4] such as obstructed labour [5], toxemia, hemorrhage, hypertension and anaemia [6], low birth weight, premature delivery, preeclampsia and anaemia [4] among others. Research has also shown that most of these maternal-related complications mentioned above can be avoided through timely access to quality antenatal health care services as it presents an opportunity to prevent or manage pregnant related risks [7–12].

According to Chama [10], antenatal care provides a platform to inform and educate expectant mothers about pregnancy and the importance of seeking skilled health care during the time before and after birth. The goal of antenatal care is to provide regular checkups that would enable doctors or midwives to screen, prevent, detect and treat potential health complications that may arise in pregnant women [3, 6]. To be specific, it provides a platform to identify and manage any maternal-related complications or risk factors [3, 4] such as pregnancy induced hypertension, malaria and anaemia which put at risk the life of both the mother and unborn baby.

In addition, antenatal care offers a conducive environment to health care providers to interact with the pregnant women on issues affecting their health and that of the unborn child because health issues are discussed at length during antenatal classes. These issues include nutrition education, information about the risk of cigarette smoking, family planning, exclusive breast feeding, immunization, care of the newborn as well as the importance of rest, hygiene and safer sex [4]. In general, studies have shown that women want and expect positive outcomes from antenatal services. These positive experiences include *maintaining physical and sociocultural normality, maintaining a healthy pregnancy for mother and baby including preventing and treating risks, illness and death, having an effective transition to positive labour and birth as well as achieving positive motherhood that includes maternal self-esteem, competence and autonomy* [3, 4].

Despite the benefits of antenatal care, adolescents are less likely to use antenatal care services compared to older women [3, 11]. The reasons for low utilisation of antenatal care services among pregnant adolescents include several issues such as, health worker judgmental attitudes and lack of training in and understanding of adolescents' reproductive needs [12]. There is also fear of humiliation and having to respond to unpleasant questions and procedures during antenatal care. Furthermore, there is lack of respect, privacy and confidentiality within the health care system [3]. Some parents and guardians for adolescent mothers maybe upset in the initial stages of the pregnancy as a result there is limited support from parents to adolescents with regard to proper guidance on attending antenatal care services. This lack of support and guidance is challenging especially in cases where adolescents depend on their parents for financial support to enable them access health care services [5, 13].

Adolescents or women friendly antenatal care services could be life saving as shown by studies that women may refuse to seek antenatal care from a health care provider who "abuses" them or one who does not treat them well, even if the health care provider is skilled in the prevention and management of pregnancy complications [6, 13].

Several maternal health-related studies have been conducted in Zambia [7, 9]. However, there is limited information specifically on the experiences of antenatal care utilization among pregnant adolescents. Therefore, a comprehensive understanding of lived experiences of pregnant adolescents with regard to the antenatal clinic environment will add value to the existing body of knowledge on issues surrounding maternal and child health in Zambia.

The specific objectives of this study were: (i) to describe the experiences of pregnant adolescents with the healthcare providers at the antenatal care clinic; (ii) to describe the experiences of pregnant adolescents with older pregnant women within the antenatal care clinic;

and (iii) to describe the experiences of pregnant adolescents with education provided at as part of antenatal care.

Methods

Study design

This study was a qualitative phenomenological study. "A phenomenological study focuses on describing what all participants have in common as they experience a phenomenon" [14]. Phenomenology provides a deep understanding of a phenomenon as experienced by several individuals. Data is collected from people who have experienced the phenomenon and develops a composite description of the experience for all the individuals. In line with the phenomenological design, this study focused on describing "what" the (adolescents) experienced and "how" they experienced it [14], as opposed to proving and disapproving a hypothesis or predicting why particular adolescents had different experiences with the health care providers or with the older pregnant women in the clinics.

This design and approach allowed the researchers to explore and develop an in-depth understanding of the experiences and perceptions of pregnant adolescents attending antenatal clinics at Kanyama and Matero Referral Clinics. In particular, the design and approach enabled the researchers to uncover details about the experiences of pregnant adolescents within the antenatal clinic environment.

Study area

The study was conducted at Kanyama and Matero Referral Clinics in Lusaka district, the Capital city of Zambia. These two clinics offer first level health care services to the surrounding communities and are both located in what are considered densely populated areas. Purposive sampling technique was used to select these two clinics based on the availability of antennal care services.

Study sample

The research participants for this study were 12 pregnant adolescents of between 15 and 19 years old who had attended two or more antenatal care visits at their respective clinics in the two research sites. The research participants were purposively selected to take part in the study from Kanyama and Matero Referral Clinics. All the names that met the inclusion criteria were identified from the antenatal care records at the clinics. Eligible pregnant adolescents were those who (a) were antenatal care attendees at the two respective research sites; (b) were between 12 to 19 years old; and (c) those who voluntarily gave consent to participate in the study. Participants were then informed about the nature of the study during the process of recruitment. For those adolescents that were below 17 years old, their parents or guardians were then contacted for parental consent.

Maximum variation sampling frame was used as a guide to determine the sample size for the study. This type of purposive sampling was applied in order to capture maximum variation in terms of age. Eight age categories of pregnant adolescents were identified (from 12 to 19 years old). From each of the eight categories, two participants, one per site, were sampled, thus bringing the total of the initial target sample size to 16 pregnant adolescents. However, only 12 participants were interviewed (7 from Matero Referral Clinic. and 5 Kanyama Referral Clinic). This was due to the fact that no new information came out from the interviews. In addition, participants from the category of 12 to 14 years old were unavailable at the time of conducting the study.

Data collection

Data were collected using semi-structured interviews. The interviews were conducted within the two clinic premises. A quiet and private room was used for the interviews. On average, the interviews lasted 30 minutes. All the interviews were audio recorded with permission from the participants.

Data analysis

The audio recorded interviews were transcribed and imported into Nvivo software version 10. The software was used to facilitate data management and analysis of emerging themes. Thematic analysis was used to analyse interview transcripts. Several broad themes were predetermined based on the questions from the interview guide on the experiences of antenatal care among pregnant adolescents. Additional themes were generated from the ideas that were coming out from the responses of participants as we read through the transcripts.

Ethical consideration

Ethical approval to conduct the study was granted by the University of Zambia Biomedical Research Ethical Committee (UNZABREC) at the University of Zambia. Approval to conduct the study at the two health facilities was also granted by the two sisters-in-charge. Voluntary written informed consent, assent and parental or guardian consent were also obtained from all the research participants.

Results

A total of 12 pregnant adolescents aged between 15 to 19 years participated in the study. The participants were receiving antenatal care services at the time of the interviews. Direct quotations from the raw data were provided to support the description of the experiences and the findings of the study. The true identities of participants were replaced with pseudonyms (the first number represented the age of the participant and the last number on the left represented the I.D number for the participant whereas letters represented the study site: K for Kanyama Referral Clinic and M for Matero referral clinic). The results were organised as follows: Experiences with service providers;

(i) Experiences with other service users;
(ii) Experiences of antenatal education; and
(iii) Health facility related challenges.

Experiences with health service providers

There were variations regarding the experiences of pregnant adolescents with health care providers at the clinics. While some adolescents had positive experiences, others had negative experiences. Below are the detailed explanations of their experiences with the health care providers.

Good reception by service providers, a motivating factor to accessing services

Most study participants from both Kanyama and Matero Referral Clinics revealed that their relationship with the health care service providers was good. This good relationship was attributed to the good reception and the general care that adolescents received from health providers. An 18 year-old participant from Kanyama Clinic explained this good relationship as follows:

> *"I have a good relationship with the nurses. They welcomed me very well the first-time l came here with my husband and they are very educative" 18-K10*

Negative health worker attitudes discouraging health service utilisation

Although some pregnant adolescents had good experiences with the health care providers, other participants encountered negative attitudes and behaviours from them during the antenatal care service. Some adolescents complained that the nurses were sometimes rude in the way they communicated with them. One participant reported that one nurse was rude in the way she spoke to her when she stated that:

> *"The first time the nurse was rude because I didn't understand her instructions clearly" 15-K8*

Another research participant echoed a similar negative experience with regards to the attitudes and behaviour of health care providers at Matero Clinic. The doctor shouted at her for not waiting for two years before conceiving the second time. Below is how the adolescent explained her situation:

> *"I had a pregnancy last year that ended up in an operation but I lost the baby. When I came back for antenatal this year I requested for a referral to go to another hospital from the in charge.. Instead, she started scolding at me for having not waited for 2 years before getting pregnant again... I was hurt with the words she used," 19-M12.*

The participants also felt that they were being discriminated against by the health care providers because of their marital status. The reasons cited for this was that health workers gave first priority to those that went with their partners for antenatal care. They complained that the nurses first attended to the couples before they attended to the adolescents despite reporting to the clinic much earlier than the said couples:

> *"I don't like the way this clinic operates because they give first priority to those women who come with their husbands... even when they come late for antenatal care" 16-K11.*

Experiences with other service users

The participants narrated different experiences with older pregnant women with whom they attended the same antenatal classes at their respective clinics. Some adolescents had positive experiences while others experienced stigma and unfriendly interactions with the older women.

The integration of adolescents and older women facilitates exchange of experiences

At both Kanyama and Matero Referral Clinics, there is no separation between adolescents and the older women in antenatal classes. The participants in this study expressed different views on how they related with the older women during antenatal care. Generally, most of the research participants reported that they had healthy relationships with older expectant mothers. Some adolescents reported that the older women provided them with advice on how to take care of their pregnancy and that they got along very well during antenatal care as one adolescent said:

> *"l ask them pregnancy related questions... They teach me on how to take care of my pregnancy such as, what to eat, not to sleep too much and carry heavy things and preparations for my delivery..... They teach me things l don't know" 19-M2.*

However, a few pregnant adolescents reported that during their interaction with the older women, they encountered negative experiences. Older women were perceived to be unfriendly or uninterested in the adolescents when they did not initiate or engage themselves in any conversations with the adolescents. Such encounters with the older women at the clinics made the adolescents feel out of place, uncomfortable, ashamed and discouraged to attend antenatal care services:

"Others don't really want to be talked to but others are very interesting and welcoming.... I feel lonely because some women are not friendly. They spend most of their time on the phone" 19-M9.

Experiences of stigma were also indicated as additional challenges faced by the adolescents at the clinic. Some adolescents complained of lack of respect by the older women. These experiences of lack of respect often arose through their contact with the older women who came for the same services. According to the adolescents, this lack of respect made them feel ashamed and uncomfortable thereby triggering stigmatization:

"I overheard some pregnant women talking in a mocking manner when I went to call my husband. This made me to feel uncomfortable and ashamed of myself. They were even laughing at me" 15-K8.

Experiences of antenatal education

There were different views on the usefulness of antenatal education by the participants. Overall, the participants highlighted their positive learning outcomes of antenatal education. These positive outcomes mainly focused on prevention, treatment as well as management of diseases.

Antenatal education very beneficial

When the issue of what was learned at antenatal was explored, the majority of the participants said that they learnt on how to take good care of themselves during pregnancy. They had learnt about HIV prevention and management, and in particular how the risk of mother to child transmission could be reduced.

"They teach us about HIV...how one can get HIV... and how to take care of ourselves when you are pregnant. I share this information with others what I learn here" 16-M1

Several other learning outcomes from the interviews were identified and these revolved around facts concerning prevention of malaria, what constitutes a healthy diet for both the mother and the unborn child, the effects of drinking or smoking on the baby and the mother and preparations for delivery.

"I learnt that a pregnant woman should not smoke or drink alcohol" 17-K6

Operating hours for antenatal care a challenge for some adolescents

Several concerns regarding the operating hours of the antenatal clinic were expressed by the study participants. Long waiting hours in the queue for consultation as well as long periods of time spent at the clinic were among the many concerns raised by the adolescents.

There are specific services that are routinely provided at Kanyama and Matero Referral Antenatal Clinics such as weight measurement, physical assessment of pregnancy, laboratory tests and immunizations. The standard operating hours for antenatal care for both Kanyama and Matero Referral Clinics is between 08:00 to 13:00 h. When asked what time, they arrived at the clinic for antenatal care, the participants gave different responses. The majority of the participants arrive at the clinic before 07:30 h, while others come at 08:00 h.

"I have to come as early as 06:00 hours" 17-K6

Pregnant adolescents also had different opinions regarding their preferred time frame to spend at the antenatal care. Some participants suggested 08:00 to 12:00 h as the most convenient time to spend at the clinic so that they could have enough time to do other things at home.

"08:30–12:00 or14:00 is ok with me so that I can go home and sleep because the fansidar we take make us drowsy" 19-M2

Too early at the health facility and yet being attended to late

Some participants complained that sometimes they could wait for about 2 to 3 h during the official antenatal clinic operating hours before they could be attended to by health workers. This was attributed to health care providers performing other tasks before attending to them.

"I wait for long hours before they begin antenatal class.... about 2 to 3 hours" 15-K8

Other research participants also complained about finishing with the clinic as late as 16:00 h in the afternoon despite them going to the clinic very early in the morning. As a result of this they felt hungry.

"I don't like it. I come around 06:00 h I sometimes have to go home at 16:00 h and I usually get very hungry" 17-K7

Health facility related challenges

Lack of adolescent specific spaces

Furthermore, all the study participants reported that the clinics did not provide separate space for antenatal care specifically for adolescents nor did they provide a waiting room for adolescents only. This meant that the pregnant adolescents utilised the same antenatal care services as the older women.

"No, the clinic has no separate space to provide services for adolescents" 18-M5

Some participants felt uncomfortable to share the same spaces with the older women.. . Adolescents also viewed this practice as a sign of lack of respect to the older women due to lack of privacy during the physical assessments of pregnancy.

"No there is no separate room for adolescents that come for antenatal care. We are mixed together with the older pregnant women....l don't like this arrangement because people lose respect. There are times were you see an older woman undressing when the nurse is conducting physical assessments of pregnancies or during delivery in the labour ward... .....Such is not a good thing to experience because she is like my mother"19-M2

"l feel shy when am with older women"18-K10

The pregnant adolescents were put in the same antenatal class as the older pregnant women. Other participants reported that the older women had the tendency of dominating the class discussions and would pass derogatory comments against the adolescents. Some participants did not feel free to participate in the lessons due to the sensitive nature of certain sexual topics. Discussing sexual issues in the presence of adults made the adolescents not to ask questions because they felt shy as attested to by a participant when she said:

"There are always embarrassing topics especially when you come with your partner... about private parts. I do not ask questions during class because I feel shy. I would only ask questions privately" 19-M9

Some participants preferred to attend antenatal classes just for adolescents. Such classes would enable them to freely express themselves and to feel comfortable because they would be with their age mates. Having a specific class for adolescents would enable them to learn more on pregnancy and the related outcomes. To support this assertion, a participant stated that:

"l would like to have a separate class specifically for adolescents because such an arrangement can make me feel free. l will be with my age mates...I am not free to ask questions because l feel shy" 17-K7

Inadequate privacy and confidentiality

Issues of privacy and confidentiality were also brought out by the adolescents. Some participants reported that the counseling and screening sessions were conducted in a private and confidential environment. They felt confident that the sensitive information that they discussed with the health care providers was not overheard or retold to other persons as indicated in the quote hereunder that:

"Yes there is privacy when we come for HIV counseling and testing. No one hears what we discuss during pre-testing and post-testing"19-M3

Other participants however reported that the counselling and examination rooms at the clinic did not guarantee privacy and confidentiality. One adolescent for example, reported that one could hear from outside what the patient and the counsellor were talking about. Lack of privacy was also raised by another participant when she reported that nurses kept on interrupting the counselling session when she said:

"The rooms are not very private because the people outside are able to hear what is being discussed between the counsellor and the patient"18-M4

Overcrowded environment

The other concern was overcrowding due to antenatal classes and children's under five clinics being conducted in the same room and at the same time. Some adolescents reported that they did not pay attention to what was being discussed in the antenatal classes because of the noise that came from the mothers and children that were being attended to as well. It was alleged that:

"We are in the same room with new recruits, the old ones and those that come for under five. This is not good because there is a lot of noise and l can't really hear what we are learning.... So they need to find another place so that we learn more. It's crowded" 19-M9

Discussion

The findings demonstrated that pregnant adolescents had both positive and negative experiences of antenatal care services. Some adolescents expressed appreciation for the healthy relationship they had with the health care providers. A study conducted in the community drop-in program for young women who were pregnant or had an infant below 6 months of age in Canada showed that providing care to adolescents in a friendly manner is important to them [15].

However, other participants felt that they were being discriminated against by health care providers especially when they gave priority to the older couples despite their reporting late. They also described some health care service providers as being rude and disrespectful in the way they communicated with the adolescents. Similar findings were reported in a study done by Duggen and Adejumo [16]. The adolescents, who were recruited from antenatal and postnatal services in South Africa, wanted health care services to be carried out in the same manner as it would be for the adult women.

Ways in which pregnant adolescents interacted with the older pregnant women were revealed. Older women were perceived to be unfriendly when they did not initiate or engage themselves in any conversations with the adolescents. Such encounters with the older women at the clinic made the adolescents feel out of place, uncomfortable, felt a sense of shame and discouraged to even to attend subsequent antenatal care visits. In such an environment, individuals may experience loneliness when they feel that their relationships with others are less satisfying than they would like them to be [6]. Similar findings were also documented [5, 17]. These authors argued that adolescents are fully aware that society tended to judge and discriminate against women who appeared to violate the perceived social or moral conventions such as having sex at a tender age. These social and moral conventions often stemmed from various societal, cultural and religious belief systems that are deeply embedded in the communities. It is therefore recommended that efforts should be made to make pregnant adolescents comfortable within the health care system that is aimed at ensuring that they continued to access appropriate care services and to minimise potential for feeling socially isolated and devalued [16].

Although there is limited information specifically on experiences of antenatal care among adolescents in Zambia, a few studies conducted in antenatal care clinics elsewhere reported findings that are consistent with those in this study [6, 16]. For example, pregnant adolescents perceived adult-oriented antenatal care to be uncomfortable because they shared the same class with the older women. Our findings suggest that pregnant adolescents were unable to freely participate in group antenatal class discussions due to the sensitive nature of certain sexual topics in the midst of adult women and their partners. Consequently, they experienced fear, embarrassment and uneasiness. According to Svanemyr et al. [18], adolescent girls are less likely than the older women to ask, obtain information, discuss and express their worries about sexual and reproductive health issues due to the culture of silence which is deeply embedded in the social norms and taboos related to sexuality in families or the communities. This is particularly the case when it comes to communication with adults either at the clinic or at home.

Some participants complained that they received antennal care services late despite arriving early at the clinic. Other participants complained of the long waiting hours at the health facility. The adolescents made suggestions on the actual time that would best suit them to spend at the clinic. The same concerns were also expressed in other studies [5, 6, 16, 19]. Addressing such delays at the clinic may motivate adolescents to regularly access antennal care services.

Strengths and limitations

This study added useful insight to the body of knowledge on issues surrounding adolescents' maternal health in Zambia. However, the study experienced methodological challenges. Firstly, the study was unable to find pregnant adolescents that represented adolescents from 12 to 14 years old. Only older adolescents (18–19 years old) were the majority participants. Therefore, this study was deprived of insights from the experiences of pregnant adolescents between the ages of 12 to 14 years as they may have had different experiences. Last but not the least, these experiences of antenatal care services among pregnant adolescents cannot be generalised because there are only limited to two health facilities. Therefore, an additional study should be conducted in other clinics outside Lusaka district to explore their experiences of antenatal care services provided to pregnant adolescents.

Conclusion

This study showed that adolescents had both positive and negative experiences with antenatal care services at Kanyama and Matero Referral Clinics. The positive experiences were attributed to a few friendly health care providers and the older expectant mothers who attended the same antenatal care services with the adolescents. Stigma and discrimination, long waiting hours at the clinic and lack of adolescent spaces were among the cited negative experiences among the research participants. Appropriate interventions targeting developing more adolescent friendly maternal health services which should integrate provision of health education to the older women to support pregnant adolescents may result in improved quality of antenatal care and subsequently increased utilisation of the services by adolescents.

Abbreviations

DHMT: University of Zambia and District Health Management Team; LMICs: Low and Middle Income Countries; SRH: Sexual and Reproductive Health; UNZABREC: University of Zambia Biomedical Research Ethical Committee; WHO: World Health Organisation

Acknowledgements

We thank all the adolescents that participated in the study. We also want to thank the Ministry of Health for the permission to use their health facilities, staff and for their support throughout the study.

Funding

The study was funded by the first author as part of her master project on experiences of antenatal care among pregnant adolescents at Kanyama and Matero Referral Clinics in Lusaka district, Zambia.

Author's contributions

BB, JMZ, DS, SB contributed towards the study design. BB and JMZ designed the interview guide. BB collected the data. BB, JMZ conducted the analysis and interpretation. BB, JMZ wrote the article and all authors critically revised the paper. All authors read and approved the final manuscript.

Authors' information

Ms. Bwalya is a student at the University of Zambia, School of Medicine, Department of Public Health Lusaka, Zambia. Dr. J M Zulu, Ms. Doreen Sitali and Prof Kumar S. Baboo are lecturers at the University of Zambia in the School of Public Health.

Competing interests

The authors declare that they have no competing interests.

Author details

[1]Ministry of Education, Matero Girls Secondary School, P.O Box 32979, Lusaka, Zambia. [2]Departments of Public Health, School of Medicine, University of Zambia, P.O. Box 50110, Lusaka, Zambia.

References

1. Morris JL, Rushwan H. Adolescent sexual and reproductive health: the global challenges. Int J Gynecol Obstet. 2015;131:S40–2.
2. Zambia Adolescent Health Strategic Plan (2011-2015), Ministry of Health, Government of the Republic of Zambia.
3. World Health Organisation. WHO recommendations on antenatal Care for a Positive Pregnancy Experience. Geneva: WHO; 2016.
4. Downe S, Finlayson K, Tunçalp Ö, Metin Gülmezoglu A. What matters to women: a systematic scoping review to identify the processes and outcomes of antenatal care provision that are important to healthy pregnant women. BJOG Int J Obstet Gynaecol. 2016;123(4):529–39.
5. Bhandari SD, Joshi S. Perception and perceived experiences about prevention and consequences of teenage pregnancy and childbirth among teenage mothers: a qualitative study. Journal of Advanced Academic Research. 2017; 3(1):164–72.
6. James S, Rall N, Strumpher J. Perceptions of pregnant teenagers with regard to the antenatal care clinic environment. Curationis. 2012;35:1–8.
7. Banda I, Michelo C, Hazemba A. Factors associated with late antenatal care attendance in selected rural and urban communities of the Copperbelt Province of Zambia. Medical Journal of Zambia. 2012;39:29–36.
8. Fernandes RFM, Meincke SMK, Thumé E, Soares MC, Collet N, Carraro TE. Characteristics of antenatal Care for Adolescents from state capitals in southern and North-Eastern Brazil. Texto and Contexto-Enfermagem. 2015;24:80–6.
9. Kyei NN, Campbell OM, Gabrysch S. The influence of distance and level of service provision on antenatal care use in rural Zambia. PLoS One. 2012;7: e46475.
10. Chama-Chiliba CM, Koch SF. Utilisation of focused antenatal Care in Zambia: examining lindividual- and community-level factors using a multilevel analysis. Health Policy Plan. 2015;30:78–87.
11. Dairo M, Owoyokun K. Factors affecting the utilisation of antenatal Care Services in Ibadan, Nigeria. Benin Journal of Postgraduate Medicine. 2010;12(1). https://www.ajol.info/index.php/bjpm/article/view/63387. Accessed 6 July 2018.
12. Atuyambe L, Mirembe F, Tumwesigye NM, Annika J, Kirumira EK, Faxelid E. Adolescent and adult first time Mothers' health seeking practices during pregnancy and early motherhood in Wakiso district, Central Uganda. Reprod Health. 2008;5(1):13.
13. Gyesaw NYK, Ankomah A. Experiences of pregnancy and motherhood among teenage mothers in a suburb of Accra, Ghana: a qualitative study. International Journal of Women's Health. 2013;5:773.
14. Lewis S. Qualitative inquiry and research design: choosing among five approaches. Health Promot Pract. 2015;16(4):473–5.
15. Peterson WE, Sword W, Charles C, Dicenso A. Adolescents' perceptions of inpatient postpartum nursing care. Qual Health Res. 2007;17:201–12.
16. Duggan R, Adejumo O. Adolescent clients' perceptions of maternity Care in Kwazulu-Natal, South Africa. Women and Birth. 2012;25:e62–7.
17. Weed K, Nicholson JS. Differential social evaluation of pregnant teens, teen mothers and teen fathers by university students. International Journal of Adolescence and Youth. 2015;20:1–16.
18. Svanemyr J, Amin A, Robles OJ, Greene ME. Creating an enabling environment for adolescent sexual and reproductive health: a framework and promising approaches. J Adolesc Health. 2015;56:S7–S14.
19. Michels TM. "patients like us": pregnant and parenting teens view the health care system. Public Health Rep. 2000;115:557.

14

Availability and use of magnesium sulphate at health care facilities in two selected districts of North Karnataka, India

Geetanjali Katageri[1], Umesh Charantimath[2*], Anjali Joshi[2], Marianne Vidler[3], Umesh Ramadurg[4], Sumedha Sharma[3], Sheshidhar Bannale[5], Beth A. Payne[3], Sangamesh Rakaraddi[6], Chandrashekhar Karadiguddi[2], Geetanjali Mungarwadi[2], Avinash Kavi[2], Diane Sawchuck[10], Richard Derman[8], Shivaprasad Goudar[2], Ashalata Mallapur[1], Mrutyunjaya Bellad[2], Laura A. Magee[7], Rahat Qureshi[9], Peter von Dadelszen[7] and the Community Level Interventions for Pre-eclampsia (CLIP) India Feasibility Working Group[2,3,9]

From 2nd International Conference on Maternal and Newborn Health: Translating Research Evidence to Practice
Belagavi, India.

Abstract

Background: Pre-eclampsia and eclampsia are major causes of maternal morbidity and mortality. Magnesium sulphate is accepted as the anticonvulsant of choice in these conditions and is present on the WHO essential medicines list and the Indian National List of Essential Medicines, 2015. Despite this, magnesium sulphate is not widely used in India for pre-eclampsia and eclampsia. In addition to other factors, lack of availability may be a reason for sub-optimal usage. This study was undertaken to assess the availability and use of magnesium sulphate at public and private health care facilities in two districts of North Karnataka, India.

Methods: A facility assessment survey was undertaken as part of the Community Level Interventions for Pre-eclampsia (CLIP) Feasibility Study which was undertaken prior to the CLIP Trials (NCT01911494). This study was undertaken in 12 areas of Belagavi and Bagalkote districts of North Karnataka, India and included a survey of 88 facilities. Data were collected in all facilities by interviewing the health care providers and analysed using Excel.

Results: Of the 88 facilities, 28 were public, and 60 were private. In the public facilities, magnesium sulphate was available in six out of 10 Primary Health Centres (60%), in all eight *taluka* (sub-district) hospitals (100%), five of eight community health centres (63%) and both district hospitals (100%). Fifty-five of 60 private facilities (92%) reported availability of magnesium sulphate.
Stock outs were reported in six facilities in the preceding six months – five public and one private. Twenty-five percent weight/volume and 50% weight/volume concentration formulations were available variably across the public and private facilities. Sixty-eight facilities (77%) used the drug for severe pre-eclampsia and 12 facilities (13.6%) did not use the drug even for eclampsia. Varied dosing schedules were reported from facility to facility.
(Continued on next page)

* Correspondence: drumesh.charantimath@gmail.com
[2]KLE Academy of Higher Education and Research's J N Medical College, Belagavi, Karnataka, India
Full list of author information is available at the end of the article

(Continued from previous page)

Conclusions: Poor availability of magnesium sulphate was identified in many facilities, and stock outs in some. Individual differences in usage were identified. Ensuring a reliable supply of magnesium sulphate, standard formulations and recommendations of dosage schedules and training may help improve use; and decrease morbidity and mortality due to pre-eclampsia/ eclampsia.

Keywords: Magnesium Sulphate, Availability, Health care facilities, Pre-eclampsia, Eclampsia, Karnataka, India

Background

Pre-eclampsia and eclampsia are a leading cause of maternal mortality, contributing to 14% of maternal deaths worldwide [1]. Every day approximately 830 women die as a result of pregnancy complications all over the world and 99% of these deaths occur in developing countries [2]. In 2015, globally there were 303,000 maternal deaths; and 45,000 (about 15%) of these were in India [3]. India has fallen short of achieving the Millennium Development Goal of reducing the national maternal mortality ratio (MMR) to 109 by 2015. Despite a substantial reduction in maternal deaths, the MMR of India stood at 174 per 100,000 livebirths in 2015 [3]. It is now necessary to focus on the newly adopted Sustainable Development Goals targeted to reduce the global MMR to 70.

Interventions targeting maternal deaths need to address pre-eclampsia and eclampsia as it is the second leading direct cause of maternal mortality, second only to haemorrhage [1]. Also, these conditions can result in major morbidity and residual complications which affect the quality of life of the woman and her family and significant economic burden.

Magnesium sulphate is the drug of choice for the prevention and treatment for the seizures of eclampsia [4]. The Magpie trial established that women receiving magnesium sulphate versus placebo were 58% less likely to have convulsions and it also led to a decreased risk of placental abruption. Follow-up studies of the participants of the Magpie trial and their babies showed no long-term harm or benefit to either [5–7]. A systematic review of the Cochrane database in 2010 found that magnesium sulphate is better than phenytoin and nimodepine in preventing convulsions and results in a non-significant decrease in maternal deaths [8]. Studies have also proven that it prevents convulsions better when compared to the other treatment regimens for eclampsia like the lytic cocktail regimen and diazepam [9, 10].

The World Health Organization's (WHO) list of essential medicines and the Indian National List of Essential Medicines (NLEM) 2015 identify magnesium sulphate as an essential commodity for maternal health [11, 12]. It is interesting to note that the NLEM lists it under S and T categories which means that it should be available at secondary and tertiary facilities, when in contrast, the Indian Public Health Standards (IPHS) Revised Guidelines 2012, specifically the IPHS guidelines for primary health centres (PHCs), state that magnesium sulphate should be present in the labour room in the PHCs [13]. The antidote to magnesium sulphate, calcium gluconate is listed on the WHO list of essential medicines and also features on the NLEM 2015 under categories P, S and T, implying that it should be present at the primary, secondary and tertiary levels.

The guidelines for skilled birth attendants in India recommend that magnesium sulphate be administered in cases of severe pre-eclampsia and eclampsia prior to referral [14]. These guidelines are meant to guide the functioning of Staff Nurses (providing services at the primary health centres and higher facilities), Auxiliary Nurse Midwives (ANMs; providing services at the subcenters) and Lady Health Visitors (LHVs) who are in a supervisory capacity for the ANMs. The guidelines also recommend that magnesium sulphate be present in the kit for home delivery and specify that the skilled birth attendants are permitted to use magnesium sulphate for both eclampsia and severe pre-eclampsia, and that arrangements for immediate referral should then be made [14]. Providing the loading dose of magnesium sulphate will stabilize a woman for safe transport to a facility, which is better equipped to handle these complications. Despite all the recommendations, use of magnesium sulphate is not universal [15].

There may be many reasons for the sub-optimal use of magnesium sulphate, such as a lack of knowledge, lack of familiarity with the drug, the large volume of the injection, apprehension of complications, widely varied doses and dosage schedules that may be confusing; among others [15]. Though there are standard regimens described in obstetric textbooks, there are concerns that the dose may be too large for the smaller built Indian woman. Hence several modified regimens are followed in practice [16–19]. In addition to this, magnesium sulphate may not be readily available in all settings [15].

We undertook an assessment of health facilities in two districts of North Karnataka to note how they were equipped in handling obstetric and neonatal care. In this study, we report the availability and use of magnesium sulphate at the facilities assessed.

Methods

This study was carried out in Belagavi and Bagalkote districts of North Karnataka. Karnataka is a south Indian state with a MMR of 133/100,000 livebirths in 2011-2013 as per the Sample Registration System. There are vast differences in health infrastructure and service delivery in the districts of northern and southern Karnataka [20]. The CLIP Feasibility Study was undertaken in 12 areas of Belagavi and Bagalkote districts (six in each district) [21]. The two adjoining districts are quite dissimilar, with poorer health indices in Bagalkote district [20]. Before the CLIP Trial (NCT01911494), the 12-month Feasibility Study was undertaken to assess the context, and identify any potential barriers and facilitators to the implementation of CLIP.

As a part of the CLIP Feasibility Study, facility assessment was undertaken to determine the capacity of facilities in the study area in the provision of maternal and newborn health services, with a focus on care of women with pre-eclampsia and eclampsia. Medical officers, in charge of provision of care at primary health centres (PHC), were asked to identify and list the health care facilities that women in their area frequent. In total, 88 facilities were identified. The survey of the facilities was undertaken between April and August 2013.

The survey was carried out by trained medical professionals from the research team from the same region, who underwent training for a day in the approach necessary for data collection. Those conducting assessments were predominantly clinicians; this provided important background knowledge for successful completion of the forms. The primary obstetric care provider at each facility was approached for a one-on-one interview to provide necessary information, with some fields being completed with inputs from pediatric care providers, laboratory technicians and review of institutional records. Consent was obtained from the respondents before proceeding.

A pre-structured questionnaire was used to document the responses received. The questionnaire recorded preliminary data about the name of the facility, location, person responding to the questionnaire, contact numbers, type of facility, usual place of referral, catchment area and population served. It also included the number of beds, availability of intensive care units, a comprehensive description of the available personnel, equipment, drugs and services, costs, transportation to and from the facility, access to blood transfusion, and the volume of patients. Questions pertaining to additional training in maternal and neonatal care were included in the format, as were those related to existence and use of facility guidelines for the management of hypertensive disorders of pregnancy. Questions regarding hypertension in pregnancy, criteria used for diagnosis of mild and severe pre-eclampsia, antihypertensive treatment, and use of magnesium sulphate were also asked. The majority of the questions in the survey tool were close-ended though a few questions requested detailed answering. Data were directly recorded on to hard copies of the questionnaire at the time of the interview. The questionnaire used in this study has been added as an appendix to this paper (Additional file 1).

All data were keyed into a locally developed Access database. The data were cleaned prior to analysis. Frequencies were run on all quantitative fields providing totals, means and standard deviations.

This study was approved by ethics review committees at the University of British Columbia, Vancouver Canada (H12-00132) and KLE University, Belgaum (Ref No: MDC/IECHSR/2013-14/A-28) India.

Results

Of the 88 facilities, 28 were public and 60 were private. Table 1 provides a description of the facilities surveyed.

The facilities assessed included 8 Community Health Centres (CHC) out of the total 24 in the two districts (33%) as reported by the Health Management Information System of the Ministry of health and Family welfare; 8 *taluka* hospitals out of the total 14 (57%), and both the district hospitals (100%). The total number of private obstetric facilities in the two districts could not be ascertained to determine the proportion assessed.

All health care facilities with magnesium sulphate at the time of assessment also reported access to the drug in the labour room. Data regarding stock outs in the preceding 6 months were collected. While the majority of the healthcare facilities did not report any stock outs, five public facilities did report stock outs at the time of assessment, one reporting multiple instances in the preceding 6 months. One private facility reported a stock out. One CHC and one private hospital reported having no availability of magnesium sulphate at any time and hence there was no response to whether stock outs occurred. One PHC medical officer reported that they did not wait for replenishment of stock through the government supply since it was not streamlined, and they bought the necessary supply through funds allocated to the PHC. Table 1 shows the different categories of health facilities surveyed, availability of magnesium sulphate at the time of assessment and stock outs in the preceding 6 months.

The availability of other essential obstetric medications was ascertained. There were differences in availability, with some facilities reporting availability of one type of a drug in a category versus another (for example betamethasone/dexamethasone, different antihypertensives etc.) and some reporting availability of all the drugs. All facilities reported the availability of uterotonics, oxytocin in particular.

Table 1 Facilities assessed, the availability of magnesium sulphate at assessment and stock outs in preceding 6 months

Type of facility		Belagavi district			Bagalkote District			Total		
		N	A	S	N	A	S	N	A	S
Public facilities	Primary Health Centre	9	5	2	1	1	0	10	6	2
	Community Health Centre	4	3	0	4	2	2	8	5	2
	Taluka Hospital	4	4	0	4	4	1	8	8	1
	District Hospital	1	1	0	1	1	0	2	2	0
Private facilities		39	35	0	21	20	1	60	55	1
All facilities		57	48	2	31	28	4	88	76	6

N Number assessed
A Magnesium sulphate available during survey
S Stock outs of magnesium sulphate in preceding six moths

Regarding the formulation of magnesium sulphate available, responses were collected from 29 facilities with magnesium sulphate at the time of assessment. Of these, 22 (6 public and 16 private) facilities reported carrying a concentration of 50% weight /volume (*w*/*v*), three (one public and 2 private) reported having 25% w/v and four (one public and 3 private) reported having both strengths available. All ampoules were of 2 ml.

Information on practices related to magnesium sulphate usage was collected, including the use of magnesium sulphate in the management of severe pre-eclampsia (Table 2). Health care professionals from 68 facilities responded that they did use it for management of severe pre-eclampsia, and notably this included five PHCs. Thirty-two providers reported differential dosing schedules for severe pre-eclampsia as opposed to eclampsia with differences in both the route and the dosage of magnesium sulphate used. Seventeen of the 68 providers reported that they did not provide a maintenance dose in cases of severe pre-eclampsia. One private practitioner reported maintenance therapy with phenytoin after the loading dose of magnesium sulphate for pre-eclampsia. All the PHCs and two private hospitals using magnesium sulphate reported immediate referral of patients with severe pre-eclampsia and eclampsia, without waiting for the maintenance dose.

Table 2 Facilities using magnesium sulphate for management of severe pre-eclampsia

Use of $MgSO_4$ for severe pre-eclampsia		
Yes	Public	17
	Private	51
	Total	68
No	Public	4
	Private	4
	Total	8
Never used $MgSO_4$ for even eclampsia	Public	7
	Private	5
	Total	12

When asked about alternative treatment strategies in eclampsia in place of magnesium sulphate amongst those using the drug, the majority of the providers mentioned use of injection diazepam or phenytoin, but only in cases where magnesium sulphate failed. Only one provider mentioned that maintenance treatment was routinely provided with phenytoin.

A notable observation was that 12 providers did not use magnesium sulphate even for eclampsia. This included 4 PHCs, 3 CHCs and 5 private facilities. Three of these 12 facilities did report availability of magnesium sulphate at the time of assessment. Four of the 12 providers mentioned the use of injectable diazepam for eclampsia.

Varied dosage schedules were reported, with 25 (3 public and 22 private) of 68 providers reporting using standard Pritchard or Zuspan regimens for severe pre-eclampsia, and 44 (13 public and 31 private) of 76 reporting use of standard Pritchard or Zuspan regimens for eclampsia. The dosages reported were very varied, with most providers who were not using standard regimens resorted to lower doses, some up to half of the Pritchard and Zuspan regimens. One obstetrician at a private facility reported the use of 2 g intramuscularly (IM) as the loading dose and 2 g IM twice a day as the maintenance dose for eclampsia. There were also some unusual responses like 100 mg intravenously (IV) every 8 h; and 25% IM. The respondents in these cases were not obstetricians by qualification but were still the primary obstetric providers in that facility. Interestingly, 10 providers said they determine the loading and maintenance doses based on the patient's condition.

The availability of calcium gluconate, the antidote to magnesium sulphate was asked for. Calcium gluconate was not available in 12 facilities, including 8 which reported availability of magnesium sulphate (Table 3).

Discussion

Despite the well-established superiority of magnesium sulphate in the management of severe pre-eclampsia and

Table 3 Non-availability of calcium gluconate by type of facility

Type of facility	Calcium gluconate not available	Calcium gluconate not available but magnesium sulphate available
PHC	2	0
Taluka Hospital	1	1
CHC	2	1
Private	7	6

eclampsia, it continues to be used sub-optimally. In our study, non-availability of magnesium sulphate was identified at several facilities. In addition, stock outs were experienced at five public facilities and one private secondary facility in the preceding 6 months but in none of the tertiary health facilities. Calcium gluconate was available in 86% of the facilities assessed but 8 facilities with availability of magnesium sulphate did not have calcium gluconate.

It was found that the health facilities had differing strengths of magnesium sulphate available, some reporting both 25% *w/v* and 50% w/v. The facilities reported varying dosage schedules, some of which may not have the required stabilizing action and may not optimally benefit the patient.

The availability of magnesium sulphate seemed to be similar across the two districts in this study. However, there were more stock outs in the preceding 6 months in Bagalkote when compared to Belagavi. Also, the stock outs were in the secondary level facilities in Bagalkote as opposed to primary health centres in Belagavi. Availability and use of magnesium sulphate across all levels of healthcare is important for ensuring favourable outcomes.

The fact that other essential medications for obstetric health were available at the facility and only magnesium sulphate seemed to be missing, points to the fact that the supply chain is generally functioning. Due importance is not given to make magnesium sulphate available. The providers at the public facilities do have funds to procure the drug through other suppliers but have to maintain a watch on the stock to see that the supply is uninterrupted.

The facilities assessed in this study were the ones most often used for delivery and it would be expected that these health facilities would have better logistics than those not providing regular obstetric services. It is probable that this assessment does not represent all facilities in the region, and that others may have poorer availability and use of magnesium sulphate. The strength of this study is that researchers were trained medical professionals and hence had a better contextualization of the study. A limitation of this study is that the health care providers self-reported the availability and use of magnesium sulphate in the facilities they served. It was not physically ascertained as to how many ampoules were present, whether the ampoules were within the date of expiry, and whether magnesium sulphate was used in the manner reported. Though the researchers encouraged practitioners to report actual practices, the fact that the researchers were fellow clinicians may have induced a bias to report favourably.

A study assessing 279 health care facilities in eight districts of northern Karnataka in 2010 revealed that magnesium sulphate was available in only 18% of PHCs, 48% of higher public facilities and 70% of private facilities [22]. In comparison, the present study found that 60% of PHCs, 72% of higher public facilities and 92% private facilities reported availability of magnesium sulphate at the time of assessment. This difference may be because we selectively sampled facilities providing regular obstetric services.

A study from Maharashtra state, India assessing 44 secondary and tertiary public health facilities in 2009-2010 found that 61% of facilities had no stock of magnesium sulphate, with the stock-out position ranging from 3 months to 3 years. The researchers ascertained whether they had the minimum of 50 ampoules recommended in the guidelines for CHCs and found that 20% facilities had less than the minimum recommended and also that 11.4% of the assessed facilities did not have enough ampoules to even provide the first dose to a single woman [23]. The stock outs in the present study were much fewer, with only five of 28 public facilities (18%) reporting stock outs in the 6 months before the survey, again perhaps due to the convenience sampling used in this study. The quantity of drug available was not assessed in this study.

Another study done in Nagpur, Maharashtra concluded that though senior gynaecologists favoured the use of magnesium sulphate especially prior to referral, its use was limited due to lack of institutional policies on dosing, timing, indications and also due to limited availability, especially in tertiary care centres [24]. In the present study too, it was found that health care providers did not have uniform policies on indications and dosing, even when the drug was available.

A 2010 WHO study that assessed emergency obstetric care across six developing countries, including India, found that only 53% of facilities with basic emergency obstetric care (BEmOC) and 86% of facilities with comprehensive emergency obstetric care (CEmOC) had IM/IV anticonvulsants [25]. The study also indicated that public facilities were unable to provide emergency obstetric care due to lack of good management systems to ensure continuous availability of drugs and supplies and emphasized the importance of strengthening the chain for procurement and distribution of basic drugs and equipment; and to improve skills of the providers to ensure at least coverage of BEmOC [25]. In the present study, in addition to the issues about availability of magnesium sulphate, we found that providers at 12 facilities did not administer magnesium sulphate even for eclampsia despite three of these facilities reporting availability. This emphasizes the need for knowledge and skill enhancement activities to improve usage practices in addition to improving the supply chain.

Even though the guidelines for skilled birth attendants [14] recommend that the ANM should administer magnesium sulphate for severe pre-eclampsia prior to referral, the medical officers (who are qualified physicians) of five of the PHCs stated that they did not use magnesium sulphate for severe pre-eclampsia and despite availability of magnesium sulphate, usage for even eclampsia was not universal. Familiarising health care professionals with treatment recommendations, and building their capacity and confidence could go a long way in optimizing the administration of magnesium sulphate.

There are standard regimens for the use of magnesium sulphate, Pritchard, Zuspan and Sibai; as well as, many other dosage schedules [16–19]. A systematic review of the studies evaluating these regimens in low- and middle-income countries was unable to establish the superiority of any regimen and the lowest effective dose is not agreed upon [26]. It was found in four studies that the administration of the loading dose only was as effective as loading plus maintenance [26]. The varied dosage schedules, however, confuse practitioners who may not be familiar with magnesium sulphate. The strength of the drug formulation also varies and achieving the correct dilution for IV administration may be prone to error and confusion [27]. In the present study, we did find that the health facilities had differing strengths available and used many differing dosing schedules. It is important that there be a standard formulation and requirement for adherence to standard dosing schedules to increase appropriate use and optimize action.

Magnesium sulphate toxicity occurs very infrequently if guidelines are followed during administration. In the event that it does occur, serious complications can usually be averted by skipping the next dose. However, in rare instances, administration of calcium gluconate is required and may be lifesaving [28]. Hence, care should be taken to ensure availability and train the providers in appropriate use. A study in Lucknow, India in 2014 found that only 33.3% *Bal Mahila Chikitsalayas* (health care facilities for women and children) which serve as first referral units had availability of calcium gluconate [29]. In our study, availability was found to be better with 86% facilities reporting the drug at the time of assessment.

The Indian guidelines are conflicting, with the NLEM recommending magnesium sulphate availability in the secondary and tertiary facilities, the IPHS guidelines for PHCs recommending availability in the labour room of the PHCs; and the guidelines for skilled birth attendants recommending that it be available at the sub-center and even in the home delivery kits [12–14]. Conflicting recommendations of this nature need to be rectified to ensure enhanced usage.

The first step to encourage enhanced magnesium sulphate use is that it should be available at all health care facilities providing for obstetric patients, without any stock-outs. It is also essential to increase the providers' comfort and confidence in using this drug. All levels of obstetric care providers need to be re-trained periodically in the benefits and use of magnesium sulphate.

Observing the appropriate use of magnesium sulphate by senior obstetric providers may enhance uptake by the other health care providers like resident doctors, ANMs and staff nurses. However, they need to be exposed to the use of this drug in a consistent manner. Standardizing the strength and dosing schedules is essential; and guidelines for referral should be developed and enforced. Identification of non-compliant facilities could be done by tracking referrals. Ascertaining the cause for deviation with corrective action and refresher training could be a solution to increase appropriate use. Cases of eclampsia could also serve as triggers for evaluating the delays and deficiencies in the health system and identifying and implementing potential remedial action.

Future research could focus on the reasons for hesitancy for use of magnesium sulphate by obstetric providers so as to inform the health system administrators about the steps necessary to increase usage.

Conclusion

This study found that there were deficiencies in the availability of magnesium sulphate in health care facilities that routinely cared for obstetric patients in north Karnataka. The public health facilities faced stock outs though they could procure the drug through funds allocated to them. This shows a poor chain of coordination between the suppliers, distributors and the users.

Addressing contradictions in the Indian national guidelines regarding place of availability, indications for use and cadre of health care professionals permitted to use magnesium sulphate is of prime importance.

The indications for which magnesium sulphate was used and the strength of drug available varied across facilities of the same type. Standardization of the drug formulation and familiarization with guidelines is important to ensure optimal use of magnesium sulphate. In addition, identification of the factors preventing use; and trainings and refresher trainings to address these issues would increase appropriate usage of magnesium sulphate.

Despite a major reduction in the maternal mortality, the Millennium Development Goals of 2015 were not met in India; nevertheless, positive action in this regard could bring us closer to attaining the Sustainable Development Goals by 2030.

Abbreviations
ANM: Auxillary nurse midwife; BEmOC: Basic emergency obstetric care; CEmOC: Comprehensive emergency obstetric care; CHC: Community Health Centre; CLIP: Community level interventions for pre-eclampsia; IM: Intramuscular; IPHS: Indian Public Health Standards; IV: Intravenous; LHV: Lady health visitor; MMR: Maternal mortality ratio; NLEM: National list of essential medicines; PHC: Primary health centre; SN: Staff nurse; *w/v*: Weight/volume; WHO: World Health Organization

Acknowledgements
This study was undertaken as a part of the PRE-EMPT (Pre-eclampsia Eclampsia Monitoring Prevention and Treatment) grant awarded to the University of British Columbia, a grantee of the Bill & Melinda Gates Foundation.
CLIP Feasibility working group: Namdev Kamble, Amit Revankar, Zulfiqar Bhutta, Sharla K Drebit, Chirag Kariya, Tang Lee, Jing Li, Mansun Lui, Asif R Khowaja, Domena K. Tu.

Funding
This study was undertaken as a part of the PRE-EMPT (Pre-eclampsia Eclampsia Monitoring Prevention and Treatment) grant awarded to the University of British Columbia, a grantee of the Bill & Melinda Gates Foundation. The funding body had no role in the design or conduct of the study or in the reporting of the results.
Publication charges for this supplement were funded by the University of British Columbia PRE-EMPT (Pre-eclampsia/ Eclampsia, Monitoring, Prevention and Treatment) initiative supported by the Bill and Melinda Gates Foundation.

Authors' contributions
GK, UC and UR were involved in the preparation of the study materials, data collection and prepared the manuscript. AJ, SB, SR, CK, GM, AK were involved in data collection. RD, SG, SS, MV, AM, MB, DS, BP, LAM were responsible for protocol preparation and overseeing the study. PVD and RQ were the Principal Investigators. All authors read the approved the final manuscript.

Competing interests
The authors declare that they have no competing interests.

Author details
[1]Department of Obstetrics and Gynaecology, S Nijalingappa Medical College, Bagalkot, Karnataka, India. [2]KLE Academy of Higher Education and Research's J N Medical College, Belagavi, Karnataka, India. [3]Department of Obstetrics and Gynaecology, University of British Columbia, Vancouver, BC, Canada. [4]Department of Community Medicine, S Nijalingappa Medical College, Bagalkot, Karnataka, India. [5]Department of Pharmacology, S Nijalingappa Medical College, Bagalkot, Karnataka, India. [6]Department of Anatomy, S Nijalingappa Medical College, Bagalkot, Karnataka, India. [7]School of Life Course Sciences, Faculty of Life Sciences and Medicine, King's College London, London, UK. [8]Global Affairs, Thomas Jefferson University, Philadelphia, USA. [9]Division of Women and Child Health, Aga Khan University, Karachi, Sindh, Pakistan. [10]Department of Research, Vancouver Island Health Authority, British Columbia, Canada.

References
1. Say L, Chou D, Gemmill A, Tuncalp O, Moller A, Daniels J, et al. Global causes of maternal death: a WHO systematic analysis. Lancet Glob Health. 2014;2:e323–33. https://doi.org/10.1016/S2214-109X(14)70227-X.
2. WHO Maternal Mortality Fact sheet Updated November 2016. http://www.who.int/mediacentre/factsheets/fs348/en/. Accessed 14 Jan 2018.
3. Alkema L, Chou D, Hogan D, Zhang S, Moller AB, Gemmill A, et al. Global, regional, and national levels and trends in maternal mortality between 1990 and 2015, with scenario-based projections to 2030: a systematic analysis by the UN maternal mortality estimation inter-agency group. Lancet. 2016;387(10017):462–74. https://doi.org/10.1016/S0140-6736(15)003-7. Epub 2015 Nov13.
4. Duley L. Magnesium sulphate in eclampsia. Eclampsia trial collaborative group. Lancet. 1998;352(9121):67–8. PMID: 9800779
5. Altman D, Carroli G, Duley L, Farrell B, Moodley J, Neilson J, et al. Do women with pre-eclampsia, and their babies, benefit from magnesium sulphate? The magpie trial: a randomised placebo-controlled trial. Lancet. 2002;359(9321):1877–90. https://doi.org/10.1016/S0140-6736(02)08778-0.
6. Magpie Trial Follow-Up Study Collaborative Group. The magpie trial: a randomised trial comparing magnesium sulphate with placebo for pre-eclampsia. Outcome for women at 2 years. BJOG. 2007;114:300–9. https://doi.org/10.1111/j.1471-0528.2006.01166.x.
7. Magpie Trial Follow-Up Study Collaborative Group. The magpie trial: a randomised trial comparing magnesium sulphate with placebo for pre-eclampsia. Outcome for children at 18 months. BJOG. 2007;114:289–99. https://doi.org/10.1111/j.1471-0528.2006.01165.x.
8. Duley L, Gülmezoglu AM, Henderson-Smart DJ, Chou D. Magnesium sulphate and other anticonvulsants for women with pre-eclampsia. Cochrane Database Syst Rev. 2010;11:CD000025. https://doi.org/10.1002/14651858.CD000025.pub2.
9. Duley L, Gülmezoglu AM, Chou D. Magnesium sulphate versus lytic cocktail for eclampsia. Cochrane Database Syst Rev. 2010;9:CD002960. https://doi.org/10.1002/14651858.CD002960.pub2.
10. Duley L, Henderson-Smart DJ, Walker GJ, Chou D. Magnesium sulphate versus diazepam for eclampsia. Cochrane Database Syst Rev. 2010;12:CD000127. https://doi.org/10.1002/14651858.CD000127.pub2.
11. 19th WHO Model List of Essential Medicines (April 2015). p.5. http://www.who.int/medicines/publications/essentialmedicines/EML2015_8-May-15.pdf. Accessed 15 Jan 2018.
12. National List of Essential Medicines (NLEM) 2015 – India. p. 11. cdsco.nic.in/WriteReadData/NLEM-2015/NLEM,%202015.pdf. Accessed 15 Jan 2018.
13. Indian Public health Standards (IPHS) Guidelines for Primary health Centres Revised 2012. Directorate General of Health Services, Ministry of Health and Family Welfare, Government of India. p. 24. https://www.karnataka.gov.in/hfw/decell/Documents/IPHS%20Guidelines%20for%20Primay%20Health%20Centres.pdf. Accessed 22 Jan 2018.
14. Guidelines for Antenatal Care and Skilled Attendance at Birth by ANMs/LHVs/SNs. Maternal Health Division, Ministry of Health and Family Welfare, Government of India April 2010. https://www.nhp.gov.in/sites/default/files/anm_guidelines.pdf. Accessed 17 Jan 2018.
15. Long Q, Oladapo OT, Leathersich S, Vogel JP, Carroli G, Lumbiganon P, et al. Clinical practice patterns on the use of magnesium sulphate for treatment of pre-eclampsia and eclampsia: a multi-country survey. BJOG. 2017;124(12):1883–90. https://doi.org/10.1111/1471-0528.14400.
16. Joshi SD, Veerendrakumar CM. 'Single dose MgSo4 regimen' for eclampsia - a safe motherhood initiative. J Clin Diagn Res. 2013;7(5):868–72. https://doi.org/10.7860/JCDR/2013/5398.2961.

17. Nagaria T, Mitra S, Banjare SP. Single loading low dose MgSo4 regimen: a simple, safe and effective alternative to Pritchard's regimen for Indian women. J Clin Diagn Res. 2017;11(8):QC08–12. https://doi.org/10.7860/JCDR/2017/26635.10453.
18. Saha PK, Kaur J, Goel P, Kataria S, Tandon R, Saha L. Safety and efficacy of low dose intramuscular magnesium sulphate (MgSO4) compared to intravenous regimen for treatment of eclampsia. J Obstet Gynaecol Res. 2017;43(10):1543–9. https://doi.org/10.1111/jog.13424.
19. Abdul MA, Nasir UI, Khan N, Yusuf MD. Low-dose magnesium sulphate in the control of eclamptic fits: a randomized controlled trial. Arch Gynecol Obstet. 2013;287(1):43–6. https://doi.org/10.1007/s00404-012-2523-z.
20. Siddu VH, Keshava Murthy KD, Revankar R. Status and infrastructure of the health sector in Karnataka. Artha J Soc Sci. 2012;11(3):15–43. https://doi.org/10.12724/ajss.22.2.
21. Khowaja AR, Qureshi RN, Sawchuck D, Oladapo OT, Adetoro OO, Orenuga EA, et al. The feasibility of community level interventions for pre-eclampsia in South Asia and sub-Saharan Africa: a mixed-methods design. Reprod Health. 2016;13(Suppl 1):56. https://doi.org/10.1186/s12978-016-0133-0.
22. Krishnamurthy J, Mony P, Ramesh BM, Thomas A, Gaikwad A, Mohan HL, et al. Assessment of facility readiness and provider preparedness for dealing with postpartum haemorrhage and pre-eclampsia/eclampsia in public and private health facilities of northern Karnataka, India: a cross-sectional study. BMC Pregnancy Childbirt. 2014;14:304. https://doi.org/10.1186/1471-2393-14-304.
23. Chaturvedi S, Randive B, Mistry N. Availability of treatment for eclampsia in public health institutions in Maharashtra, India. J Health Popul Nutr. 2013; 31(1):86–95. PMID: 23617209
24. Barua A, Mundle S, Bracken H, Easterling T, Winikoff B. Facility and personnel factors influencing magnesium sulfate use for eclampsia and pre-eclampsia in 3 Indian hospitals. Int J Gynaecol Obstet. 2011;115(3):231–4. https://doi.org/10.1016/j.ijgo.2011.07.016. Epub 2011 Sept 17.
25. Ameh C, Msuya S, Hofman J, Raven J, Mathai M, van den Broek N. Status of emergency obstetric care in six developing countries five years before the MDG targets for maternal and newborn health. PLoS One. 2012;7(12): e49938. https://doi.org/10.1371/journal.pone.0049938.
26. Gordon R, Magee LA, Payne B, Firoz T, Sawchuck D, Tu D, et al. Magnesium sulphate for the management of preeclampsia and eclampsia in low and middle income countries: a systematic review of tested dosing regimens. J Obstet Gynaecol Can. 2014;36(2):154–63. https://doi.org/10.1016/S1701-2163(15)30662-9.
27. Reducing the risk of medication errors with intravenous magnesium sulfate. Bulletin prepared by Wessex Academic Health Science Network. http://wessexahsn.org.uk/img/projects/Magnesium%20Sulfate%20Safety%20Bulletin.pdf. Accessed 1 Feb 2018.
28. Lu JF, Nightingale CH. Magnesium sulphate in eclampsia and pre-eclapmsia pharmacokinetic principles. Clin Pharmacokinet. 2000;38:305. https://doi.org/10.2165/00003088-200038040-00002.
29. Sahu K, Manar M, Singh S. Assessment of health care facilities for maternal and child health care at Bal Mahila chikitsalyas in Lucknow district, India. IJBAR. 2014;5(1):26–8. https://doi.org/10.7439/ijbar.v5i1.615.

Associations of gestational weight gain with offspring thinness and obesity: by prepregnancy body mass index

Nianqing Wan[1†], Li Cai[1†], Weiqing Tan[2], Ting Zhang[1], Jiewen Yang[2*] and Yajun Chen[1*]

Abstract

Background: Previous studies indicated that excessive gestational weight gain (GWG) was positively associated with offspring obesity. Nevertheless, little is known about the effect of GWG on offspring thinness. This study aimed to assess the association of GWG with childhood weight status across the full range of weight status by prepregnancy body mass index (BMI).

Methods: We used data from a retrospective study of 33,828 Chinese children aged 6–18 years and their mothers. Children's weight and height were objectively measured. Maternal GWG and other information were collected by using self-reported questionnaires. Multivariate linear regressions and logistic regressions were applied.

Results: Overall, the prevalence of thinness and overweight/obesity in children were 12.9 and 17.3% respectively ($p < 0.05$). Children's BMI z-score was on average 0.021 higher for every 1-kg greater GWG. For mothers who were underweight or normal weight before pregnancy, excessive GWG was positively associated with offspring overweight/obesity [OR (95% CI): 1.51 (1.21, 1.90) and 1.30 (1.17, 1.45)], whereas inadequate GWG was associated with increased risk of offspring thinness [OR (95% CI): 1.24 (1.05, 1.46) and 1.17 (1.04, 1.32)]. Similar but non-significant associations were found in prepregnancy overweight mothers. Notably, there was a very high prevalence of child overweight/obesity (30.2%) in prepregnancy overweight subgroup regardless of GWG status.

Conclusions: Inadequate GWG was associated with an increased risk of offspring thinness, whereas excessive GWG was associated with an increased risk of offspring overweight and obesity among prepregnancy underweight and normal weight mothers only.

Keywords: Gestational weight gain, Maternal prepregnancy BMI, Childhood thinness, Childhood obesity, Epidemiology

Plain English summary

Gestation period is considered as a crucial time for growth, development, and physiological changes in children. Excessive gestational weight gain (GWG) was suggested to be positively associated with offspring obesity. Nevertheless, little is known about the effect of GWG on offspring thinness. This study aimed to assess the association of GWG with childhood weight status across the full range of weight status by prepregnancy body mass index (BMI).

* Correspondence: 360449586@qq.com; chenyj68@mail.sysu.edu.cn
†Nianqing Wan and Li Cai contributed equally to this work.
[2]Health Promotion Centre for Primary and Secondary Schools of Guangzhou Municipality, Guangzhou 510000, China
[1]Department of Maternal and Child Health, School of Public Health, Sun Yat-sen University, Guangzhou 510000, China

The weight and height of 33,828 Chinese children were objectively measured. These children and their mothers were asked to fill in a self-reported questionnaire which included socio-demographic data, maternal prepregnancy weight (kg) and height (cm), as well as mother's weight (kg) at delivery and so on.

Overall, the prevalence of thinness and overweight/obesity in children were 12.9 and 17.3% respectively. For mothers who were underweight or normal weight before pregnancy, excessive GWG was positively associated with offspring overweight/obesity, whereas inadequate GWG was associated with increased risk of offspring thinness. Similar but non-significant associations were found in prepregnancy overweight mothers. Notably, there was a very high prevalence of child overweight/obesity (30.2%) in prepregnancy overweight subgroup regardless of GWG status. In addition, children's BMI z-score was on average 0.021 higher for every 1-kg greater GWG in the overall group.

In conclusion, inadequate GWG was associated with an increased risk of offspring thinness, whereas excessive GWG was associated with an increased risk of offspring overweight and obesity among prepregnancy underweight and normal weight mothers only.

Background

Childhood obesity has been a serious public health problem worldwide [1]. The global prevalence of childhood overweight and obesity increased rapidly, for example in developed countries, from 16.9% of boys in 1980 to 23.8% in 2013 [2]. Previous of evidences have demonstrated that obesity is linked to medical, neurocognitive and psychological abnormalities which impact children's health and quality of life [3–5]. Despite the rapidly increasing prevalence of obesity, thinness [i.e. low body mass index (BMI) for age] remains a health concern among children in many countries [6–8]. A global survey of 12–18-year-old girls from 40 countries indicated that the prevalence of moderate/severe thinness was 7.6%, especially with higher levels in Asia [9]. It has been suggested that thinness may affect physical growth of children, lower immunity and increase risk of infection [10–12]. Therefore, prevention of childhood thinness should also be taken into account when it comes to the design and implementation of child weight control programs.

Gestation period is considered as a crucial time for growth, development, and physiological changes in children. Previous studies showed that gestational weight gain (GWG) was positively associated with offspring's birth weight [13] and BMI in childhood [14, 15], adolescence [16, 17], and adulthood [18]. These associations are complex [19, 20], consequently, epidemiologic studies assessing the association between GWG and child weight status are supposed to control for lifestyle and genetics factors between mother and child to reduce bias. Considering the influence of maternal nutritional status before pregnancy, in 2009, the Institute of Medicine (IOM) recommended ranges of BMI-specific weight gain during pregnancy to achieve optimal pregnancy outcomes. However, whether the effect of inappropriate GWG on child weight status also varies in different maternal prepregnancy BMI category is controversial.

Although many of the previously published studies had investigated the relationship of excessive GWG with offspring obesity [21–23], very few reported the long-term impact of inadequate GWG on child weight status in terms of category structure and limited focused on the adolescent population. One longitudinal study consisted of 3600 participants found that excess GWG was associated with an increase in child BMI z-score in early childhood among normal and overweight mothers, whereas low GWG was not associated with child BMI z-score among all pregnancy BMI groups [24]. Furthermore, to the best of our knowledge, no previous study has investigated the association of inadequate GWG with childhood thinness.

Thus, using data from a large population-based, retrospective study, we aimed to examine the association between GWG and weight status across the full range of weight status in offspring aged 6–18 years, and whether these associations differ by mother's prepregnancy BMI.

Methods

Data were obtained from a retrospective study, conducted between September 2015 and June 2016 in Guangzhou, a large city in South China. Multistage cluster sampling method was adopted in the recruitment of participants. In the first stage, 30 schools were randomly selected from 12 districts of Guangzhou using probability proportional to size sampling method. In the second stage, all the children in selected schools and their mothers were invited to participate in our survey. A total of 56,096 mother-child pairs participated in our study, 54,395 children completed physical examination and 42,049 children (with 75% response rate) completed the questionnaire with their mothers. In the study, those with missing information about age, gender, BMI, maternal prepregnancy BMI, or GWG were excluded. Lastly, 33,828 mother-child pairs remained in the analyses.

Study variables and measurements

Children and their mothers were asked to fill in a self-reported questionnaire which included socio-demographic data, maternal prepregnancy weight (kg) and height (cm), as well as mother's weight (kg) at delivery. Data of children's birth and feeding situation, personal and family medical history were also collected. Additionally, children's daily physical activity/sedentary behavior were reported. Trained staff checked the integrity of completed questionnaires upon returned.

Prepregnancy BMI

Prepregnancy BMI (kg/m^2) was calculated by dividing weight (kg) by the square of height (m^2). We adopted the Chinese standard [25] to categorize maternal prepregnancy weight status as underweight (prepregnancy BMI < 18.5 kg/m^2), normal weight (prepregnancy BMI 18.5–23.9 kg/m^2), and overweight (including obesity: prepregnancy BMI ≥ 24.0 kg/ m^2).

Gestational weight gain

GWG (kg) was calculated as the difference between maternal weight before delivery and weight before pregnancy. According to Chinese standard for prepregnancy BMI categories [25] and IOM recommendations [26], adequate GWG was defined as: 12.5–18.0 kg for initially underweight women (< 18.5 kg/m^2); 11.5–16.0 kg for normal weight women (18.5–23.9 kg/m^2); 7.0–11.5 kg for overweight women (24.0–27.9 kg/ m^2); and 5.0–9.0 kg for obese women (≥ 28 kg/m^2). Inadequate and excessive GWG were defined as below and above these ranges within each prepregnancy BMI category, respectively.

Child weight status

Children's height (cm) and weight (kg) were measured by qualified technicians according to a standardized protocol. Height was measured to the nearest 0.1 cm using a free-standing stadiometer, with each child wearing no shoes. Weight was measured to an accuracy of 0.1 kg using a calibrated digital scales, with each child wearing only underwear and standing at ease. Age- and sex-specific child BMI z-scores were calculated using the WHO's Growth Reference. Child overweight and obesity were defined based on the age- and gender-specific BMI cutoffs for school-aged children developed by the Working Group on Obesity in China [27]. Thinness was defined by the age- and gender-specific cutoffs of malnutrition for Chinese children [28].

Covariates

Mothers provided information about their education level, family income, gestational diabetes mellitus (yes/no), child's gestational age (i.e., preterm, full-term, or post-term), birth weight (kg), and feeding patterns in the first 6 months (i.e., exclusive breast feeding, mixed feeding, or exclusive artificial feeding). Physical activity was reported by children, with their mothers' assist if needed. Physical activity of children was estimated using the International Physical Activity Questionnaire-Short Form (IPAQ-SF) [29]. Children were asked to reported the frequency (days) and

Table 1 Characteristics of mothers and children by gestational weight gain

	N	GWG categories			Overall	*P*[*]
		Inadequate	Adequate	Excessive		
Maternal characteristics						
Prepregnancy BMI, kg/m^2	33,828	20.1 ± 2.1	20.1 ± 2.2	20.2 ± 2.6	20.1 ± 2.3	0.0136
Gestational weight gain, kg	33,828	8.1 ± 2.4	13.7 ± 1.9	20.2 ± 4.0	12.9 ± 5.6	< 0.0001
GDM, %	33,643	1.3	2.0	2.8	1.9	< 0.0001
Education, %	33,044					< 0.0001
Junior high school or below		37.1	23.3	17.5	27.9	
Senior high school or above		27.2	25.6	25.1	26.2	
College or above		35.7	51.1	57.4	45.9	
Family monthly income, %	33,025					< 0.0001
< 8000 RMB		52.1	47.3	43.3	48.4	
8000~ 15,000 RMB		18.4	22.5	24.5	21.2	
≥ 15,000 RMB		9.2	12.3	15.3	11.7	
Refuse to answer		20.3	17.9	16.9	18.7	
Child characteristics						
Boy, %	33,828	47.7	49.6	51.8	49.3	< 0.0001
Age, year	33,828	12.9 ± 3.5	11.7 ± 3.4	11.2 ± 3.3	12.1 ± 3.5	< 0.0001
Feeding pattern in the first 6 months, %	32,826					< 0.0001
Breast feeding		41.7	38.4	36.6	39.4	
Mixed feeding		45.3	46.8	47.3	46.2	
Artificial feeding		13.0	14.8	16.2	14.4	
Birth weight, kg	32,674	3.0 ± 0.5	3.0 ± 0.5	3.1 ± 0.5	3.0 ± 0.5	< 0.0001
Child BMI, kg/m^2	33,828	18.3 ± 3.5	18.0 ± 3.6	18.2 ± 3.8	18.2 ± 3.6	< 0.0001
MVPA≥60 min	27,182	35.3	37.4	38.5	36.8	< 0.0001

Values are presented as mean ± SD or percentages

GWG gestational weight gain, *BMI* body mass index, *GDM* gestational diabetes mellitus, *MVPA* moderate-to-vigorous physical activity

[*]Differences of continuous and categorical variables between gestational weight gain categories were evaluated by using One-way ANOVA and Chi-square test, respectively

duration (hours and minutes in each of those days) of each of the following activities during the last 7 days: 1) vigorous-intensity activity; 2) moderate-intensity activity; 3) walking; and 4) sitting.

Statistical analysis

Data were analyzed using SAS 9.2. Descriptive statistics were conducted for all variables by GWG categories. Continuous variables were presented as mean and standard deviation (SD), and categorical variables were presented as percentage. One-way ANOVA test and Chi-square test were applied to evaluate the differences of continuous and categorical variables, respectively. Multiple linear regression model was used to examine the association between GWG and children's current BMI or BMI z-score in each prepregnancy BMI subgroup, and multiple logistic regression analyses were performed to assess the association of GWG (inadequate, adequate, or excessive) with children's thinness and overweight (including obesity), with adjustment for the potential confounders. Adjusted odds ratio (OR) and 95% confidence interval (CI) were calculated from the logistic regression analyses. In addition, we used the Cochran-Armitage test and linear regression to assess trends of maternal prepregnancy BMI and gestational weight gain between 1996 and 2009. p value less than 0.05 was considered statistically significant in all analyses.

Results

Table 1 presents the general characteristics of mothers and children by GWG. Of the 33,828 participating mothers, the proportion of inadequate, adequate, and excessive GWG in mothers was 44.2, 30.9 and 25.0%, respectively. Overall, the mean maternal GWG was 12.9 ± 5.6 kg, and mean prepregnancy BMI was 20.1 ± 2.3 kg/m^2. Compared with mothers with inadequate GWG, mothers with adequate or excessive GWG had significantly higher maternal education level and family income. Children whose mothers had excessive GWG were younger and were more likely to be boys, to have higher birth weight, and to be artificially fed during the first 6 months (All $P < 0.0001$).

As shown in Table 2, the prevalence of overweight and obesity was higher in children of mothers who had excessive GWG (12.7 and 9.9%) than that in those of mothers had adequate (11.0 and 6.8%) or inadequate GWG (8.8 and 5.1%). Whereas the prevalence of offspring thinness was higher in the inadequate GWG group (14.4%) than that in adequate (12.6%) or excessive GWG group (10.6%). This trend also existed within each prepregnancy BMI subgroup. Mothers with prepregnancy overweight, regardless of GWG category, were more likely to have overweight or obese offspring and less likely to have normal weight offspring compared with those with prepregnancy normal weight or underweight. In particular, among the prepregnancy overweight group, there was very high combined prevalence

Table 2 Children's weight status by GWG stratified by prepregnancy BMI categories

GWG categories	Children weight status (%)				P^*
	Thinness	Normal	Overweight	Obesity	
Overall	12.9	69.8	10.5	6.8	< 0.0001
Inadequate	14.4	71.6	8.8	5.1	
Adequate	12.6	69.7	11.0	6.8	
Excessive	10.6	66.7	12.7	9.9	
Prepregnancy underweight	19.0	69.3	7.4	4.3	< 0.0001
Inadequate	21.0	68.5	7.2	3.4	
Adequate	18.0	71.0	6.9	4.1	
Excessive	16.6	68.5	8.6	6.3	
Prepregnancy normal weight	11.4	70.5	11.0	7.1	< 0.0001
Inadequate	12.6	72.6	9.3	5.5	
Adequate	11.3	69.9	11.8	6.9	
Excessive	9.4	67.1	13.4	10.1	
Prepregnancy overweight	6.5	63.3	15.8	14.4	< 0.0001
Inadequate	8.0	72.4	11.0	8.6	
Adequate	6.5	62.4	16.7	14.3	
Excessive	5.4	58.2	18.2	18.2	

Values are presented as percentages

GWG gestational weight gain

*Differences of child weight status between gestational weight gain categories were evaluated by using Chi-square test

of offspring overweight and obesity in both the adequate (around 31%) as well as the excessive GWG group (around 36%).

As a continuous variable, GWG was positively associated with children's mean BMI after adjustment for all confounding factors, though the effect size was small (0.049 kg/m^2 change in children's mean BMI per 1-kg change in GWG). After stratified by prepregnancy BMI categories, the association remained statistically significant only in the prepregnancy underweight and normal weight subgroup. Similar associations were also observed between GWG and offspring BMI z-score (Table 3).

In logistic regression models, after adjustment for confounders, excessive GWG was associated with increased risk of offspring overweight/obesity [OR (95% CI): 1.31 (1.20, 1.43)] and lower risk of thinness [OR (95% CI): 0.80 (0.72, 0.90)] compared with adequate GWG (Table 4). In contrast, inadequate GWG was associated with elevated risk of offspring thinness [OR (95% CI): 1.18 (1.08, 1.30)] and lower odds of overweight/obesity [OR (95% CI): 0.86 (0.79, 0.94)] compared with adequate GWG. After stratified by prepregnancy BMI categories, we found positive associations between excessive GWG and offspring overweight/obesity, as well as between inadequate GWG and childhood thinness only among prepregnancy underweight and normal weight mothers. There was also a negative relation of inadequate GWG and risk of offspring overweight/obesity in prepregnancy normal weight and overweight/obese mothers.

Table 5 presents the trend of maternal prepregnancy BMI and GWG between 1996 and 2009. The average prepregnancy BMI decreased slightly from 20.4 kg/m^2 in 1996 to 20.1 kg/m^2 in 2009 ($P < 0.001$) (Fig. 1a). Accordingly, the prevalence of prepregnancy underweight increased from 22.7 to 24.8% ($P < 0.0001$). Especially noteworthy is that the average GWG increased significantly from 10.5 kg to 14.4 kg ($P < 0.001$) (Fig. 1b), with the prevalence of excessive GWG rising from 16.2 to 31.8%. Meanwhile, the prevalence of inadequate GWG decreased from 58.7 to 33.4% between 1996 and 2009. The increasing trend of GWG remained significant within each prepregnancy BMI category.

Table 4 Association between GWG and child weight status stratified by prepregnancy BMI categories

GWG categories	Childhood thinness		Childhood overweight/obesity	
	OR (95% CI)	*P*	OR (95% CI)	*P*
Overall				
Inadequate	1.18(1.08, 1.30)	0.0004	0.86(0.79, 0.94)	0.0009
Adequate	1.00		1.00	
Excessive	0.80(0.72, 0.90)	0.0002	1.31(1.20, 1.43)	< 0.0001
Prepregnancy underweight				
Inadequate	1.24(1.05, 1.46)	0.01	1.19(0.96, 1.47)	0.1127
Adequate	1.00		1.00	
Excessive	0.91(0.74, 1.11)	0.3458	1.51(1.21, 1.90)	0.0004
Prepregnancy normal weight				
Inadequate	1.17(1.04, 1.32)	0.0071	0.80(0.72, 0.89)	< 0.0001
Adequate	1.00		1.00	
Excessive	0.76(0.66, 0.88)	0.0002	1.30(1.17, 1.45)	< 0.0001
Prepregnancy overweight				
Inadequate	1.20(0.69, 2.09)	0.5243	0.55(0.39, 0.79)	0.0013
Adequate	1.00		1.00	
Excessive	0.84(0.48, 1.47)	0.5363	1.16(0.87, 1.54)	0.3214

Adjusted for child's age, gender, school, gestational age, birth weight, feeding patterns in the first 6 months, child's physical activities, maternal prepregnancy BMI, maternal education level, family monthly income and gestational diabetes mellitus
GWG gestational weight gain, *BMI* body mass index, *OR* odds ratio, *CI* confidence interval

Discussion

In this study, heterogeneity of relationship between GWG and offspring weight status stratified by prepregnancy BMI categories was observed. For mothers with prepregnancy underweight or normal weight, inadequate GWG increased the risk of thinness, while excessive GWG increased the risk of overweight/obesity in children aged 6–18 years, compared with mothers with adequate GWG. However, such associations were not found in children whose mothers were overweight/obese before pregnancy.

The positive overall association between excessive GWG and increased risk of children overweight/obesity in our study was consistent with previous studies [30–32]. Nevertheless, results from different studies

Table 3 Association between GWG and children's BMI stratified by prepregnancy BMI categories

GWG, kg	Children's BMI, kg/m^2			Children's BMI z-score		
	Coefficient	Standardized coefficient	*P*	Coefficient	Standardized coefficient	*P*
Overall	0.049	0.075	< 0.0001	0.021	0.090	< 0.0001
Prepregnancy underweight	0.037	0.063	< 0.0001	0.017	0.078	< 0.0001
Prepregnancy normal weight	0.058	0.088	< 0.0001	0.025	0.105	< 0.0001
Prepregnancy overweight	0.024	0.034	0.2096	0.008	0.033	0.2429

Adjusted for child's age, gender, school, gestational age, birth weight, feeding patterns in the first 6 months, child's physical activities, maternal prepregnancy BMI, maternal education level, family monthly income and gestational diabetes mellitus
GWG gestational weight gain, *BMI* body mass index

Table 5 Trends for maternal prepregnancy BMI and gestational weight gain during 1996 ~ 2009

	1996~ 2000	2001~ 2005	2006~ 2009	Overall	P^* for trend
Prepregnancy BMI categories[§]					
Underweight	22.7	23.1	24.8	23.5	0.0001
Normal weight	71.0	71.4	70.1	70.8	0.0784
Overweight	6.3	5.6	5.0	5.6	< 0.0001
GWG categories					
Overall[#]					
Inadequate	58.7	42.1	33.4	44.2	< 0.0001
Adequate	25.2	31.9	34.7	30.9	< 0.0001
Excessive	16.2	26.0	31.8	25.0	< 0.0001
Prepregnancy underweight[#]					
Inadequate	58.6	42.6	34.9	44.5	< 0.0001
Adequate	24.9	32.3	37.1	31.8	< 0.0001
Excessive	16.6	25.1	28.0	23.7	< 0.0001
Prepregnancy normal weight[#]					
Inadequate	61.0	43.2	34.2	45.6	< 0.0001
Adequate	23.8	31.5	33.9	30.0	< 0.0001
Excessive	15.2	25.3	31.9	24.5	< 0.0001
Prepregnancy overweight[#]					
Inadequate	32.4	25.9	15.1	24.9	< 0.0001
Adequate	42.0	36.3	35.1	37.8	0.0069
Excessive	25.6	37.8	49.8	37.2	< 0.0001

Values are presented as percentages
GWG gestational weight gain, *BMI* body mass index
[*]The Cochran-Armitage trend test were used for comparing the prevalence of each prepregnancy BMI and GWG category in different years
[#]Significant proportions ($P < 0.0001$) of GWG category during different period
[§]Significant proportions ($P < 0.0001$) of prepregnancy BMI category during different period

on the prepregnancy BMI-specific associations between excess GWG and child weight status have been inconsistent. Hinkle et al. [24] found a positive association between excess GWG and child BMI Z-score among normal and overweight mothers only, whereas Wrotniak et al. [33] found that the impact of excess GWG on offspring overweight was greatest in prepregnancy underweight women. Notably, we observed such association only among mothers who were underweight or normal weight, but not among overweight/obesity mothers. This result may reflect that there are many factors contributing to obesity among children born to overweight or obese mothers. These children may have already at increased risk of overweight/obesity because of genetic predisposition or familial lifestyle factors [20]. Indeed, we observed that both the prevalence of overweight and obesity were alarmingly high in children born to mothers with prepregnancy overweight, regardless of GWG status. A systematic review also lends support that prepregnancy overweight was associated with an increased risk of offspring overweight/obesity, compared with mothers with normal weight [34]. Therefore, in addition to preventing excess GWG, these findings further highlight the importance of avoiding prepregnancy overweight for the prevention of childhood overweight/obesity.

Research evaluating the relationship between inadequate GWG and childhood overweight/obesity has produced mixed conclusions. Two studies [30, 35] found that low GWG was associated with an increase in obesity risk, whereas another study [36] found no association between low GWG and child obesity in any prepregnancy BMI group. In contrast, we found a negative association between inadequate GWG and child overweight/obesity among prepregnancy non-underweight mothers. Our findings are intriguing for further studies to explore the reasons for such variation in different populations.

Our work also extends previous studies in which it examined the effect of maternal GWG on offspring thinness and found that inadequate GWG increased the risk of offspring thinness among mothers who were underweight or normal weight before pregnancy. Sarah et al. [37] found that low GWG during the first trimester of pregnancy was associated with reduced child BMI at age 4.5 years, independent of prepregnancy BMI and birth size, which provided some support for our findings. This suggests the need to promote adequate GWG for the

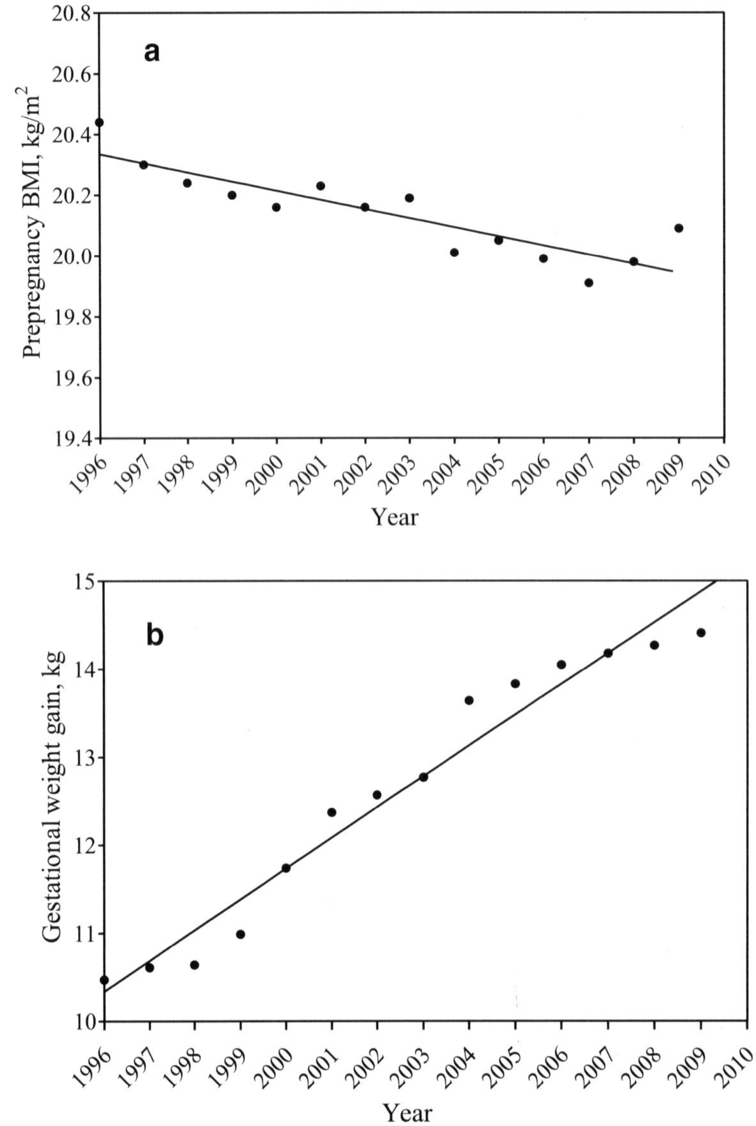

Fig. 1 **a** Trend of the mean maternal prepregnancy BMI during 1996–2009. **b** Trend of the mean maternal gestational weight gain during 1996–2009

prevention of not only childhood overweight/obesity but also thinness.

Interestingly, we found a negative association between excess GWG and offspring thinness, especially among normal weight mothers. This should be interpreted with caution and future studies are warranted to confirm the present finding. In the other hand, when considering the genetic variation among populations, the appropriate GWG may vary by ethnic group. The IOM category has been recommended by the Chinese Society of Nutrition and was applied in our study. However, the IOM recommended levels of pregnancy weight gain might not be optimal for Chinese women, especially for those with prepregnancy overweight women ($BMI \geq 24$ kg/m^2). Hence, further studies are required to access the applicability of IOM guidelines and to investigate whether new GWG classification guidelines are needed in China.

There are several important potential pathways by which GWG may relate to offspring BMI later in life. GWG is suggested to exert an indirect effect on child's weight status through birth weight [24]. However, despite the positive association of birth weight with later BMI [16], we found that the associations between GWG and child weight status remained fairly robust after adjusted for child's birth weight and other confounders.

Furthermore, measuring maternal nutrition or GWG is recognized as a proxy of the fetal nutrition environment [37]. Changes in fetal nutrition status or endocrine system may induce lasting alterations in physiology, metabolism, or organ structure of individuals, predisposing them to later metabolic disorders [38, 39]. Therefore, inadequate or excessive GWG may lead to partially nutritional modification of intrauterine exposures of the fetus. Firstly, intrauterine exposures may have sustained influence on offspring weight by determining fetus's body composition and programming of hypothalamic appetite regulation centers [40, 41]. Secondly, maternal over-nutrition may overstimulate fetal pancreatic Beta-cells and accordingly bring about fetal hyper-insulinism, which may have permanent effects on offspring pancreatic structure and function, resulting in impaired glucose tolerance and obesity in adolescence [40, 42]. Thirdly, central leptin sensitivity in offspring may also be affected by prenatal over-nutrition [43]. Changes in leptin levels during key periods of hypothalamic development may induce long-term and potentially irreversible effects on metabolism in later life [41]. It is not likely to test these possibilities based on this study, but these findings support that intrauterine exposures may mediate the relations of GWG and offspring weight status. Thus, promoting measures to ensure appropriate GWG is important for the prevention of childhood thinness and obesity regardless of maternal prepregnancy BMI.

Although achieving adequate GWG plays an important role in the long-term health of offspring, the average maternal GWG and the prevalence of excessive GWG were significantly increased during 1996 to 2009. It is noteworthy that the prevalence of excessive GWG during 2006–2009 was approximately twice as high as during 1996–2000. In contrast, both the percentage of women gaining above IOM recommendations and mean GWG in America only slightly increased from 2000 through 2009 [44]. The rapid economic development, improvement of food environment, as well as low level of physical activity may account for the increasing prevalence of excessive GWG women in China. Nevertheless, other reasons for this trend warrant further investigation. These trends suggest that it is important for policymakers and health professionals to develop practical strategies for healthy weight management during pregnancy.

There are several strengths of this study. Firstly, we related GWG to the risk of offspring thinness in childhood and adolescence. Our findings not only support other evidences suggesting to avoid excess weight gain during pregnancy but also emphasis the negative impact of inadequate GWG. Secondly, we considered the broad age spectrum of children (6–18 years). Finally, this is the first study to report the recent secular trends in prepregnancy BMI and maternal GWG among Chinese women. A rapidly increasing trend in GWG was identified and warranted more attention from researchers and clinicians.

A major limitation in our study is that the prepregnancy BMI and maternal GWG were assessed based on self-reported data rather than objective measurement, which may result in recall bias. However, previous studies found that self-reported weight and height were generally valid for identifying associations in epidemiological studies [45, 46]. Besides, a potential selection bias can't be excluded in this study, because children who didn't respond to questionnaire survey were more likely to be boys (55.4% vs. 49.9%) and be older (13.24 year vs. 12.32 year) than those who completed the questionnaire. To account for this, we additionally carried out subgroup analyses by gender and age. Results show that the associations between inappropriate GWG and offspring weight status were similar in different age group, and were slightly stronger in boys than in girls. Therefore, the associations we report here are possible to be underestimated, but not overestimated.

Conclusions

Our study suggested that inadequate GWG was associated with an increased risk of offspring thinness at 6–18 years of age, whereas excessive GWG was associated with an increased risk of offspring obesity. The adverse effects of inadequate or excessive GWG on offspring weight status were only found for initially underweight and normal-weight mothers, but not for overweight/obese mothers. More attention should be paid to the influences of maternal weight change during pregnancy on childhood weight status to prevent the inter-generational cycle of thinness and obesity.

Abbreviations

BMI: Body mass index; CI: Confidence interval; GDM: Gestational diabetes mellitus; GWG: Gestational weight gain; IOM: the Institute of Medicine; MVPA: Moderate-to-vigorous physical activity; OR: Odds ratio

Acknowledgments

We acknowledged the participation of all participants, as well as the efforts of doctors and nurses in anthropometric measurement and data collection.

Funding

This study is sponsored by Guangdong Science and Technology Program (No.2014A0202-20002). LC and NW's contribution were also supported by the National Natural Science Foundation of China (No. 81602862) and the Natural Science Foundation of Guangdong Province, China (No. 2016A030310150).

Authors' contributions

LC and YC conceived and designed the study; JY, NW, TZ and WT collected the data; LC and NW analyzed the data; JY and WT contributed materials; LC and NW wrote the draft. All authors read and approved the final manuscript.

Competing interests

The authors declare that they have no competing interests.

References

1. Han JC, Lawlor DA, Kimm SY. Childhood obesity. Lancet. 2010;375:1737–48.
2. Ng M, Fleming T, Robinson M, Thomson B, Graetz N, Margono C, Mullany EC, Biryukov S, Abbafati C, Abera SF, et al. Global, regional, and national prevalence of overweight and obesity in children and adults during 1980-2013: a systematic analysis for the Global Burden of Disease Study 2013. Lancet. 2014;384:766–81.
3. Pulgaron ER. Childhood obesity: a review of increased risk for physical and psychological comorbidities. Clin Ther. 2013;35:A18–32.
4. Owens S, Galloway R. Childhood obesity and the metabolic syndrome. Curr Atheroscler Rep. 2014;16:436.
5. Sweat V, Yates KF, Migliaccio R, Convit A. Obese adolescents show reduced cognitive processing speed compared with healthy weight peers. Child Obes. 2017;13:190–6.
6. Noh JW, Kim YE, Park J, Oh IH, Kwon YD. Impact of parental socioeconomic status on childhood and adolescent overweight and underweight in Korea. J Epidemiol. 2014;24:221–9.
7. Martinez-Vizcaino V, Solera MM, Notario PB, Sanchez LM, Garcia-Prieto JC, Torrijos NC, Arias PN, Salcedo AF, Rodriguez-Artalejo F. Trends in excess of weight, underweight and adiposity among Spanish children from 2004 to 2010: the Cuenca study. Public Health Nutr. 2012;15:2170–4.
8. Lee G, Ham OK. Factors affecting underweight and obesity among elementary school children in South Korea. Asian Nurs Res. 2015;9:298–304.
9. Candler T, Costa S, Heys M, Costello A, Viner RM. Prevalence of thinness in adolescent girls in low- and middle-income countries and associations with wealth, food security, and inequality. J Adolesc Health. 2017;60:447–54.
10. Wolnicka K, Jarosz M, Jaczewska-Schuetz J, Taraszewska AM. Differences in the prevalence of overweight, obesity and underweight among children from primary schools in rural and urban areas. Ann Agric Environ Med. 2016;23:341–4.
11. Schaible UE, Kaufmann SH. Malnutrition and infection: complex mechanisms and global impacts. PLoS Med. 2007;4:e115.
12. Gaayeb L, Sarr JB, Cames C, Pincon C, Hanon JB, Ndiath MO, Seck M, Herbert F, Sagna AB, Schacht AM, et al. Effects of malnutrition on children's immunity to bacterial antigens in northern Senegal. Am J Trop Med Hyg. 2014;90:566–73.
13. Goldstein RF, Abell SK, Ranasinha S, Misso M, Boyle JA, Black MH, Li N, Hu G, Corrado F, Rode L, et al. Association of gestational weight gain with maternal and infant outcomes: a systematic review and meta-analysis. JAMA. 2017;317:2207–25.
14. Guo L, Liu J, Ye R, Liu J, Zhuang Z, Ren A. Gestational weight gain and overweight in children aged 3-6 years. J Epidemiol. 2015;25:536–43.
15. Leonard SA, Petito LC, Rehkopf DH, Ritchie LD, Abrams B. Weight gain in pregnancy and child weight status from birth to adulthood in the United States. Pediatr Obes. 2017;12(Suppl 1):18–25.
16. Oken E, Rifas-Shiman SL, Field AE, Frazier AL, Gillman MW. Maternal gestational weight gain and offspring weight in adolescence. Obstet Gynecol. 2008;112:999–1006.
17. Laitinen J, Jaaskelainen A, Hartikainen AL, Sovio U, Vaarasmaki M, Pouta A, Kaakinen M, Jarvelin MR. Maternal weight gain during the first half of pregnancy and offspring obesity at 16 years: a prospective cohort study. BJOG. 2012;119:716–23.
18. Mamun AA, O'Callaghan M, Callaway L, Williams G, Najman J, Lawlor DA. Associations of gestational weight gain with offspring body mass index and blood pressure at 21 years of age: evidence from a birth cohort study. Circulation. 2009;119:1720–7.
19. Lawlor DA, Lichtenstein P, Fraser A, Langstrom N. Does maternal weight gain in pregnancy have long-term effects on offspring adiposity? A sibling study in a prospective cohort of 146,894 men from 136,050 families. Am J Clin Nutr. 2011;94:142–8.
20. Branum AM, Parker JD, Keim SA, Schempf AH. Prepregnancy body mass index and gestational weight gain in relation to child body mass index among siblings. Am J Epidemiol. 2011;174:1159–65.
21. Mamun AA, Mannan M, Doi SA. Gestational weight gain in relation to offspring obesity over the life course: a systematic review and bias-adjusted meta-analysis. Obes Rev. 2014;15:338–47.
22. Fraser A, Tilling K, Macdonald-Wallis C, Sattar N, Brion MJ, Benfield L, Ness A, Deanfield J, Hingorani A, Nelson SM, et al. Association of maternal weight gain in pregnancy with offspring obesity and metabolic and vascular traits in childhood. Circulation. 2010;121:2557 64.
23. Mourtakos SP, Tambalis KD, Panagiotakos DB, Antonogeorgos G, Alexi CD, Georgoulis M, Saade G, Sidossis LS. Association between gestational weight gain and risk of obesity in preadolescence: a longitudinal study (1997–2007) of 5125 children in Greece. J Hum Nutr Diet. 2017;30:51–8.
24. Hinkle SN, Sharma AJ, Swan DW, Schieve LA, Ramakrishnan U, Stein AD. Excess gestational weight gain is associated with child adiposity among mothers with normal and overweight prepregnancy weight status. J Nutr. 2012;142:1851–8.
25. Chen C, Lu FC. The guidelines for prevention and control of overweight and obesity in Chinese adults. Biomed Environ Sci. 2004;17(Suppl):1–36.
26. to IOMU, Guidelines RIPW. Weight gain during pregnancy: reexamining the guidelines. Washington (DC): National Academies Press (US); 2009.
27. Group of China Obesity Task Force. Body mass index reference norm for screening overweight and obesity in Chinese children and adolescents. Zhonghua Liu Xing Bing Xue Za Zhi. 2004;25:97–102.
28. China NHAF. Screening standard for malnutrition of school-age children and adolescents. 2014. http://www.moh.gov.cn/zwgkzt/pqt/201407/38b15c0a1ed444e8908e12752decaffa.shtml. Accessed 4 July 2014.
29. Lee PH, Macfarlane DJ, Lam TH, Stewart SM. Validity of the international physical activity questionnaire short form (IPAQ-SF): a systematic review. Int J Behav Nutr Phys Act. 2011;8:115.
30. Stuebe AM, Forman MR, Michels KB. Maternal-recalled gestational weight gain, pre-pregnancy body mass index, and obesity in the daughter. Int J Obes. 2009;33:743–52.
31. Ensenauer R, Chmitorz A, Riedel C, Fenske N, Hauner H, Nennstiel-Ratzel U, von Kries R. Effects of suboptimal or excessive gestational weight gain on childhood overweight and abdominal adiposity: results from a retrospective cohort study. Int J Obes. 2013;37:505–12.
32. Shao T, Tao H, Ni L, Sun Y, Yan S, Gu C, Cao H, Huang K, Hao J, Tao F. Maternal pre-pregnancy body mass index and gestational weight gain with preschool children's overweight and obesity. Zhonghua Yu Fang Yi Xue Za Zhi. 2016;50:123–8.
33. Wrotniak BH, Shults J, Butts S, Stettler N. Gestational weight gain and risk of overweight in the offspring at age 7 y in a multicenter, multiethnic cohort study. Am J Clin Nutr. 2008;87:1818–24.
34. Yu Z, Han S, Zhu J, Sun X, Ji C, Guo X. Pre-pregnancy body mass index in relation to infant birth weight and offspring overweight/obesity: a systematic review and meta-analysis. PLoS One. 2013;8:e61627.
35. Crozier SR, Inskip HM, Godfrey KM, Cooper C, Harvey NC, Cole ZA, Robinson SM. Weight gain in pregnancy and childhood body composition: findings from the Southampton Women's survey. Am J Clin Nutr. 2010;91:1745–51.
36. von Kries R, Ensenauer R, Beyerlein A, Amann-Gassner U, Hauner H, Rosario AS. Gestational weight gain and overweight in children: results from the cross-sectional German KiGGS study. Int J Pediatr Obes. 2011;6:45–52.
37. Wilcox SK. Risk factors for maternal low weight gain during pregnancy and associations with offspring body size and fat distribution. Atlanta: Emory University. Health Sciences, Public Health. 2006. p. 104–7.
38. Barker DJ. In utero programming of chronic disease. Clin Sci (Lond). 1998;95:115–28.
39. Godfrey KM, Barker DJ. Fetal nutrition and adult disease. Am J Clin Nutr. 2000;71:1344S–52S.
40. Oken E, Gillman MW. Fetal origins of obesity. Obes Res. 2003;11:496–506.
41. Bouret SG. Early life origins of obesity: role of hypothalamic programming. J Pediatr Gastroenterol Nutr. 2009;48(Suppl 1):S31–8.
42. Silverman BL, Rizzo TA, Cho NH, Metzger BE. Long-term effects of the intrauterine environment. The Northwestern University diabetes in pregnancy center. Diabetes Care. 1998;21(Suppl 2):B142–9.
43. Ferezou-Viala J, Roy AF, Serougne C, Gripois D, Parquet M, Bailleux V, Gertler A, Delplanque B, Djiane J, Riottot M, Taouis M. Long-term consequences of maternal high-fat feeding on hypothalamic leptin sensitivity and diet-induced obesity in the offspring. Am J Physiol Regul Integr Comp Physiol. 2007;293:R1056–62.
44. Johnson JL, Farr SL, Dietz PM, Sharma AJ, Barfield WD, Robbins CL. Trends in gestational weight gain: the pregnancy risk assessment monitoring system, 2000-2009. Am J Obstet Gynecol. 2015;212:801–6.
45. Spencer EA, Appleby PN, Davey GK, Key TJ. Validity of self-reported height and weight in 4808 EPIC-Oxford participants. Public Health Nutr. 2002;5:561–5.
46. Stommel M, Schoenborn CA. Accuracy and usefulness of BMI measures based on self-reported weight and height: findings from the NHANES & NHIS 2001-2006. BMC Public Health. 2009;9:421.

Health-related quality of life among Chinese adolescent girls with Dysmenorrhoea

Cho Lee Wong

Abstract

Background: Primary dysmenorrhoea is common in girls who have begun menstruating. However, few studies have examined its effect on the quality of life of a young population. The study aimed to evaluate the quality of life of adolescent girls with dysmenorrhoea in Hong Kong.

Methods: The study adopted a cross-sectional descriptive approach. A convenience sample of 653 girls aged 13 to 19 years old was recruited from three secondary schools in Hong Kong. The 36-item Short-Form Health Survey was used to examine the health-related quality of life of the participants. The severity of dysmenorrhoea was assessed using a 10-point visual analog scale.

Results: Girls suffering from dysmenorrhoea reported high pain prevalence and intensity. However, the majority of girls with dysmenorrhoea did not seek medical advice (93.2%) or self-medicate (82%). The role-physical, bodily pain, general health and social functioning domain scores of girls with dysmenorrhoea were significantly lower than those without dysmenorrhoea. Moreover, girls with severe dysmenorrhoea had a significantly lower quality of life in the bodily pain domain than those with mild and moderate forms of condition.

Conclusions: Findings suggest that dysmenorrhoea is highly prevalent among adolescent girls in Hong Kong. Girls may suffer severe pain, which degrades their quality of life.

Keywords: Adolescent, Dysmenorrhoea, Quality of life

Plain English summary

Dysmenorrhoea not only affects girls' physical health, but also affects their daily lives and social activities. These effects, in turn, likely affect the emotional and social functions of girls with dysmenorrhoea. Some studies have examined quality of life as a specific construct among university students and women with dysmenorrhoea. However, the influence of dysmenorrhoea on the quality of life of adolescent Chinese girls has been poorly studied. This study describes and compares the quality of life of adolescent Chinese girls with or without dysmenorrhoea. A total of 653 girls were recruited from three secondary schools in Hong Kong. The prevalence of dysmenorrhoea was 65.5% in this group. Over 90% of the participants did not seek medical advice, and some participants reported self-medicating with an incorrect dose or unknown medication. In addition, girls with dysmenorrhoea have significantly lower quality of life than those without dysmenorrhoea. Healthcare professionals should be made aware that adolescent girls who suffer from dysmenorrhoea are likely to have a lower quality of life. Adolescent girls should be screened for dysmenorrhoea symptoms and promptly provided with appropriate interventions. Moreover, the understanding of self-medication among Chinese adolescent girls should be improved. Appropriate educational interventions related to dysmenorrhoea, with the correct administration of self-medication as an essential component, should be developed and provided.

Correspondence: jojowong@cuhk.edu.hk
The Nethersole School of Nursing, Faculty of Medicine, The Chinese University of Hong Kong, Room 824, Esther Lee Building, Shatin, New Territories, Hong Kong

Background

Primary dysmenorrhoea is one of the most common menstrual problems among adolescent girls [1] and is defined as painful menstruation in the absence of abnormal pelvic anatomy and ovulation [2]. It often commences six to twelve months post-menarche, and its symptoms appear a few hours prior to or with the onset of menstrual flow. Symptoms of dysmenorrhoea include cramping pain that often radiates to the lower back or anterior thigh from the lower abdomen [3]. Pain is most intense during the first 24 to 36 h and lasts for two to three days [4]. Some girls may experience nausea, vomiting, headache, loose bowel movements or dizziness as well [5]. Dysmenorrhoea is highly prevalent among adolescent girls: worldwide, approximately 20 to 90% of adolescent girls suffer from dysmenorrhoea [6–8]. Its prevalence progressively decreases with age [9]. To date, no extensive epidemiological study has investigated the prevalence of dysmenorrhoea among adolescent girls in Hong Kong. One local study indicated that 68.7% of 5609 secondary-school girls aged 11 to 20 suffer from dysmenorrhoea [10].

Dysmenorrhoea affects adolescent girls' academic, social and physical activities [3, 11]. Other studies have quantified the effect of dysmenorrhoea in terms of days of lost work or school absenteeism [8, 12–15]. Dysmenorrhoea results in the loss of 600 million working hours and two billion dollars' worth of productivity leach year in the United States [12]. Dysmenorrhoea also negatively affects sufferers' quality of life [16–18]. A study in Hong Kong utilised the Short-Form Health Survey (SF-36) to compare the effects of different menstrual problems, such as dysmenorrhoea, amenorrhea (absence of a menstrual period in a girl with reproductive age), menorrhagia (periods with abnormally heavy or prolonged bleeding) and eumenorrhoeic (normal periods), on 235 adolescents [18]. Results showed that adolescents with dysmenorrhoea had the lowest quality of life scores in the bodily pain domain. Moreover, their scores in the general health and social functioning domains were significantly lower than those of girls without menstrual problems. However, the above results should be treated with caution given the small sample size of subjects with dysmenorrhoea ($n = 43$).

Currently, few studies have examined quality of life as a specific construct among university students and women with dysmenorrhoea [16, 19]. However, the influence of dysmenorrhoea on the quality of life among adolescent Chinese girls has been poorly studied. Therefore, this study aimed to examine the effects of dysmenorrhoea on the quality of life of adolescent girls in Hong Kong. In this study, dysmenorrhoea was defined in accordance with a review conducted by the World Health Organization [1]. It was defined as painful menses within the last three months [8]. It is hypothesised that adolescent girls with dysmenorrhoea will report a lower quality of life than those without dysmenorrhoea.

Methods

Sample and setting

The study sample was recruited from Hong Kong secondary schools and was randomly selected. The sample was recruited from secondary schools given that all girls in their early adolescence are in Forms 1 to 3 in accordance with the compulsory education policy of Hong Kong; moreover, according to a previous government report, approximately 85% of students aged 15–16 are in Forms 4 or 5 [20]. Boys-only and international schools were excluded.

Given that the mean age of menarche among Hong Kong adolescent girls is 12.3 [10], and girls experience dysmenorrhoea at six to twelve months after menarche when ovulatory cycles are established [21], a convenience sample of students from Forms 2 to 7 (13 to 19 years old) were recruited to avoid having large numbers of pre-menarche girls. Information about dysmenorrhoea was collected from those who indicated that they had experienced dysmenorrhoea within the last three month [8, 22]. Girls who (1) were pre-menarche, (2) had a previous history of gynecological disease or surgery or (3) had a severe condition such as heart or malignant disease, were excluded.

Outcome measures

The demographic and menstrual characteristics questionnaire

A 19-item questionnaire for the demographic and menstrual characteristics of adolescents was developed by the researcher given the lack of an appropriate questionnaire. The questionnaire was developed on the basis of available literature [23].

The Pain Visual Analogue Scale (PVAS) was used to assess the average intensity of dysmenorrhoea pain experienced within the last three months [24, 25]. The PVAS consists of a 10 cm horizontal line with verbal descriptors at either end (0 = "no pain"; 10 ="worst possible pain"). Subjects were instructed to place a cross on the line that represent the average intensity of their pain. Scores ranged from 0 to 10, with high scores indicating high pain intensity. The scale has well-established reliability and validity with a Cronbach's alpha of 0.94 [26]. Scores between 1 and 3.9 were classified as mild dysmenorrhoea, those between 4 and 7.9 as moderate dysmenorrhoea, and those between 8 and 10 as severe dysmenorrhoea [27].

Health-related quality of life

The HRQOL of the participants were assessed using the 36-item SF36 [28]. The form consists of 36 questions that measure eight HRQOL domains: physical functioning, role-physical, bodily pain, general health, vitality, social functioning, role-emotional and mental health.

Item scores in each domain were summed to yield domain scores, which were transformed into a range of 0 to 100. A high score indicated superior HRQOL. The eight domain scores were summed to form the physical and mental component summary scores. The Chinese (HK) SF-36v2 used in this study had undergone validity testing and was normalised to the general Chinese population in Hong Kong [29, 30].

Procedure

A letter was sent to schools inviting their students to join the study. Students who showed interest received written information. In a classroom or hall setting, a female research assistant explained details of the study. Girls who agreed to participate were asked to complete the informed consent forms and questionnaires, which included the structured demographic and menstrual characteristics and the Chinese (HK) version SF-36v2 questionnaires. During the data collection process, the researcher answered queries about the questionnaires.

Statistical analyses

SPSS 22.0 (SPSS, Chicago, IL) was used to analyse data and descriptive statistics to present the participants' characteristics and HRQQL scores. For each outcome variables, an independent sample t-test or chi-square test was performed to identify differences between girls with or without dysmenorrhoea. Linear regressions were used to compare HRQOL between the two groups with adjustments for significantly different socio-demographics. A one-way analysis of variance or a Kruskal-Wallis test was used to compare menstrual characteristics and quality of life scores among the mild, moderate and severe dysmenorrhoea groupings. All statistical tests were two-tailed, and the level of statistical significance was set at 5%.

Ethical approval

Ethical approval from the study institution and permission to use the study instruments were obtained. This study was carried out in accordance with the Declaration of Helsinki. Participants were informed that their participation was voluntary, and they could withdraw from the study at any time. They were also told that all the information collected would be kept confidential.

Results

Six secondary schools were approached and three agreed to participate in the study with a participation rate of 50%. A total of 704 girls from the three schools participated, 51 of them were excluded (two with gynecological disease, 21 were pre-menarche and 28 produced incomplete item responses). The final sample consisted of 653 girls.

Demographic and menstrual characteristics

The ages of the participants ranged from 13 to 19 years (mean = 15.67, SD = 1.54). The average body mass index of the participants was 19.00 (SD = 2.63). Nearly 40% (n = 251) had a family income of more than HK$20,000. Their age at menarche ranged from 10 to 16 (mean = 12.07, SD = 2.23). Over 70% (n = 504) of the participants had a menstrual cycle of between 21 and 35 days, with a mean menstruation period of 5.60 days (SD = 1.08). A majority had moderate menstruation (n = 528). The prevalence of dysmenorrhoea in the recruited group was 65.5% (n = 428). Participants with dysmenorrhoea were significantly older than those without dysmenorrhoea ($p < 0.001$). The demographics and menstrual characteristics of the participants are shown in Table 1.

Menstrual characteristics of girls with dysmenorrhoea

Participants with dysmenorrhoea reported an average pain intensity over the previous three menstrual cycles of 5.43 (SD = 2.13). Of the participants, 27.1% reported mild pain, 60.8% reported moderate pain and 12.1% reported severe pain. The most common area of pain was the lower abdomen (83.9%) and lumbar region (6.1%). Fatigue (37.5%) and breast tenderness (16.1%) were other common complaints. Nearly 40% of the subjects first experienced dysmenorrhoea six months to a year after menarche. More than half (51.6%) of the participants reported that the onset of dysmenorrhoea occurred on the first day of their menstrual cycle, and 34.8% reported that their dysmenorrhoea symptoms disappeared on the third day of their cycle. A total of 239 girls (55.8%) reported that dysmenorrhoea only slightly affected their daily activities. Approximately 16% (n = 68) of the participants were absent from class in the current half year because of dysmenorrhoea. Approximately half of the participants (56.8%) had received menstrual education. The person most commonly consulted on the subject of dysmenorrhoea was their mother (n = 201) or a friend (n = 73). The menstrual characteristics of adolescent girls with dysmenorrhoea are shown in Table 2.

A majority of girls did not seek medical advice (93.2%) or self-medicate (82%) during the last three cycles, whereas 16.6% took modern medicine and 1.4% took Chinese herbs or traditional remedies for their pain (Table 2). The medication and dosage the participants used were revealed through open-ended questions. A total of 62 participants took one to three tablets of paracetamol, and one took poston, a non-steroidal anti-inflammatory drug. One girl reported taking a few tablets of paracetamol, which is used to treat pain and fever, each time she experienced pain. One girl mentioned using famotidine, which is used to inhibit stomach acid production. Other girls reported taking one tablet of an unknown medication. Among those using Chinese herbs

Table 1 Demographic and menstrual characteristics of the participants

	Total sample ($n = 653$)	With dysmenorrhea ($n = 428$)	Without dysmenorrhea ($n = 225$)	p-value
Age (years)				
Mean (SD)	15.67 (1.54)	15.82 (1.56)	15.40 (1.50)	< 0.001[a]
Height (cm)				
Mean (SD)	159.32 (5.79)	159.39 (5.66)	159.16 (6.04)	0.62[a]
Weight (kg)				
Mean (SD)	48.25 (7.24)	48.10 (7.14)	48.53 (7.44)	0.48[a]
BMI				
Mean (SD)	19.00 (2.63)	18.91 (2.47)	19.12 (2.91)	0.25[a]
Family income (HK$)				
< 5000	20 (3.1)	12 (2.8)	8 (3.6)	0.27[b]
5001–10,000	136 (20.8)	80 (18.7)	56 (24.9)	
10,001–20,000	246 (37.7)	166 (38.8)	80 (35.6)	
20,001–30,000	146 (22.4)	94 (22.0)	52 (23.1)	
> 30,001	105 (16.1)	76 (17.8)	29 (12.9)	
Age at menarche (years)				
Mean (SD)	12.07 (2.23)	12.06 (1.00)	12.14 (1.07)	0.33[a]
Menstrual cycle (days)				
16–20	47 (7.2)	29 (6.8)	18 (8.0)	0.44[b]
21–25	137 (21.0)	97 (22.7)	40 (17.8)	
26–30	262 (40.1)	165 (38.6)	97 (43.1)	
31–35	105 (16.1)	74 (17.3)	31 (13.8)	
36-40	45 (6.9)	31 (7.2)	14 (6.2)	
≥ 40	57 (8.8)	32 (7.5)	25 (11.1)	
Menstruation duration (days)				
Mean (SD)	5.60 (1.08)	5.60 (1.10)	5.61 (1.12)	0.93[a]
Amount of menstruation				
Small	42 (6.4)	24 (5.6)	18 (8.0)	0.30[b]
Moderate	528 (80.9)	345 (80.6)	183 (81.3)	
Large	83 (12.7)	59 (13.8)	24 (10.7)	

Data is presented as frequencies (percentages)
SD standard deviation
[a] independent sample t-test
[b] chi-square test

or remedies, two took Bak Foong pill, which is used to relieve menstrual discomfort. Three took Gu Sao pill to relieve menstrual discomfort. However, one girl was unable to name the medication she took.

Menstrual characteristics of adolescent girls with different severities of dysmenorrhoea

Compared with adolescent girls with mild or moderate dysmenorrhoea, girls with severe dysmenorrhoea were significantly more likely to have higher pain intensity ($p < 0.001$), more limited daily activities ($p = 0.002$), and a higher absence rate ($p < 0.001$). They were more likely to consult others ($p < 0.001$) and self-medicate ($p < 0.001$). However, they were less likely to have received menstrual education ($p = 0.016$) (Table 3).

Health-related quality of life

No difference was reported between the average SF-36 scores of girls with and without dysmenorrhoea, except for that in role-physical ($p = 0.04$), bodily pain ($p < 0.001$), general health ($p = 0.02$), and social functioning ($p = 0.003$) domains. The comparative difference in the mental component summary between the two groups was non-significant ($p = 0.17$), whereas the difference in the physical component summary was significant ($p < 0.001$) after adjusting for age (Table 4). The scores in the bodily

Table 2 Menstrual characteristics of adolescent girls with dysmenorrhea

	With dysmenorrhea (*n* = 428)
Pain intensity	
Mean (SD)	5.43 (2.13)
Area of dysmenorrheal pain	
Upper abdomen	17 (4.0%)
Lower abdomen	359 (83.9%)
Pelvic region	17 (4.0%)
Lumbar region	26 (6.1%)
Inner thigh	5 (1.2%)
Other	4 (0.9%)
Other discomforts	
Breast tenderness	85 (16.1%)
Swelling of lower limbs	17 (3.2%)
Fatigue	197 (37.5%)
Nausea	35 (6.7%)
Headache	43 (8.2%)
Diarrhea	33 (6.3%)
Anxiety	38 (7.2%)
Palpitations	4 (0.8%)
Skin problems	57 (10.8%)
Other	17 (3.2%)
First experience of dysmenorrhea	
In the first menarche	82 (19.2%)
6 months to a year after menarche	161 (37.6%)
1 to 2 years after menarche	93 (21.7%)
2 years after menarche	68 (15.9%)
Other/ forgotten	24 (5.6%)
Onset of dysmenorrhea	
Day before menstrual cycle	109 (25.5%)
First day of cycle	221 (51.6%)
Second day of cycle	80 (18.7%)
Other	18 (4.2%)
End of dysmenorrhea	
First day of menstrual cycle	54 (12.6%)
Second day of menstrual cycle	135 (31.5%)
Third day of menstrual cycle	149 (34.8%)
Fourth day of menstrual cycle	56 (13.1%)
Fifth day of menstrual cycle	22 (5.1%)
Others	12 (2.8%)
Limitation of daily activities due to dysmenorrhea	
None	52 (12.1%)
Slightly affected	239 (55.8%)
Moderately affected	108 (25.2%)
Seriously affected	29 (6.8%)
Absence from class in this half year due to dysmenorrhea (days)	
0	360 (84.1%)
1	43 (10%)
2	15 (3.5%)
3	6 (1.4%)
≥ 4	4 (0.9%)
Received menstrual education	
No	185 (43.2%)
Yes	243 (56.8%)
Others consulted about dysmenorrheal	
No one	174
Mother	201
Father	3
Sister	42
Friend	73
Teacher	4
Nurse	2
Medical consultation for dysmenorrhea	
None	399 (93.2%)
Chinese practitioner	9 (2.1%)
Modern practitioner	20 (4.7%)
Self-medication for dysmenorrhea in the last 3 months	
None	351 (82%)
Chinese herbs/ medicine	6 (1.4%)
Modern medicine	71 (16.6%)

pain domain of girls with severe dysmenorrhoea were significantly lower than those of girls with mild or moderate dysmenorrhoea (Table 5).

Discussion

This is the first large-scale study to examine HRQOL among Chinese adolescent girls with dysmenorrhoea in Hong Kong. Results found that the prevalence of dysmenorrhoea was 65.5%, and the mean dysmenorrhoeal pain score of the girls, as measured by PVAS, was 5.43 (SD = 2.13). The majority of participants reported that dysmenorrhoea limited their daily activities. Besides, adolescent girls with dysmenorrhoea not only had a reduced quality of life in the role-physical, bodily pain and general health domains, but also in the social functioning domain compared with those without dysmenorrhoea. However, most of the girls (93.2%) did not seek medical advice despite the significant effect of dysmenorrhoea on their lives. Only approximately 18% of the participants in this study self-medicated.

Table 3 Menstrual characteristics of adolescent girls with different severity rates of dysmenorrhea

	Mild dysmenorrhea (*n* = 116)	Moderate dysmenorrhea (*n* = 260)	Severe dysmenorrhea (n = 52)	p-value
Pain intensity				
Mean (SD)	2.75 (0.78)	5.94 (1.10)	8.87 (0.81)	< 0.001[a]
Limitation of daily activities due to dysmenorrhea				
None	24 (20.7)	26 (10)	2 (3.8)	0.002[b]
Affected	92 (79.3)	234 (90)	50 (96.2)	
Absence from class in this half year due to dysmenorrhea (day)				
No	113 (97.4)	215 (82.7)	32 (61.5)	< 0.001[b]
Yes	3 (2.6)	45 (17.3)	20 (38.5)	
Received menstrual education				
No	38 (32.8)	119 (45.8)	28 (53.8)	0.016[b]
Yes	78 (67.2)	141 (54.2)	24 (46.2)	
Consulted others on dysmenorrhea				
No	64 (55.2)	101 (38.8)	9 (17.3)	< 0.001[b]
Yes	52 (44.8)	159 (61.2)	43 (82.7)	
Medical consultation for dysmenorrhea				
No	110 (94.8)	241 (92.7)	48 (92.3)	0.72[b]
Yes	6 (5.2)	19 (7.3)	4 (7.7)	
Self-medication for dysmenorrhea in the last 3 months				
No	109 (94)	210 (80.8)	32 (61.5)	< 0.001[b]
Yes	7 (6)	50 (19.2)	20 (38.5)	

Data is presented as frequencies (percentages)
SD, standard deviation
[a] one-way analysis of variance
[b] Kruskal-Wallis test

Prevalence, symptoms, and effect

The prevalence of dysmenorrhoea found in this study (65.5%) corresponded with the results of a previous local study [10]. The worldwide prevalence of dysmenorrhoea ranges from 20 to 90% [6, 8]. Different operational definitions of dysmenorrhoea may account for the differences in reported prevalence. Some empirical studies defined dysmenorrhoea as any subjective report of pain [4, 31] or pain during the previous menstrual cycle with a score higher than 5 on the 0-to-10 point PVAS [32]. The

Table 4 Average SF-36 scores of girls with or without dysmenorrhea

	Total Sample n = 653	With dysmenorrhea n = 428	Without dysmenorrhea n = 225	p-value (unadjusted)[a]	*p*-value (adjusted)[b]
Health-related quality of life (SF-36)					
Physical functioning	85.75 (17.97)	86.27 (16.93)	84.76 (19.82)	0.33	0.41
Role-physical	65.62 (37.70)	63.14 (38.16)	70.33 (36.45)	< 0.001	0.04
Bodily pain	64.79 (21.94)	59.58 (20.38)	74.71 (21.43)	< 0.001	< 0.001
General health	56.69 (18.33)	55.31 (18.32)	59.33 (18.10)	< 0.001	0.02
Vitality	56.37 (18.81)	55.88 (18.48)	57.31 (19.42)	0.36	0.63
Social functioning	72.48 (19.19)	70.82 (18.74)	75.64 (19.67)	< 0.001	0.003
Role-emotional	52.99 (41.90)	50.78 (41.47)	57.19 (42.48)	0.07	0.15
Mental health	60.55 (17.50)	59.77 (17.63)	62.04 (17.19)	0.11	0.15
Physical component summary (PCS) score	50.29 (7.96)	49.48 (8.03)	51.83 (7.62)	< 0.001	< 0.001
Mental component summary (MCS) score	38.39 (12.01)	37.82 (12.04)	39.54 (11.90)	0.08	0.17

Data is presented as frequencies (percentages)
[a] Unadjusted comparisons between girls with or without dysmenorrhea were made using independent t-tests
[b] Adjusted comparisons between girls with or without dysmenorrhea were made using linear regression with adjustment for age

Table 5 Severity of dysmenorrhea and mean scores of SF-36 domains

	Severity of dysmenorrheal			
	Mild dysmenorrhea (n = 116)	Moderate dysmenorrhea (n = 260)	Severe dysmenorrhea (n = 52)	p-value[a]
Health-related quality of life (SF-36)				
Physical functioning	85.56 (18.31)	86.13 (16.75)	88.56 (14.53)	0.77
Role-physical	62.07 (39.77)	63.65 (37.62)	62.98 (37.86)	0.91
Bodily pain	63.28 (19.97)	59.53 (20.40)	51.60 (21.38)	0.005
General health	57.06 (18.00)	54.76 (17.90)	54.13 (20.97)	0.44
Vitality	56.29 (16.19)	55.98 (19.10)	54.42 (20.36)	0.92
Social functioning	73.60 (17.35)	70.10 (19.40)	68.30 (17.93)	0.17
Role-emotional	47.41 (39.35)	51.92 (42.56)	52.56 (40.88)	0.60
Mental health	61.00 (15.38)	59.57 (20.40)	58.00 (21.22)	0.83
Physical component summary (PCS) score	50.05 (8.32)	49.39 (8.08)	48.71 (7.15)	0.52
Mental component summary (MCS) score	37.78 (10.61)	37.88 (12.48)	37.32 (13.00)	0.93

Data is presented as frequencies (percentages)
[a] independent samples t-test

present study defined dysmenorrhoea as any subjective report of menstrual pain within the last three months. This definition is consistent with that provided by the World Health Organization [1]. The duration used to define or investigate dysmenorrhoea may also affect the reported prevalence. Ohde and colleagues revealed that only 15.8% of 823 Japanese women aged 18 to 51 years old experienced dysmenorrhoea within the previous month [33]. However, this figure was lower than that reported by another study, which reported that more than 70% of 3941 Japanese women suffered from dysmenorrhoea over the previous six months [22]. The high prevalence in that study may have been caused by recall bias given its relatively long investigation period. On the other hand, the use of a short period for reporting pain may also introduce bias because of the spontaneous resolution of symptoms [34].

The findings of this study revealed that girls with dysmenorrhoea were significantly older ($p < 0.001$) because the condition occurs when the ovulatory cycle matures [21]. The mean age at menarche of the participants in this study was 12.07 (SD = 2.23), which is close to the mean age of 12.15 reported in Singapore [35], 12.6 in Taiwan [23] and 12.0 in the United States [6] but lower than the mean age of 13.38 recently reported in Turkey [16]. These differences may be attributed to socio-economic or nutritional status and living conditions in different countries [36]. The better living conditions and nutritional status of girls in developed countries favour the early onset of menarche [36].

The mean dysmenorrhoeal pain score of the girls reported in this study echoed with previous local [10, 37] and international studies [8, 25]. Most of the girls (84%) reported that their pain localised in the lower abdomen. Participants also revealed that they experienced numerous symptoms, such as fatigue, breast tenderness and skin problems. Fatigue, headache and backache are the most common dysmenorrhoea-associated symptoms reported by 664 secondary school students in Egypt [38], whereas girls in another study reported sweating, loss of appetite and headache [39].

Over 80% of participants reported that dysmenorrhoea limited their daily activities. The results consistent with a study of 417 Taiwanese students which showed that dysmenorrhoea affects the participants' mood (74.8%), daily activities (73.1%), academic performance (64.6%) and social life (50.1%) [11]. However, only 16% of the participants in current study missed classes within the previous half year. This result was comparatively lower than the sick leave rate of 44% reported in previous studies [6, 15]. O'Connell and colleagues reported that 39% of female students aged 19 or younger are usually absent from school for one day each month, and an additional 14% are usually absent for two or more days because of dysmenorrhoea [15]. The low sick leave rate among adolescent girls in Hong Kong may be attributed to the importance of academic achievement in Chinese society. In Chinese culture, academic achievement represents an intrinsic advancement. This attribute is particularly notable in Hong Kong, where the tight teaching schedule and stressful academic environment probably make girls reluctant to apply for sick leave [40].

Health-related quality of life

Present findings reflected that girls perceived that not only their physical aspects but also the psychological and social aspects were affected by dysmenorrhoea. Previous studies have shown that girls commonly complain that dysmenorrhoea affects their physical aspect [16, 41]. This result is understandable because dysmenorrhoea symptoms restrict physical function. Unsal and colleagues compared the health-related quality of life (HRQOL) in Turkish university students with or without dysmenorrhoea, and the two groups exhibited differences in physical functioning, role-physical, bodily pain, general health and vitality domains. A study conducted in Australia also showed that girls with dysmenorrhoea have a lower physical functioning score in quality of life than those with other menstrual problems [17]. The results of this study likely because dysmenorrhoea primarily affects the physical health but also the daily lives and social activities of sufferers [11], thereby affecting their emotional and social functioning domains as well.

Interestingly, our findings noted that scores on the physical functioning and role-emotional domains increased with the severity of dysmenorrhoea. These differences were non-significant, indicating that girls with severe dysmenorrhoea were likely to have a better quality of life in these aspects. One possible explanation is that girls with severe dysmenorrhoea receive more concern from other people or from their friends or mothers. In particular, in Chinese culture, mothers are responsible for their daughters and manage all aspects of their care [42]. As a result, daughters who suffer from dysmenorrhoea would receive constant concern from their mothers, thus receiving better emotional support.

Medical consultation and self-medication

Most of the girls (93.2%) did not seek medical advice despite the significant effect of dysmenorrhoea on their lives. Local and international studies reported similarly low rates for medical consultation among females with dysmenorrhoea [10, 35, 37, 38]. The impression that many girls experience pain may reinforce the concept of normality, which in turn discourages girls from questioning the significance of their pain and considering medical consultation [43]. Only approximately half the participants in this study had received menstrual education, reflecting the inadequacy of the education provided to them and the likelihood that insufficient knowledge on the physiology of menstruation contributes to the low rate of medical consultation [10]. Previous studies in Australia and England have shown that women fail to seek medical help for menstrual symptoms because they encounter difficulty in differentiating between normal and pathological symptoms [44, 45]. All these factors suggest the importance of not only educating girls about what constitutes an "abnormal" menstrual period, but also of the need for open conversation about dysmenorrhoea to raise public awareness of its problems.

Only approximately 18% of the participants in this study self-medicated. By contrast, previous studies have reported moderate to high rates of self-medication among adolescent girls with dysmenorrhoea (60 to 80%) [19, 32]. The result of the present study is in line with a study that reported that local secondary school girls seldom take analgesics to manage dysmenorrhoea [10]. In addition, the present findings further support previous studies maintaining that self-medication is not part of the construct of self-care among adolescent Chinese girls with dysmenorrhoea [46–48]. The low rate of self-medication may be attributed to the perception of girls that self-medication require a prescription or at least medical advice and should not be self-initiated. Without a prescription, girls would not take medication or buy it from a pharmacy. This interpretation explains why self-medication is not relevant to the self-care construct among adolescent girls with dysmenorrhoea.

Although relatively few girls self-medicated for dysmenorrhoea, those who did used medication inappropriately. Some girls reported taking three or 'a few' paracetamol tablets each time they experienced pain, and one girl mentioned using famotidine, a drug that inhibits stomach acid production, to relieve dysmenorrhoea. Others could not name what medication they took. Girls did not know the medication they used, used it inconsistently or took less than the recommended dose. These behaviours imply that girls lacked knowledge of self-medication and raise the possibility of adverse health effects of inappropriate self-medication [15, 35]. The findings highlighted the need for improving the understanding of self-medication among adolescent girls in Hong Kong. They also shed light on the need to develop and provide appropriate educational interventions related to dysmenorrhoea, with the correct administration of self-medication as an essential component. Girls should also be reminded to use self-medication only after receiving proper education.

Strengths and limitations

The strengths of this study included examining the quality of life of Chinese adolescent girls with dysmenorrhoea, whereas previous studies mainly focused on Western university students or other women [16, 19] or else only examined the influence of dysmenorrhoea on the daily lives and school performance of adolescents but not their quality of life [19, 27]. This study also expands previous findings that compare the quality of life of Chinese girls with or without dysmenorrhoea and with different severity levels of the condition. However, the results of the current study should be interpreted with caution given its limitations. First, girls were recruited from secondary schools because a school-based sample is convenient for a researcher who wants to recruit a large number of participants within a short period of time. However, such a sample could not represent girls who left or dropped out of school. This recruitment method can only reasonably be expected to represent the majority of, but not all, adolescent girls in Hong Kong. Second, this study excluded secondary dysmenorrhoea on the basis of the participants' responses. However, dysmenorrhoea was not clinically verified. Although only nearly 10% of girls have severe secondary dysmenorrhoea, the current study did not employ ultrasound or pelvic examination to prove the absence of secondary dysmenorrhoea during the recruitment process given their expense [49]. The possibility of including a girl with a secondary cause of dysmenorrhoea cannot be completely avoided, but girls who reported a history of gynecological disease (such as endometriosis, ovarian cysts or pelvic inflammation) or gynecological surgery, which are both potential causes of secondary dysmenorrhoea [50], were excluded from this study. Nevertheless, as a history of fever during periods is a good way to exclude pelvic inflammatory disease or pathology and thus can be used to differentiate between primary and secondary dysmenorrhoea, future studies should ask girls if they experienced fevers during periods. Finally, data were collected from retrospective self-reports, perhaps leading to recall bias. In addition, the retrospective nature of self-reporting may amplify the cyclicity of pain variation. Nevertheless, retrospective reports of pain severity have a reasonable standard of accuracy [51].

Implications to clinical practice

The findings of this study expand understanding of HRQOL of adolescent Chinese girls with dysmenorrhoea. Healthcare professionals should be made aware that adolescent girls with dysmenorrhoea are likely to have a lower quality of life. Screening should be carried out for the early identification of girls with dysmenorrhoea and for timely interventions. In addition, a brief educational intervention to enhance knowledge of appropriate medications could reduce the severity of dysmenorrhoea and enhance the quality of life among adolescent girls [52]. Clearly, effective educational interventions should be developed and provided to this group of girls.

Conclusions

This study confirms the findings of previous works showing that dysmenorrhoea is a widespread problem and identifies its detrimental effect on adolescent girls. The consequences of dysmenorrhoea appear to be substantial. Thus, adolescent girls should receive assistance to manage and reduce the effects of dysmenorrhoea. Effective interventions for symptom relief should be identified and provided to this vulnerable group to improve their quality of life. Such interventions would not only benefit adolescent girls but society as a whole.

Abbreviations

HRQOL: health-related quality of life; PVAS: The Pain Visual Analogue Scale; SF-36: Short-Form Health Survey

Acknowledgements

The author would like to thank the secondary school students who participated in the study for their help and support.

Author's contribution

CL developed the project, undertook the literature review, collected, analysed and managed the data. CL also draft the paper. The author read and approved the final manuscript.

Competing interests

The authors declare that they have no competing interests.

References

1. Latthe P, Latthe M, Say L, Gülmezoglu M, Khan KS. WHO systematic review of prevalence of chronic pelvic pain: a neglected reproductive health morbidity. BMC Public Health. 2006;6:177.
2. Dawood MY. Primary dysmenorrhea: advances in pathogenesis and management. Obstet Gynecol. 2006;108(2):428–41.
3. Hillen TI, Grbacac SL, Johnston PJ, Straton JA, Keogh JM. Primary dysmenorrhea in young western Australian women: prevalence, impact, and knowledge of treatment. J Adolesc Health. 1999;25(1):40–5.
4. Robertson C. Differential diagnosis of lower abdominal pain in women of childbearing age. Lippincotts Prim Care Pract. 1998;2(3):210–29.
5. Granot M, Yarnitsky D, Itskovitz-Eldor J, Granovsky Y, Peer E, Zimmer EZ. Pain perception in women with dysmenorrhea. Obstet Gynecol. 2001; 98(3):407–11.
6. Banikarim C, Chacko MR, Kelder SH. Prevalence and impact of dysmenorrhea on Hispanic female adolescents. Arch Pediatr Adolesc Med. 2000;154:1226–9.
7. Davis AR, Westhoff CL, O'Connell K, Gallagher N. Oral contraceptives for dysmenorrhea in adolescent girls: a randomized trial. Obstet Gynecol. 2005;106(1):97–104.
8. Ortiz MI. Primary dysmenorrhea among Mexican university students: prevalence, impact and treatment. Eur J of Obstet Gynecol Reprod Biol. 2010;152(1):73–7.
9. Weissman AM, Hartz AJ, Hansen MD, Johnson SR. The natural history of primary dysmenorrhoea: a longitudinal study. BJOG. 2004;111(4):345–52.
10. Chan SS, Yiu KW, Yuen PM, Sahota DS, Chung TK. Menstrual problems and health-seeking behavior in Hong Kong Chinese girls. Hong Kong Med J. 2009;15(1):18–23.
11. Chang YT, Chen YC. Menstrual health care behavior and associated factors among female elementary students in the Hualien region. J Nurs Res. 2008;16:8–16.
12. Coco AS. Primary dysmenorrhea. Am Fam Physician. 1999;60(2):489–98.
13. Burnett MA, Antao V, Black A, Feldman K, Grenville A, Lea R, Lefebvre G, Pinsonneault O, Robert M. Prevalence of primary dysmenorrhea in Canada. J Obstet Gynaecol Can. 2005 Aug;27(8):765–70.

14. Cakir M, Mungan I, Karakas T, Girisken I, Okten A. Menstrual pattern and common menstrual disorders among university students in Turkey. Pediatr Int. 2007;49:938–42.
15. O'Connell K, Davis AR, Westhoff C. Self-treatment patterns among adolescent girls with dysmenorrhea. J Pediatr Adolesc Gynecol. 2006;19(4):285–9.
16. Unsal A, Ayranci U, Tozun M, Arslan G, Calik E. Prevalence of dysmenorrhea and its effect on quality of life among a group of female university students. Ups J Med Sci. 2010;115(2):138–45.
17. Nur Azurah AG, Sanci L, Moore E, Grover S. The quality of life of adolescents with menstrual problems. J Pediatr Adolesc Gynecol. 2013;26(2):102–8.
18. Yang TM. To WWK. Comparison of quality of life scores in adolescents with menstrual dysfunction. Hong Kong J Gynecol Obstet. Midwifery. 2006;6:24–31.
19. Al-Jefout M, Seham AF, Jameel H, Randa AQ, Ola AM, Oday AM, Luscombe G. Dysmenorrhea: prevalence and impact on quality of life among young adult Jordanian females. J Pediatr Adolesc Gynecol. 2015;28:173–85.
20. Education Bureau, Hong Kong. Report on Review of 9-year compulsory October 1997 Education (Revised Version). Available at http://www.edb.gov.hk/en/about-edb/publications-stat/major-reports/consultancy-reports/9-year-compulsory-edu-review-report/ch9.html. Accessed 31 May 2016.
21. Loto OM, Adewumi TA, Adewuya AO. Prevalence and correlates of dysmenorrhea among Nigerian college women. Aust N Z J Obstet Gynecol. 2008;48(4):442.
22. Osuga Y, Hayashi K, Kobayashi Y, Toyokawa S, Momoeda M, Koga K, Yoshino O, Tsutsumi O, Hoshiai H, Terakawa N, Taketani Y. Dysmenorrhea in Japanese women. Int J Gynecol Obstet. 2005;88(1):82–3.
23. Chiou MH, Wang HH. Predictors of dysmenorrhea and self-care behavior among vocational nursing school female students. J Nurs Res. 2008;16(1):17–25.
24. Proctor ML, Farquhar CM. Dysmenorrhea. Clin Evid. 2006 Jun;15:2429–48.
25. Chen HM, Chen CH. Effects of acupressure at the Sanyinjiao point on primary dysmenorrhea. J Adv Nurs. 2004;48(4):380–7.
26. Mcdowell I, Newell C. Measuring health – a guide to rating scales and questionnaires 2nd edn. New York: Oxford University Press; 1996.
27. Potur DC, Bilgin NC, Komurcu N. Prevalence of dysmenorrhea in university students in Turkey: effect on daily activities and evaluation of different pain management methods. Pain Management Nursing. 2014;15(4):768–77.
28. Ware JE Jr. SF-36 health survey update. Spine (Phila Pa 1976). 2000; 25(24):3130–9.
29. Lam CL, Gandek B, Ren XS, Chan MS. Tests of scaling assumptions and construct validity of the Chinese (HK) version of the SF-36 health survey. J Clin Epidemiol. 1998;51(11):1139–47.
30. Lam ETP, Lam CLK, Lo YYC, Grandek B. Psychometrics and population norm of the Chinese (HK) SF-36 health survey version 2. Hong Kong Pract. 2008; 30:185–98.
31. Campbell MA, McGrath PJ. Non-pharmacological strategies used by adolescent girls for the management of menstrual discomfort. Clin J Pain. 1999;15:313–20.
32. Campbell MA, McGrath PJ. Use of medication by adolescents for the management of menstrual discomfort. Arch Pediatr Adolesc Med. 1997; 151(9):903–13.
33. Ohde S, Tokuda Y, Takahashi O, Yanai H, Hinohara S, Fukui T. Dysmenorrhea among Japanese women. Int J Gynecol Obstet. 2008;100(1):13–7.
34. Latthe P, Mignini L, Gray R, Hills R, Khan K. Factors predisposing women to chronic pelvic pain: systematic review. BMJ. 2006;332:749–55.
35. Agarwal A, Venkat A. Questionnaire study on menstrual disorders in adolescent girls in Singapore. J Pediatr Adolesc Gynecol. 2009;22:365–71.
36. Thomas F, Renaud F, Benefice E, de Meeüs T, Guegan JF. International variability of ages at menarche and menopause: patterns and main determinants. Hum Biol. 2001;73(2):271–90.
37. Chia CF, Lai JH, Cheung PK, Kwong LT, Lau FP, Leung KH, Leung MT, Wong FC, Ngu SF. Dysmenorrhoea among Hong Kong university students: prevalence, impact, and management. Hong Kong Med J. 2013 Jun;19(3):222–8.
38. El-Gilany AH, Badawi K, El-Fedawy S. Epidemiology of dysmenorrhoea among adolescent students in Mansoura, Egypt. East Mediterr health J. 2005 Jan-Mar;11(1–2):155–63.
39. Eryilmaz G, Ozdemir F. Evaluation of menstrual pain management approaches by northeastern Anatolian adolescents. Pain Manag Nurs. 2009; 10(1):40–7.
40. Salili F, Lai MK. Leung SSK (2004). The consequences of pressure on adolescents students to perform well in school. Hong Kong J Pediatr. 2004; 9:329–36.
41. Iacovides S, Avidon I, Bentley A, Baker FC. Reduced quality of life when experiencing menstrual pain in women with primary dysmenorrhea. Acta Obstetr Gynecol Scand. 2014;93(2):213–7.
42. Park M, Chesla C. Revisiting Confucianism as a conceptual framework for Asian family study. J Fam Nurs. 2007;13(3):293–311.
43. Markovic M, Manderson L, Warren N. Endurance and contest: women's narratives of endometriosis. Health (London). 2008;12(3):349–67.
44. Cox H, Henderson L, Andersen N, Cagliarini G, Ski C. Focus group study of endometriosis: struggle, loss and the medical merry-go-round. Int J Nurs Pract. 2003;9(1):2.
45. Ballard K, Lowton K, Wright J. What's the delay? Fertil Steril. 2006;5: 1296–301.
46. Wong CL, Ip WY, Choi KC, Lam LW. Examining self-care behaviors and their associated factors among adolescent girls with dysmenorrhea: an application of Orem's self-care deficit nursing theory. J Nurs Scholarsh. 2015; 47(3):219–27.
47. Wong CL, Ip WY, Choi KC, Shiu TY. Translation and validation of the Chinese-Cantonese version of the adolescent Dysmenorrhic self-care scale in Hong Kong adolescent girls. J Clin Nurs. 2013;22(11–12):1510–20.
48. Wong CL, Ip WY, Lam LW. Self-care strategies among Chinese adolescent girls with dysmenorrhea: a qualitative study. Pain Manag Nurs. 2016;17(4):262–71.
49. Fenning NR. Dysmenorrhea. Curr Obstet Gynaecol. 2005;15:394–401.
50. Harel Z. Dysmenorrhea in adolescents and young adults: an update on pharmacological treatments and management strategies. Expert Opin on Pharmacother. 2012;13(15):2157–70.
51. Nunnink S, Meana M. Remembering the pain: accuracy of pain recall in endometriosis. J Psychosom Obstet Gynecol. 2007;28(4):201–8.
52. Jung HS, Lee J. The effectiveness of an educational intervention on proper analgesic use for dysmenorrhea. Eur J Obstet Gynecol Reprod Biol. 2013; 170(2):480–6.

17

Partner influences on young women's risky drug and sexual behavior

Miriam Clark[1], Rohanna Buchanan[1*], Rachel Kovensky[2] and Leslie D. Leve[2]

Abstract

Background: Adolescent girls with a history of maltreatment are at heightened risk for health-risking behaviors, including unsafe sexual behaviors and drug use. However, few studies have examined the views of this population in regard to sexual partner choice, sexual behaviors, and decisions to use drugs with sexual partners.

Methods: We conducted 15 semistructured, open-ended qualitative interviews with young women ages 18–24 with a history of maltreatment and asked them to reflect on their experiences as adolescents. We used the constant comparison method to group the qualitative coded data into themes.

Results: Analysis of the interviews suggested that adolescent girls with maltreatment histories often report that they chose partners who are promotive of risky drug and sexual behavior. The interviews also provided insight into why this population is likely to use drugs with their partner and why they might be hesitant to talk about or practice safe sex with their partner.

Conclusion: The young women's feedback highlighted five areas where adolescent girls with maltreatment histories could benefit: (a) provision of information about partner characteristics that are promotive of both risky behavior and those that are linked to healthy relationships, (b) provision of information about how one's partner can influence one's own drug use, (c) practice talking about safe sex with partners, (d) provision of information about safe sex practices and the risks associated with unsafe sex, and (e) provision of information about the risks associated with drug use and unsafe sexual behavior to adolescent boys.

Keywords: Drug use, Health-risking sexual behavior, Adolescent experiences, Partner influence, Qualitative interview

Plain english summary

In our study we talked to young women who had been maltreated as adolescents and were subsequently placed in out-of-home treatment (foster care or treatment facilities). This population is at heightened risk for unsafe sexual behavior and drug use. We asked the young women how their romantic relationships influenced their sexual behavior and drug use when they were adolescents. The women told us how the partners they chose as adolescents often encouraged unsafe sex and drug use, and that they were often hesitant to talk to their partners about these issues. Through these interviews, we received insight into topics for practitioners to focus on when working with adolescents. The women's stories highlight that adolescent girls could benefit from knowing about partner characteristics that are likely to lead to risky sex and drug use, and learning more about how to talk about and practice safe sex with their partners.

* Correspondence: rohannab@oslc.org
[1]Oregon Social Learning Center, 10 Shelton McMurphey Blvd, Eugene, OR 97401, USA
Full list of author information is available at the end of the article

Background

Adolescents with a history of maltreatment are at heightened risk for engaging in multiple forms of health-risking behaviors, including unsafe sexual behaviors and drug use [1–6]. Unsafe sexual behaviors and drug use (via needle injection) are highly correlated with sexually transmitted diseases, including HIV/AIDS and other negative health consequences [https://www.cdc.gov/pwud/]. Young women in this population often bear more health burdens than do their male counterparts because of specific health consequences, including unwanted pregnancies, ectopic pregnancies and infertility [7]. In addition, adolescent girls are also more likely than adolescent boys to become addicted to drugs [8, 9], experience intimate partner violence [10], and contract sexually transmitted infections (STI's) [11].

Romantic partners (defined as dating or sexual partners) have a significant impact on the sexual behaviors and drug use of adolescent girls with maltreatment histories [12, 13]. Despite high rates of romantic relationships in this population [14], very few studies have focused on the role of partners on adolescent girls' drug use and sexual behaviors. To help fill this gap, we sought to learn retrospectively about the partner experiences of adolescent girls with a history of maltreatment. Using a semistructured qualitative interview format, we asked young women to reflect on their experiences as adolescents and discuss the relationships they had with their partners. We asked questions about how they chose their partners and the impact their partners had on their sexual behavior and drug use. We also explored reasons why adolescent girls with a history of maltreatment used drugs and/or engaged in unsafe sexual behaviors with their partners.

Health-risking behaviors in adolescent girls

Problem behavior theory [15] suggests that young people who engage in one type of risky behavior in youth (such as drug use, early or risky sexual behavior, and delinquent behaviors) are more likely to also engage in other types of risky behavior. Findings from longitudinal studies of adolescents and young adults have confirmed that young people who engage in risky or problem behavior often engage in multiple types of such behavior [15, 16]. This theory guided the current study questions and our qualitative interview process to jointly focus on a range of health-risking behaviors, including drug use and sexual behavior.

Health-risking behaviors, such as unprotected sex and drug use, often emerge in adolescence and peak during young adulthood [17], resulting in immediate developmental consequences and deleterious health outcomes that can persist across the lifespan. According to the Centers for Disease Control and Prevention [18], individuals between ages 15 and 24 comprise half of the nearly 20 million newly diagnosed sexually transmitted infections (STIs) in the United States every year. Further, more than 1.2 million people are currently living with HIV in the United States, and approximately 19% of those who are newly diagnosed with HIV are women. Of women diagnosed, 87% have contracted HIV from heterosexual contact and 13% from needle injection [19].

The National Center on Addiction and Substance Abuse [20] reports that 76% of high school students have used one or more addictive drugs. Although prevalence of STIs and drug use is relatively evenly distributed among adolescent boys and girls [11, 18, 21], adolescent girls often bear disproportionate health consequences (e.g. life-threatening ectopic pregnancy, infertility, unwanted pregnancy) and are biologically predisposed to be more susceptible to certain STI's [11]. In addition, adolescent girls have a heightened risk for sexual violence [10] and addiction once drug use is initiated [8, 9]. Adolescent and adult women with a history of childhood maltreatment are a subgroup at particularly high risk for participating in unsafe sexual behavior [2, 4–6]. Using a large nationally representative sample of young adult women, Hahm, Lee, Ozonoff, and Van Wert [22] found a significant cumulative relationship between increased exposure to multiple types of maltreatment and increased risk for STI diagnosis and early sexual contact. Adults with a history of child maltreatment are also more likely to engage in unprotected sex with casual partners [2].

Adolescent girls and adult women with a maltreatment history are also more likely to have problems with drug use than their non-maltreated counterparts. For example, Fettes, Aarons, and Green [3] compared two nationally representative samples of adolescents and found that adolescents with a maltreatment history were significantly more at risk for drug use involvement than were those without a maltreatment history. These findings are consistent with research that has documented higher rates of drug use disorders among adolescents with a maltreatment history [1]. Drug use and unsafe sexual behavior are linked, with adolescents and adults with a history of maltreatment being more likely to have sex while drinking alcohol or using drugs, which often leads to unprotected, casual sex [4–6]. Although the elevated risks and serious consequences of unsafe sexual behavior and drug use are fairly well established among adolescent girls with a history of maltreatment, relatively little is known about pathways to these health-risking behaviors among this population [23] and about pathways to healthy sexual behavior in this population [24].

The United Nations Educational, Scientific and Cultural Organization (UNESCO) recently published a resource detailing the core elements of sexual education programs [25]. The UNESCO resource advocates teaching young people—through skill based learning—how to recognize relationship power dynamics, how to seek help and support, and how to negotiate safe sex practices [25]. Findings from a review of programs to promote positive youth development (PYD) suggests that safer sexual behavior tends to be correlated with other positive psychosocial behaviors (such as sports, academic activities, and goal setting) and that effective PYD programs that target one of these often affect the others [24]. In addition, the findings from this review of PYD programs suggest that including training and activities related to goal setting, social skills, and engagement in positive social activities can enhance sexual education programs [24].

Partner influences on drug use and sexual behavior

One potential pathway linking drug use and sexual behaviors among adolescent girls and young women with a maltreatment history is the influence of their romantic partners. A large body of evidence suggests that child maltreatment is associated with problematic romantic relationships later in life [26]. Specifically, McLeod, Fergusson, & Horwood [27] found a significant association between childhood maltreatment and elevated negative partner relationships, interpersonal violence-related victimization and perpetration, and choosing partners with social problems related to alcohol use and illegal behavior in their 30-year longitudinal study of a large New Zealand birth cohort. Adolescent girls who select partners who are involved in antisocial behavior, such as drug use and delinquency, appear to be at particular risk for engaging in these behaviors themselves. For instance, Rhoades, Leve, Harold, Kim, & Chamberlain [28] found that among a sample of women with juvenile justice and child welfare history, drug use was significantly associated with their partners' use. Silverman, Raj, Mucci, & Hathaway [13] found that adolescent girls who were in violence-prone dating relationships were significantly more likely to use substances (e.g., alcohol, tobacco, cocaine), engage in risky sexual behavior (e.g., early sexual debut, multiple partnering), and seriously consider or attempt suicide.

Additionally, research shows adolescent girls are more likely to participate in risky sexual behavior when partners are older than them [29, 30], when they are driven by a sense of need to be in a relationship [31], or when they rely heavily on their partner for emotional or financial support [32]. Conversely, self-regulation (ability to regulate behavior, attention, and emotions) is associated with lower sexual risk taking in adolescents, as is parental control and lower levels of negative peer pressure [33].

Despite the known associations between childhood maltreatment and young women's sexual behavior, there is very little research on the association between childhood maltreatment and young women's feelings about safe sex. In one of the few studies on this topic, women filled out a childhood sexual abuse questionnaire and then read a sexual scenario involving either alcohol or no alcohol. Results indicated that childhood sexual abuse was a predictor of the women's perception of the partner's motives and intentions, which was then a predictor of the likelihood she would report she would engage in unprotected sex [34]. The authors suggested that women with maltreatment histories might make decisions in different ways than would their non-maltreated peers. Although not specific to a sample of participants with maltreatment histories, a quantitative study examining women living in high poverty, crime, and drug use environments reported that the women's attitudes about condom use are quite variable [35]. For example, although the majority of the women said that condoms did *not* reduce sexual pleasure, a quarter of the women still listed reduction in sexual pleasure as a reason they did not use condoms. Because of the variability of women's responses, further research is needed to more fully understand women's opinions of condom use and how their opinions are influenced by their partner.

Although evidence points to the influential role partners play in determining whether or not adolescent girls engage in drug use and sexual behaviors, little is known about the mechanisms underlying partner choice or the degree to which specific partner traits predict health-risking behaviors in the relationship [12]. To fill this gap in the literature, Rhule-Louie & McMahon [36] suggest that qualitative interviews could be particularly effective for clarifying the factors that underlie partner selection and for informing interventions to influence adolescent partner selection.

This study

We conducted 15 semistructured, open-ended qualitative interviews with young adult women with a documented history of maltreatment that had resulted in placement in foster care or other out-of-home care setting during childhood and/or adolescence. The interviews focused on the adolescents' experiences with regard to sexual partner choice decisions to engage in safe or unsafe sexual behavior, and decisions to use alcohol and drugs with sexual partners. Qualitative interviews and analyses were guided by two research questions: (1) How do adolescent girls who have experienced maltreatment choose romantic partners? (2) What influence do romantic partners have on adolescent drug use and sexual behavior in this population? Our goal for the current study was to learn about malleable relationship-based processes that could be targeted in future preventive interventions with high-risk adolescent and young adult female populations, including those who have experienced maltreatment.

Methods

Participants

Participants were 15 women with a history of maltreatment. Participants were selected based on having had a childhood history of maltreatment (ascertained via child welfare case worker report) and having engaged in sexual behavior as an adolescent (ascertained via responses to a questionnaire administered when the participants were adolescents). Ethics approval for the study was granted by the University of Oregon Institutional Review Board (IRB; 10,312,013.040). For the current study, all of the young women participated in an informed consent procedure that was individually administered.

Study participants were women ages 18 to 24 (M = 20.93, SD = 2.09) at the time of the interview. They identified as White or Caucasian (60%), American Indian/Alaska Native (7%), or more than one race (33%). Overall, 20% identified as Hispanic/Latina. One participant reported that she was married, 6 were living with a partner and unmarried, and 8 were dating or seeing someone but not living together or married. Participants reported a range of educational attainment, including having completed the eighth grade (n = 1), completed some high school (n = 4), received a GED (n = 3), received a high school diploma (n = 5), and completed some college (n = 2). The sample was generally unemployed and low income, with only 4 women employed for pay and a median annual income ranging from \$5000 to \$9999.

Measures

Interview guide

We used an individually administered, semistructured, and open-ended qualitative interview format and conducted one interview with each participant. Interviews were scheduled for 2 h in duration though the average length was 102 min and ranged from 66 to 136 min. The interview guide included broad, general questions designed to prompt respondents to think retrospectively about their adolescent years and to solicit information about the topics most important to them. The initial interview questions focused on the women's prior treatment and intervention experiences (see Clark, Buchanan, & Leve, 2018 [37] for details). To gain a broad understanding of how adolescent girls choose romantic partners and partners' influence on drug use and sexual behavior, we next asked general or hypothetical questions to create a pressure-free environment and provide an opportunity for respondents to give concrete examples. Example questions included, "What do you think adolescents look for in a partner?" and, "We know from previous research studies that when a girl's partner uses drugs, she's more likely to use drugs too. Why do you think this might be?" Interviewers were trained in techniques to elicit information from participants, remain neutral to a range of responses, and move the discussion through the semistructured format.

Demographic survey

Immediately prior to the qualitative interview, participants were given a demographic survey that included items related to their age, race/ethnicity, current relationship status, highest education level completed, current occupation and employment status, and current gross annual household income.

Analysis

All interviews were audio recorded and transcribed verbatim. The transcriptions were then reviewed by the interviewer for accuracy and completeness. Participants and other individuals identified in the transcripts were assigned an identification number to protect confidentiality, increase cross-group comparisons, and reduce subjectivity in the analyses [38]. After reviewing all the interviews, the authors met and discussed broad themes identified across all transcripts. Using NVIVO software [39], the first author completed an initial coding of the broad themes for each interview. Next, a codebook emerged as the first author coded sections of text (ranging in size from short phrases to long discussions) by hand into more specific emergent subthemes and then compared the coded content across each interview. The constant comparison method [40] was used to group codes into themes. All authors met to discuss findings related to the broad themes and subthemes and to identify representative quotes.

Results

Participants were candid in their responses to questions in the interview guide and included stories and examples from their own and their peers' experiences as adolescents. The broad themes and subthemes that emerged from the interviews were grouped under two general topics: adolescent's partner choices and partner influences. The two themes are described in the following subsections.

Partner choice

Responses to questions about characteristics adolescent girls look for when choosing a partner varied based on the personal interests of the participating women, and they are reviewed in the following subsections. Table 1 displays subthemes with regard to desirable partner characteristics. We identified four themes promotive of risky behavior: "partner is rebellious," "partner emotional and financial support," "wants a boyfriend," and "partner is older/experienced." The other four themes focused on positive partner characteristics, such as personality traits or interests in specific activities.

Partner is rebellious

The theme of adolescent girls looking for rebellious partners emerged in 6 of the 15 interviews. Respondents identified that, as adolescents, they looked for partners who were "reckless," "dangerous," "rebellious," "trouble," and who were "bad boys." The women said that, as adolescents, they looked for partners who used drugs and alcohol and "beat people up." For example, when one respondent was asked what she thought adolescent girls looked for in a partner, she responded, "Horrible things.

Table 1 Desired Partner Characteristics

Subtheme	*n*	Sample Quote
Partner is rebellious	6	"I always looked for the bad boys...the ones that were doing the exact same thing I was...going out and smoking weed and at times, you know when I would drink or when I used to use meth."
Emotional and financial support	5	"I think that girls want to find a man who can support them and who can um who has a job and who has a good head on their shoulders."
Wants a boyfriend	5	"Usually girls just want a boyfriend just to have a boyfriend. You know, just for cuz I mean to have someone through high school is awesome..."
Partner is older or experienced	3	"The way that they got to do whatever they wanted. I think, like it seemed like they were a lot more free to do as they pleased. And that was somehow attractive."
Positive partner characteristics	14	"Somebody who's, like, popular, and good looking, and has a lotta friends."

I don't think teen girls have the best decision making when it comes to their partners...I didn't. I had no standards...I think a lot of teenage girls now look for who's a little bit rebellious." Other participants echoed similar opinions, and one woman summed up her feedback by saying, "Me and my friends dated all those types of douchebags."

One participant said that she liked the rebellious adolescent boys because of the commonalities they shared: "I always looked for the bad boys...the ones that were doing the exact same thing I was...going out and smoking weed and at times, you know when I would drink or when I used to use meth."

Another participant explained that she had found rebelliousness attractive because of the sense of freedom it brought: "Nobody wants to go to school. General consensus, nobody wants to go to school. So when a boy kind of skips school one day, it shows some of, like, freedom that he has and it might attract you...." Another participant explained the attraction to rebellious partners a different way, saying, "I read once in a good book is you go for the love you think you deserve." She went on to explain that "a lot of girls who have had a hard time, who are in foster care, or had bad relationships, go back to those bad relationships. Which is not healthy." In general, these 6 participants talked candidly about how, in retrospect, they regretted that they had been interested in rebellious partners as adolescents.

Partner emotional and financial support

Five respondents mentioned that adolescent girls looked for a partner who could support them, to help compensate for support they lack at home. The women defined this kind of partner support in various ways, including attention, comfort, or advice; help feeling good about themselves; and the potential of financial support. For example, one respondent described the attention she sought as an adolescent in this way: "They [adolescent girls] look for somebody who gives them attention.... Girls like me who have had crazy childhoods, or you know, you know like not the most picture perfect childhoods...but I think [they look for] someone who pays attention to them." Another respondent talked about how she sought a partner who could give her support, given her past experiences, saying, "I want someone who can relate to me. Who's had some issues and who can comfort me and give me advice on how they went through things that so that way we can both go through it..." A third respondent talked about financial support in addition to emotional support, saying, "I think that girls want to find a man who can support them and who can ... who has a job and who has a good head on their shoulders."

Wants a boyfriend

Five respondents mentioned that adolescent girls just want a boyfriend and seem less concerned with the adolescent boy's other characteristics. One participant put it simply, saying, "Usually girls want a boyfriend just to have a boyfriend. You know? Just for, cuz, I mean to have someone through high school is awesome..." Another woman talked about how she was shy ("I was always really shy when it came to boys"), and although she wanted a boyfriend ("there's not like a how-to book to get a boyfriend"), she seemed to care little about who that person was as long as they "make the first move."

Another participant said that adolescent girls are just looking "to hang out" with male partners because "maybe they're lonely." Later she talked about how she thought adolescent girls commit to long-term relationships "...cuz they wanting to grow up because their life was so miserable when they were younger and they wanna have a better life so they're going to find this first guy that they really love."

Partner is older/experienced

Three participants mentioned that they thought adolescents were into older or more experienced partners. For example, one participant said she looked for "someone that's been in long-term relationships or long relationships, like longer than a week." Another participant explained that being older was another sign of the partner's freedom, saying, "The way that they got to do whatever they wanted. I think, like it seemed like they were a lot more free to do as they pleased. And that was somehow attractive." She went on to explain that it might also be because of the issues she and her peers faced as adolescents: "Maybe had somethin' to do with being like some sort of like a father figure. I don't know. Lots of daddy issues."

Positive partner characteristics

When talking about positive partner characteristics, the descriptions were brief and included less detail than the women's descriptions of the qualities promotive of risky behavior. Fourteen women mentioned the importance of a potential partner's social status or attractiveness. One woman's comment about looking for "somebody who's, like, popular, and good looking, and has a lotta friends" was representative of the types of things said by the other participants. Seven of the women used individual words or short phrases when identifying positive personality traits that they looked for in a partner such as, "funny," "humor," "somebody they can probably share their emotions with or trust," "someone who is open and communicates," "reliable," "has plans and goals for their future," "kind," "respectful," "fun," "patient," "honest," "understanding," "soft-spoken," "sweet," "adventurous," and "a good friend." Three women also mentioned that they looked for partners interested in specific positive activities, including "art," "music," "outdoors," "sports," or "physical activity."

Partner influence

Most responses to questions about partner influence on adolescent girls related to drug use, talking about safe sex, and practicing safe sex. Each of these subthemes is reviewed in the following subsections. Table 2 displays themes and subthemes about partner influence on adolescent girls' drug use, talking about safe sex, and practicing safe sex.

Partner influence on drug use

During the interviews, all 15 women identified that they had used drugs as adolescents. The women identified 6 general reasons an adolescent girl might be more likely to use drugs when her partner uses drugs. These reasons included being accepted or fitting in, pressure, a desire for a common experience, to keep the guy or improve the relationship, the proximity and access to drugs, and curiosity.

Fitting in Five respondents explained that using drugs with a partner is a way to fit in. Participants used words stating that they wanted to be "accepted," "cool," and to "fit in with his crowd." Most participants described wanting to fit in with a simple sentence before moving on to a different idea. For example, one participant simply said, "Maybe just to be accepted...I mean to be cool, I guess..." Another said, "Like say if I was with someone that was using drugs, um, and if they used them around me, I would want to feel cool or whatever. Um, and just kind of like fit in with his crowd."

Pressure Nine participants talked about how adolescent girls often feel pressure to use drugs when their partner is using. Several participants briefly explained that adolescent girls often felt "peer pressure" from their partners. For example, one participant explained, "Because her partner feels guilty about doing 'em [drugs] and to justify what he's doing and make himself feel better about himself...they [the boyfriend] pretty much get their partner to do it [use drugs] with them..." Another participant said, "They make it seem cool or make it seem right, make it to where that's what they're supposed to be doing. It's pressuring." A few of the women went into more detail about pressure they or their peers felt from partners to use drugs. One participant told a story about how her boyfriend convinced her to use methamphetamine:

> I originally started using meth because my boyfriend at the time used to use it and he loved it and my excuse for not wanting to use it was I didn't wanna go find it. I didn't know where it was, I didn't have the money for it. But, at the same time he knew I wanted to use it because it would get me skinny. And I've always have had an unhappy weight and it's always been a weakness of mine and he knew that and so he took advantage of it and he went and got meth. Went and got everything we needed and then brought it to me and so at that point it was really hard for me to say no.

Another participant talked about how a partners' pressure to use drugs can be related to the cost of drugs and hope for help in paying for them: "I know a first-hand story I just got yesterday of someone who started heroin for the first time and she was with her boyfriend and she had a job and he didn't. And so what he did is he filled up a syringe of heroin and stuck it in her thigh. And then she's like, 'You know why? Because I had a job and he didn't and now I'm addicted and so now I can buy his shit too.'"

A common experience Nine of the women described how doing drugs together gives a couple something in common and an ability to communicate on the same level. For example, one participant described it this way: "And um you want to bond with each other! [laughs]" She went on to explain in more detail, saying, "...like, of course you don't wanna be with somebody that's getting

Table 2 Partner Influences

Subtheme	*n*	Sample Quote
Theme: Partner Influence on Drug Use		
Fitting in	5	"Like say if I was with someone that was using drugs um, and if they used them around me I would want to feel cool or whatever. Um, and just kind of like fit in with his crowd."
Pressure	9	"…they make it seem cool or make it seem right, make it to where that's what they're supposed to be doing. It's pressuring."
A common experience	6	"…my sister had done it here and there, you know, she'd once in a while but she never really did it all the time. And she started dating her, and uh, whenever she uses something, it doesn't matter if it's pot, alcohol, what she has to use it when she uses it cuz they say that, she says she don't want her to be high and her not cuz then they might not communicate the same way."
Improve or maintain the relationship	4	"I didn't want them to break up with me. You know I, I oh well if I do this with him, he won't break up with me."
Proximity or access	5	"Because they're around each other and they wanna do what each other are doing."
Theme: Talking About Safe Sex		
Awkward or uncomfortable	10	"It's not gonna be like some made out scene like how they say in Sex Ed, because really, in all reality, it's not. You don't think, hey we're gonna have sex in two hours let's talk about this for an hour and then cuddle for 15 min and then you know, do all this other stuff for you know another 45, and then we could have sex."
Nervous, scared, or unsure	3	"Neither partner is really actually has developed a close relationship with each other and they're not actually comfortable enough with each other to talk about things that could be awkward or embarrassing and serious."
Theme: Practicing Safe Sex		
Not thinking about consequences	10	"…they don't have a condom but they wanna do it now, so they just do it…"
Don't like condoms/birth control	7	"Because it feels better [without a condom]. Or they just don't wanna wear that. Or they're allergic… The way that it hurts their area or whatever"
Alcohol or drugs	6	I didn't really take the time to get to know any of em. So it was like extremely uncomfortable. I was always on drugs. You know or alcohol or something. So I didn't, I really never connected to em. So it made it extremely awkward to talk to anybody.
Partner is dishonest	3	"…and then after we slept together my aunt found out and told me that he had herpes and I didn't even know because he didn't tell me. And I got really upset…"
Male pressures female	4	"I was raped one time. Well, a couple of times, but this one stands out the most because I was young. It was with a boyfriend and I had told him no and he forced it on me anyway and he was a lot stronger than I was. And there was no fighting him off."
Unrealistic expectations	5	"Just because he says he cares about you before doesn't mean that he still will afterwards. I've seen that way too many times…He'll just leave or that's all you will do afterwards, when you refuse to, he breaks it off with you. That happened to a very good friend of mine."
Putting on a condom is awkward	1	"I think sex in itself is a pretty awkward when you're doing it with somebody you don't really know, and so to have to put on a condom or to put in a female condom or to do something like that in the middle of sex its already awkward just makes it 10 times more awkward. And then you kinda just don't want to do it anymore. Or it's just like you're embarrassed."

high without you, you know? ...cuz if not, they're just gonna be like high all over the place and you're gonna be sittin' there like, whoa!" Although most of these participants explained a similar desire for a common experience, another participant went into more detail with a story about her sister:

> My sister had done it [used drugs] here and there, you know. She'd [used drugs] once in a while but she never really did it all the time. And she started dating her [partner], and uh, whenever she uses something, it doesn't matter if it's pot, alcohol, what she has to use it when she uses it cuz they say that, she says she don't want her [partner] to be high and her [the sister] not, cuz then they might not communicate the same way. They're very, very codependent on each other…

Improve or maintain the relationship Four participants said that they felt adolescent girls used with their partners because of a hope that it would improve their relationship. For example, one participant explained her experience this way: "I didn't want them to break up with me. You know I, 'oh well, if I do this with him, he won't break up with me.' And that's what started it all." Another participant talked about how not using together could lead to problems in the relationship if the partner was using, explaining, "Uh, and maybe the drugs can make the relationship harder and so you, maybe your mind would think, 'well if I do the drugs with him maybe our relationship will be better.'"

Another participant talked about how her boyfriend seemed to be interested in her only when they were using together:

> There was a couple times that, like, the guy that I was doing heroin with, that got me into it, there was times that when we were high together he would...spill out everything, all of his feelings to me. That he was really in love with me and that kinda stuff. And then once he got sober he was the complete opposite. And like, he didn't wanna look at me, he didn't wanna sit in the same room as me. There's a lot of swishy-washy when you do drugs and are trying to have a relationship. And there's a lot of co-dependent on each other.

Similarly, another participant explained she had used drugs with her partner for a long time, and the relationship ended when she decided to stop using:

> She [the partner] was using and I was using with her, and I told her, "You know, I don't want to do this all the time. I don't care if I do it, you know, maybe one night a year or something, but I don't wanna do it all the time because..." I showed her a picture. I said, "This is me at fourteen. I look thirty." Cuz I was on meth. And it just was horrible. Sunken face, messed up teeth, and I was like, "I don't wanna look like that ever again. And I don't wanna lose my mind. And I have permanent heart and lung damage from using and I just, who know." You know? And I told her, "It's either my heart or a bag of dope," and she chose meth. So I left her...

Proximity or access Five participants said it is simply a matter of proximity or access to drugs. Most participants put it directly like this participant, who said, "Because they're around each other and they wanna do what each other are doing." Another respondent explained the impact of proximity in terms of doing the same things as the people around her: "I think it's cuz when you love somebody, it's just you want to do the same things that they're doing. If your partner's being productive I think it encourages you to be more productive yourself. But when they're doing drugs you're obviously okay with it so you're obviously gonna start doing it too."

Talking about safe sex

During the interviews, participants shared experiences and opinions about talking about safe sex. The women overwhelmingly agreed that talking about safe sex for an adolescent can be hard. When participants explained why talking about safe sex can be difficult for adolescents, two subthemes emerged: (a) it is awkward or uncomfortable, and (b) the adolescent is nervous, scared, or unsure about how to talk about safe sex. One participant–interviewer discussion illustrated the challenges faced by adolescent girls when talking with partners about safe sex:

> Respondent: I'd say the majority of them talk to their home girls and their best friends.
>
> Interviewer: Okay, so they talk to friends, but do they talk to their partners?
>
> Respondent: Not as probably much as it should be talked about I guess. Unless they're like, in a serious committed relationship. Then you're gonna talk to them [the partner]. But if you've only been dating this guy, for like, let's say two or three weeks, or even a month or two, you're not gonna be like, "Hey dude, I wanna boil this down and we can talk about, you know, well, I don't wanna get chlamydia and I don't know if you've ever seen but it really is, really bad you know? And I wanna baby someday and I just hope that we could use a condom right now and every time that we have sex and I would really..." No dude! They [adolescent girls] ain't gonna do that. It's gonna be like, you know, "Hey, lets fuck, no I'm okay [don't have an STI], c'mon." You know? And then they'd [the adolescent girl] be like, "Oh, okay, let's get this condom." "No I'm not using that." "Well you know I feel better if we could use condoms cuz I don't wanna get pregnant." "Well then get on birth control." You know? It's gonna be, you know, short little. It's not gonna be like some made out scene like how they say in Sex Ed, because really, in all reality, it's not. You don't think, hey we're gonna have sex in two hours let's talk about this for an hour and then cuddle for 15 minutes and then you know, do all this other stuff for you know another 45, and then we could have sex.

Awkward or uncomfortable Feeling awkward, embarrassed, or uncomfortable during talks about safe sex was mentioned in 10 interviews. "I know for me," explained one respondent, "that [safe sex] was a pretty uncomfortable topic." Most of the women just mentioned that it was uncomfortable, but a few respondents went on to explain why they felt uncomfortable. For example, some women talked about how, as adolescents, they were not very close to their sexual partners, so talking about a serious topic like safe sex was uncomfortable. One participant put it this way: "I feel like some of them [adolescent girls] don't really have a relationship that is in any way permanent. It's very temporary. Neither partner is really actually has developed a close relationship with each other and they're not actually comfortable enough with each other to talk about things that could be awkward or embarrassing and serious." Another participant gave a similar explanation about why she felt uncomfortable talking about safe sex: "Um, just because uhh, just because, you know, I mean, it wasn't, it wasn't a long-term boyfriend."

Nervous, scared, or unsure Seven of the women explained that they were nervous, scared, or unsure of how to talk to their partner about safe sex. One respondent described the reason for adolescent girls' nervousness this way: "Uh, well I think that when you're young, and you have that whole like, uh, you don't really know a lot about it and you haven't really done it too much yet so you're kinda nervous and, and um. Maybe the guy laughs at you, I don't know." Other participants said similar things, such as, "Girls are scared the guy might laugh, the guy won't like her anymore, and are scared of what the guy might say." "They're afraid that they'll feel hurt by the response, or that they will offend the guy by asking about STIs," and "Some girls don't know what to say in a conversation."

One participant said that fear keeps adolescent girls from talking about sex with their partners. When asked what they fear, she said, "Talking about it. Fear of what their partner will do. Um, fear of what their partner will say." Another participant described adolescent girls fear as "...being scared of that person. Um, [the partner] not liking her anymore, or, you know, not getting attention from that person anymore."

Although participants said that adolescent girls feel nervous or scared, they also talked about the importance of getting over that nervous feeling. One participant expressed regret that she's 24 and pregnant with her third child and talked about how uncomfortable she has felt talking to partners about safe sex. She went on to say that adolescent girls need to remember the consequences of unsafe sex when they are nervous to bring it up with their partners:

> They [adolescent girls] are gonna get nervous [to talk to their partners about safe sex], yeah. But in all reality they have to be reminded that they're gonna be the ones who be miserable [if they don't talk about safe sex]. Yeah, it's gonna be cool, but in all reality if you're sitting there taking care of one kid, and this guy's having sex with your best friend, and you just got pregnant by him and you don't know what to do, and you don't want an abortion. You're gonna be sitting there crying because you're gonna have to take care of a baby in 9 months. And then your whole life is gonna be ruined. And then you can't go to college, you know? It just boils everything all crazy like.

Practicing safe sex

In addition to discussing the difficulty of talking about safe sex, respondents talked about why practicing safe sex is also difficult for adolescent girls. Nine subthemes related to these barriers, illustrating a wide range of reasons adolescent girls might engage in unsafe sexual behavior.

Not thinking about consequences Ten of the women said that it's easy not to think about the consequences of unsafe sexual behavior while in the moment. Six of those 10 women mentioned that often they can fail to practice safe sex because they are in a hurry to have sex and do not think about using protection. Participants talked about how often couples are engaged in sexual activity, want to have intercourse, and do not have protection, so go ahead without thought of the future. One participant talked about how adolescents can be impulsive in the moment so they don't practice safe sex, saying, "They don't have a condom but they wanna do it now, so they just do it..." Other respondents echoed similar stories about unsafe sexual behavior occurring as a result of being in a hurry. One participant explained how she had been taught since middle school by her mother to carry protection, because sexual partners would typically not think about consequences in the moment:

> I carried 'em [condoms] because I never knew. And I wanted to make sure if I get in a situation I have something, because, you know, my mom always told me when I was younger, "You know men don't care. They're gonna just do it. If they want to get their dick wet, they're gonna do it, so you better carry one just in case and tell him he's puttin' it on or you ain't doin' it."

When asked why she thought male partners pressured adolescent girls not to use condoms during sex, the respondent said, "Cuz they're stupid. Cuz it feels better to have sex without a condom." Another participant related how she thinks men's attitudes toward women and impulsivity about sex are linked to men not thinking about the consequences of unsafe sexual behavior, saying, "And all they [her male friends] talk about is, 'I'm gonna fuck this bitch and I wanna fuck that bitch.' And, you know, 'That girl's so hot.'" When she hears this kind of talk, she said that she often tells her male friends what she thinks about the consequences of their actions:I tell

> them straight up... "You know, you think it's cool, really. But in all reality, do you wanna tell your mom, 'Hey I got this girl pregnant. Now I have to pay child support'? Because I'm [the male] 15 years old and she's 14, or vice versa? Dude! You're fuckin' 18 or 17 and this girl's fuckin' 13? You're going to fuckin' jail when you're 18, you know? You're going to prison and you're gonna have to be a sex offender for the rest of your life."

Don't like condoms or birth control Seven respondents noted that men do not like to use condoms and many of the men they knew chose not to use condoms. One women said simply, "The guys aren't [using condoms]. A majority of them don't want to." When asked why men did not want to use condoms, one participant was sympathetic to the men, saying, "Because it feels better. Or they just don't wanna wear that. Or they're allergic... The way that it hurts their area or whatever...But I wouldn't wanna wear that either, you know what I mean?"

Another respondent seemed skeptical of men who say they don't want to use condoms or for their female partners to use birth control. Her skepticism was illustrated in this discussion with the interviewer:

> Respondent: Guys refusing to wear protection...or not wanting their girlfriends to be on birth control.
>
> Interviewer: Okay. And do you hear of that happening a lot?
>
> Respondent: I've heard of it, yes.
>
> Interviewer: Okay. And do you know maybe some reasons that guys don't want their girlfriends to wear condoms or use birth control?
>
> Respondent: For the condoms because it feels better without [said sarcastically]. I used quotations; sorry, you didn't see my hands [laughs]. And the birth control, like hormones and stuff like that, because a lot of the times it can make your hormones go crazy.
>
> Interviewer: Okay. So are the boys concerned about the girl's hormones? Or?
>
> Respondent: [Nods head yes.] Sometimes. I've heard guys say that...I heard my friend's ex-boyfriend say that to her...because it made her crazy. [Said sarcastically]

Alcohol and drugs Six of the women talked about the prevalence and negative ramifications of drugs and alcohol in their adolescent sexual behavior. Participants said alcohol or drugs obscure judgment—either their own or their partners'. One participant said that being under the influence of drugs or alcohol led her to have sex without ever getting to know or talk with her partner: "I didn't really take the time to get to know any of 'em. So it was like extremely uncomfortable. I was always on drugs. You know, or alcohol or something. So I didn't, I really never connected to 'em. So it made it extremely awkward to talk to anybody."

Related to drugs or alcohol increasing sexual risk, one participant said, "It does change your judgment. Alcohol is one of the biggest judgment changers, you know? You know, especially with sexual activities. You know somebody can get you all drunk and then try to take advantage." Another participant talked about how she "didn't really take the time to get to know any of 'em [male sexual partners]. So it was like extremely uncomfortable [to talk to the partner about safe sex]. I was always on drugs." A third participant described the influence of alcohol on her own unsafe sexual behavior experiences like this: "Well, when I did alcohol, I would black out all the time...But I would get so wasted and I'd puke a lot sometimes. It was all fun and games and when I was dating a guy like, I'd hit on all his friends. Maybe make out with a couple of them. You know? Maybe go a little further and regret it in the morning and not even remember. Yeah, that happened a few times."

Partner is dishonest Three participants explained that sexual partners can lie about or fail to give partners information about their STI status, which they defined as a barrier to practicing safe sex. One participant said that men will lie about their health, saying, "We don't need it [a condom], it's okay. I've only been with one other girl...I'm clean." Two participants talked about instances when a male sexual partner had omitted such health information. One respondent talked about how a friend contracted HIV/AIDS from a male partner who did not disclose his health status, saying, "...I knew a girl who waited until she was 19 years old to have sex and had sex with her boyfriend of a year and a half and he had AIDS and he spread it to her...She even calls me crying, 'The one time I have sex, I get AIDS.'"

Another respondent talked about a personal experience when she found out that a sexual partner had an STI and didn't tell her:

> I don't think that the individuals who do have the STD are being honest because I've had that incident where I had a family friend who was really, really close to my aunt and he ended up wanting to sleep with me. And I slept with him. And then after we slept together, my aunt found out and told me that he

> had herpes and I didn't even know because he didn't tell me. I got upset that he didn't tell me and then I found out.

Male pressures female Four participants described the pressure male partners put on adolescent girls to engage in unsafe sexual behavior. Three participants discussed this pressure in broad terms, with one saying, "Like they just pressure you not to [use condoms]...they say it either feels better [without a condom] or they have nothing to worry about [they do not have an STI] or... somethin'. They say whatever they got to [laughs]." The fourth participant talked about a personal experience with forced sex, describing a time when her boyfriend raped her: "I was raped one time. Well, a couple of times, but this one stands out the most because I was young. It was with a boyfriend and I had told him 'no,' and he forced it on me anyway. And he was a lot stronger than I was. And there was no fighting him off."

Unrealistic expectations Five respondents talked about how adolescent girls can have unrealistic expectations about their sexual relationships, such as thinking they are ready to start a family as adolescents or that they would be loved by the partner and the relationship would last. For example, one participant said, "Just because he says he cares about you before doesn't mean that he still will afterwards. I've seen that way too many times...He'll just leave or that's all you will do afterwards, when you refuse to, he breaks it off with you. That happened to a very good friend of mine."

One participant described her own experience getting pregnant at a very young age, saying,

> But he seemed really sweet at first. Really kind, really understanding. Everything I looked for. But only being with him for two months, I found out that it was just a façade. He put on a mask pretty much just to snag me, I guess...Basically he was just a really conniving, deceitful person who was trying to get me in bed with him. And being so young, like, I trusted him. I believed everything he said. There was no precaution, there was no taking any caution at all with him. It was just go, go, go pretty much.

Putting on a condom is awkward Though many respondents had mentioned that it is awkward to talk about safe sex, only one participant said it was awkward to use condoms. She talked about her experience this way: "I think sex in itself is a pretty awkward when you're doing it with somebody you don't really know. And so to have to put on a condom, or to put in a female condom, or to do something like that in the middle of sex is already awkward. Just makes it 10 times more awkward. And then you kinda just don't want to do it anymore. Or it's just like you're embarrassed."

Discussion

The women in the study candidly shared their own and their friends' experiences from their adolescent years that illustrate the connection between drug and alcohol use and sexual behavior for adolescent girls with maltreatment histories. Many of the women in our study talked about how they did not think about the future when making risky decisions about drug use or sexual behavior as adolescents. In addition, most of the women said they regretted that using drugs or alcohol led to sexual experiences that they would not have wanted to engage in sober.

Many adolescents lack the long-term perspective that contributes to healthy decision making [41]. Recent research has shown that adolescence is marked by dramatic growth in brain activity associated with puberty that peaks in early adulthood [42]. Notably, multiple studies indicate that adolescence is a period during which the brain might be more sensitive to learning through experience than during other developmental periods [42]. Specifically, brain imaging studies have shown that adolescents are less likely to engage in risky behavior if they perceive that there will be a negative consequence for their behavior and, conversely, adolescents are more likely to engage in risky behavior if they deem the outcome to result in a reward [43]. Some researchers argue that although this period of rapid growth and development may be a time when adolescents are particularly vulnerable to engaging in risky behavior (e.g., drug use, unsafe sexual behavior), it can also be an opportunity for positive intervention [44]. This brain development research provides insight into opportunities for intervention with adolescents.

Implications for practice

The experiences and feelings shared by the women in this study highlight the urgent public health need for at-risk adolescent girls to be empowered with more information and skills related to drug use and safe sex practices [45]. Further, although we did not interview young men, several of the women's interviews provided insight into things that they wished their male counterparts had known. Based on the information shared in the qualitative interviews and current recommendations for comprehensive sexuality education [25], we propose six key implications for education and intervention programs: (1) adolescent girls could benefit from learning about partner characteristics that are promotive of risky behavior and partner characteristics that increase the potential for healthy relationships, (2) adolescent girls could benefit from receiving information about how romantic or sexual partners can influence their own drug use, (3) adolescent girls could benefit from practice talking about safe sex with partners so that they are more likely to do so with a new partner, (4) adolescent girls could benefit from receiving information about safe sex practices and the risks associated with unsafe sexual behavior, (5) adolescent boys could benefit from receiving information about the risks associated with drug use and unsafe sexual behavior, and (6) implications 1–5 could be integrated into comprehensive sexuality education for adolescents.

Partner choice

Data from a diverse national study show that adolescents choose romantic and sexual partners with similar characteristics (race, age, socioeconomic status) and similar interests [46]. Many of the women in this study mentioned that, as adolescents, they often sought relationships that led to risky behavior in an attempt to feel cool, independent, cared about, or free. Many of the women also said that, as adolescents, they sought a partner who would support them emotionally or financially [32]. However, when a young woman relies on the support of a partner to survive (either emotionally or physically), the relationship can easily develop into one that is unhealthy or codependent [47]. Similarly, the desire to have a partner or staying in a relationship to have a partner can be associated with adolescent girls' increased risk for contraction of sexually transmitted infections [31]. This is particularly true for relationships that include abuse and a power imbalance with the partner [31]. Including a component in intervention programs for at-risk adolescent girls to identify negative or risky partner characteristics (e.g., partner uses drugs or alcohol, partner is controlling) and identify partner characteristics that are promotive of a healthy relationship might reduce adolescent girls' later drug use or unsafe sexual behavior. Several women talked about positive personality traits or interests in specific activities that they had looked for in a relationship as an adolescent. Intervention programs could help at-risk adolescent girls not only identify negative partner characteristics, but also explicitly define the positive characteristics they seek in a partner. Although identifying risky or positive characteristics is no guarantee that adolescents will find or connect with safe, healthy partners, building their skills in this way could reduce the prevalence of unsafe sexual behavior in this population.

Partner influence on drug use

Consistent with findings from prior research [48], the women reported that partners had an influence on their adolescent drug use. The women identified several reasons why they or their peers would use drugs and alcohol with a partner. A potential strategy for intervention programs is to provide at-risk adolescent girls with information and skills about partner influence and associated risks. Because recent brain research shows that adolescents often learn best through experience [42], pairing information with explicit practice about how to respond to partner pressure to use drugs could reduce the prevalence of their drug use [28]. For example, several of the women in the study said that they thought adolescent girls use drugs to try to improve the relationship they have with their using partner. Understanding such influences could help those who develop intervention programs customize the message and associated practice to be relevant to the unique influences faced by this vulnerable population.

Talking about safe sex

Women in the sample emphasized that talking with a partner about safe sex practices is awkward or uncomfortable for adolescents. The women's descriptions of feeling nervous, scared, or unsure about talking about safe sex underscore the need for adolescents to be taught how to have these conversations. In addition, our findings suggest that there is a need for adolescent girls to learn how talking with a partner about safe sex practices directly benefits their own health and future opportunities. Consistent with the UNESCO recommendations for skill-based learning [25], intervention programs could teach adolescent girls practical skills for talking with partners about safe sex practices and provide a relatable rationale. An intervention approach that combines skills practice and information incorporates both experiential learning and risk/benefit evaluation, both of which are effective strategies to promote learning in adolescents [25, 42, 43].

Practicing safe sex

Many of the women talked about not using safe sex practices for a variety of reasons, including that putting on a condom can be awkward, they thought providing protection was the male partner's job, they had trusted their partners when they said they did not have an STI, or they did not feel comfortable insisting on safe sex. Other women talked about direct pressure not to use safe sex practices, including the partner using sexual coercion tactics or refusing to use condoms. As a result of engaging in unsafe sexual behavior, many of the women had stories about early pregnancy and/or contracting STIs. In addition, many of the women's stories illustrated the link between drug use and unsafe sexual behavior during adolescence. Our findings suggest that intervention programs for at-risk adolescent girls could benefit from including developmentally appropriate and comprehensive sex education that incorporates information about the relationship between drug use and unsafe sexual behavior, strategies for responding to pressure from partners, and the rationale and skills for talking with a partner about the safe sex practices described in the "Talking About Safe Sex" subsection.

Interventions for adolescent boys

Although we did not talk directly to men in this study, several themes emerged from the women's interviews that are applicable for adolescent boys. The women in this study confirmed that, as adolescents, their male partners regularly used drugs and/or alcohol and engaged in a range of sexual coercion tactics that promoted unsafe sexual behavior. As would adolescent girls, adolescent boys would likely benefit from sex education intervention programs that combine information and skills practice, including talking about safe sex, practicing safe sex, recognizing and avoiding sexually coercive behavior, and the relationship between drug use and unsafe sexual behavior. As described previously, recent brain research suggests that females and males learn best through a combination of experiential learning and risk/benefit evaluation [25, 42, 43].

Comprehensive sexuality education

Due to the study context and population, the implications discussed in this report focus on support and education for adolescents at heightened risk for health-risking behaviors. In addition, the current UNESCO guidelines for comprehensive sexuality education worldwide emphasize a holistic and developmental approach that includes a wide range of topics and life skills to facilitate healthy choices [25]. These guidelines are consistent with positive youth development research linking safer sexual behavior to other positive psychosocial behaviors [24]. Within the comprehensive sexuality education framework, complex concepts and skills related to gender equity, gender norms, consent, intimate relationships, communication, conflict resolution, self esteem, physical and mental health and wellness, emotional development, and socio-cultural norms are as essential as traditional sexual education topics such as puberty, reproduction, and unsafe sexual practices [25]. Specifically, education and intervention programs could incorporate the suggestions outlined in the paragraphs above within a more comprehensive framework that includes a broad spectrum of life skills for a lasting impact. For girls in particular, it is critical to recognize and address the contextual challenges that may impede girls' ability to adopt safer sexual behaviors such as gender inequality and gender-based violence. Comprehensive sexual education provides girls with the opportunity to explore how socio-cultural norms about gender and sexuality affect how they experience and navigate their own sexuality, identify barriers to accessing services or practicing protected sex (e.g., gender-based violence), and acquire critical knowledge, skills, and values for negotiating such barriers and pursuing relationships based upon mutual respect and equality.

Limitations and future directions

Despite the study strengths, several limitations should be noted. First, the sample was relatively homogenous. Study participants were recruited from a community in the Pacific Northwest, a region that is predominantly White. Future qualitative research with a more diverse sample recruited from other regions of the United States could expand and potentially enhance the generalizability of findings. Second, because our study focused on the experiences of young women, the sample included only females. Interviewing male participants with a history of maltreatment could provide additional insights into tailoring intervention programs based on gender. Third, we conducted the qualitative interviews at one time point. Our interviews were designed to ask the women to reflect retrospectively on their experiences as adolescents. Asking adolescent participants to reflect on their experiences and then following up with later interviews in young adulthood could illustrate the development of their thinking about these issues over time. Fourth, our interviews focus on only women with maltreatment histories. It would be beneficial to compare their motivations/decision making processes with women who do not have maltreatment histories. This comparison could provide insight into common influences for adolescents as well as those specific to the study population. Finally, further exploration on other factors that contribute to adolescents' decision making processes would be beneficial. Factors such as socioeconomic status, education, and other social influences are likely to be relevant influencers.

The qualitative interviews in our study were designed to elucidate factors that influence the decision-making processes for adolescent girls with a maltreatment history in regard to partner selection, drug use, and sexual behavior. Examining these factors can provide interventionists and researchers with valuable information to fill a gap in the literature and better understand the experiences of this vulnerable population.

Conclusion

This qualitative study substantiates the need for additional support for adolescent girls with histories of maltreatment. Five key targets for intervention emerged from the interviews: First, adolescent girls could benefit from receiving information about partner characteristics promotive of healthy relationships, including how to recognize power dynamics in relationships and how to seek out help and support. Second, adolescent girls could benefit from information about how romantic partners can influence their own drug use. Third, adolescent girls could benefit from instruction on how to discuss safe sex with partners. This includes giving adolescents opportunities to practice through role play. Fourth, adolescent girls could benefit from knowing details about what safe sex is and knowing how to identify their needs and desires. Finally, adolescent boys might also benefit from learning about these same risks and practicing these skills. By gearing intervention programs to focus on these key elements, adolescents with histories of maltreatment will be better equipped to navigate romantic relationships promotive of healthy sexual behavior in the context of a social environment where some youth are engaging in drug use. These intervention targets are consistent with the UNESCO recommendations on the core elements of sexual education programs [25].

Acknowledgements

The authors thank the women who participated in the interviews; Lawrence Palinkas for support on the development of the interview guide and training protocol; Danielle Guerrero for project coordination; Aliya Khan for conducting the interviews in partnership with the third author; Michelle Bauman, Sadie Baratta, Amala Shetty, Emily Kavanagh-Martin, Sophie Kreitzberg, Mariam Admasu, and Tim Matthews for transcribing the interviews; and Caroline Dennis and Cheryl Mikkola for editorial support.

Funding

Support for this research was provided by the following grants: R01 DA024672, R01 DA032634, R21 DA027091, and P50 DA035763 from the Division of Epidemiology, Services, and Prevention Research, NIDA U.S. PHS.

Authors' contributions

MC coded and analyzed the qualitative data and took primary responsibility for writing the manuscript. LL was the Principal Investigator and RB was a Co-Investigator on this study and both contributed to writing and editing the manuscript. RK conducted many of the interviews and contributed to the writing. All authors read and approved the final manuscript.

Competing interests

The authors declare that they have no competing interests.

Author details

[1]Oregon Social Learning Center, 10 Shelton McMurphey Blvd, Eugene, OR 97401, USA. [2]Prevention Science Institute, 6217 University of Oregon, Eugene, OR 97403, USA.

References

1. Aarons GA, James S, Monn AR, Raghavan R, Wells RS, Leslie LK. Behavior problems and placement change in a national child welfare sample: a prospective study. J Am Acad Child Adolesc Psychiatry. 2010;49:70–80.
2. Banducci AN, Hoffman EM, Lejuez CW, Koenen K. The impact of childhood abuse on inpatient substance users: specific links with risky sex, aggression, and emotion dysregulation. Child Abuse Negl. 2014;38(5):928–38.
3. Fettes DL, Aarons GA, Green AE. Higher rates of adolescent substance use in child welfare versus community populations in the United States. J Stud Alcohol Drugs. 2013;74(6):825.
4. Oshiri A, Tubman JG, Burnette ML. Childhood maltreatment histories, alcohol and other drug use symptoms, and sexual risk behavior in a treatment sample of adolescents. Am J Public Health. 2012;102(Suppl 2): S250–7.
5. Parkhill MR, Norris J, Cue Davi K. The role of alcohol use during sexual situations in the relationship between sexual revictimization and women's intentions to engage in unprotected sex. Violence Vict. 2014;29(3):492–505.
6. Walsh K, Latzman NE, Latzman RD. Pathway from child sexual and physical abuse to risky sex among emerging adults: the role of trauma-related intrusions and alcohol problems. J Adolesc Health. 2014;54(4):442–8. https://doi.org/10.1016/j.jadohealth.2013.09.020.
7. Kost K. Unintended Pregnancy Rates at the State Level: Estimates for 2002, 2004, 2006 and 2008. New York: Guttmacher Institute; 2013. http://www.guttmacher.org/pubs/StateUP08.pdf. Accessed 16 Mar 2018.
8. Anker JJ, Carroll ME. Females are more vulnerable to drug abuse than males: evidence from preclinical studies and the role of ovarian hormones. In: Neill JC, Kulkarni J, editors. Biological basis of sex differences in psychopharmacology. Berlin, Heidelberg: Springer; 2010. p. 73–96.
9. Ridenour TA, Lanza ST, Donny EC, Clark DB. Different lengths of times for progressions in adolescent substance involvement. Addict Behav. 2006; 31(6):962–83.
10. Reed E, Silverman JG, Raj A, Decker MR, Miller E. Male perpetration of teen dating violence: associations with neighborhood violence involvement, gender attitudes, and perceived peer and neighborhood norms. J Urban Health. 2011;88(2):226–39.
11. Kaushic C, Roth KL, Anipindi V, Xiu F. Increased prevalence of sexually transmitted viral infections in women: the role of female sex hormones in regulating susceptibility and immune responses. J Reprod Immunol. 2011; 88(2):204–9.
12. Furman W, Simon VA. Homophily in adolescent romantic relationships. In: Prinstein MJ, Dodge KA, editors. Understanding peer influence in children and adolescents. New York: Guilford Press; 2008. p. 203–24.
13. Silverman JG, Raj A, Mucci LA, Hathaway JE. Dating violence against adolescent girls and associated substance use, unhealthy weight control, sexual risk behavior, pregnancy, and suicidality. JAMA. 2001; 286(5):572–9.
14. Collins WA, Welsh DP, Furman W. Adolescent romantic relationships. Annu Rev Psychol. 2009;60:631–52.
15. Jessor R, Jessor SL. Problem behavior and psychosocial development: a longitudinal study of youth. New York: Academic Press; 1977.
16. Donovan JE, Jessor R. Structure of problem behavior in adolescence and young adulthood. J Consult Clin Psychol. 1985;53(6):890.
17. Arnett JJ. Emerging adulthood: a theory of development from the late teens through the twenties. Am Psychol. 2000;55:469–80.
18. Centers for Disease Control and Prevention Web site. https://www.cdc.gov/std/. Accessed 1 June 2017.
19. Centers for Disease Control and Prevention Web site. http://www.cdc.gov/hiv/statistics/overview/ataglance.html. Accessed 5 June 2017.
20. The National Center on Addiction and Subst Abus Web site. http://www.centeronaddiction.org/. Accessed 25 May 2017.
21. Substance Abuse and Mental Health Services Administration. Results from the 2013 National Survey on Drug Use and Health: Mental Health Findings. NSDUH Series H-49, HHS Publication No. (SMA) 14–4887. Rockville: Substance Abuse and Mental Health Services Administration; 2014.
22. Hahm HC, Lee Y, Ozonoff A, Van Wert MJ. The impact of multiple types of child maltreatment on subsequent risk behaviors among women during the transition from adolescence to young adulthood. J Youth Adolesc. 2010; 39(5):528–40.
23. Kim HK, Pears KC, Leve LD, Chamberlain P, Smith DK. Intervention effects on health-risking sexual behavior among girls in foster care: the role of placement disruption and tobacco and marijuana use. J Child Adolesc Subst Abuse. 2013;22(5):370 87.

24. Gavin LE, Catalano RF, David-Ferdon C, Gloppen KM, Markham CM. A review of positive youth development programs that promote adolescent sexual and reproductive health. J Adoles Health. 2010;46(3):S75–91.
25. UNESCO. International technical guidance on sexuality education: an evidence-informed approach. Paris: United Nations Educational, Scientific and Cultural Organization (UNESCO); 2018.
26. Trickett PK, Negriff S, Ji J, Peckins M. Child maltreatment and adolescent development. J Res Adolesc. 2011;21(1):3–20.
27. McLeod GFH, Fergusson DM, Horwood LJ. Childhood physical punishment or maltreatment and partnership outcomes at age 30. Am J Orthop. 2014; 84:307–15.
28. Rhoades KA, Leve LD, Harold GT, Kim HK, Chamberlain P. Drug use trajectories after a randomized controlled trial of MTFC: associations with partner drug use. J Res Adolesc. 2014;24(1):40–54.
29. Morrison-Beedy D, Xia Y, Passmore D. Sexual risk factors for partner age discordance in adolescent girls and their male partners. J Clin Nurs. 2013; 22(23–24):3289–99.
30. Oudekerk BA, Guarnera LA, Reppucci ND. Older opposite-sex romantic partners, sexual risk, and victimization in adolescence. Child Abuse Negl. 2014;38(7):1238–48.
31. Raiford JL, Seth P, DiClemente RJ. What girls won't do for love: human immunodeficiency virus/sexually transmitted infections risk among young African-American women driven by a relationship imperative. J Adoles Health. 2013;52(5):566–71.
32. Paxton KC, Williams JK, Bolden S, Guzman Y, Harawa NT. HIV risk behaviors among African American women with at-risk male partners. J AIDS Clin Res. 2013;4(7):221.
33. Raffaelli M, Crockett LJ. Sexual risk taking in adolescence: the role of self-regulation and attraction to risk. Dev Psychol. 2003;39(6):1036.
34. Masters NT, George WH, Davis KC, et al. Women's unprotected sex intentions: roles of sexual victimization, intoxication, and partner perception. J Sex Res. 2014;51(5):586–98.
35. Sterk CE, Klein H, Elifson KW. Predictors of condom-related attitudes among at-risk women. J Women's Health. 2004;13(6):676–88.
36. Rhule-Louie DM, McMahon RJ. Problem behavior and romantic relationships: assortative mating, behavior contagion, and desistance. Clin Child Fam Psychol Rev. 2007;10(1):53–100.
37. Clark M, Buchanan R, Leve LD. Young women's perspectives of their adolescent treatment programs: a qualitative study. Int J Environ Res Public Health. 2018;15(2):373.
38. Padgett DK. Qualitative methods in social work research. 2nd ed. Thousand Oaks: Sage Publications Inc.; 2008.
39. QSR International. NVivo qualitative data analysis Software, Version 10. Cambridge: QSR International Pty Ltd; 2012.
40. Glaser B, Strauss AL. The discovery of grounded theory: strategies for qualitative research. Chicago: Aldine Publishing; 1967.
41. Weller JA, Leve LD, Kim HK, Bhimj J, Fisher PA. Plasticity of risky decision making among maltreated adolescents: evidence from a randomized controlled trial. Dev Psychopathol. 2015;27(02):535–51.
42. Blakemore SJ, Choudhury S. Development of the adolescent brain: implications for executive function and social cognition. J Child Psychol Psychiatry. 2006;47(3–4):296–312.
43. Galvan A, Hare T, Voss H, Glover G, Casey BJ. Risk-taking and the adolescent brain: who is at risk? Dev Sci. 2007;10(2):F8–F14.
44. Dahl RE. Adolescent brain development: a period of vulnerabilities and opportunities. Keynote address. Ann N Y Acad Sci. 2004;1021(1):1–22.
45. Markham CM, Peskin MF, Shegog R, Baumler ER, Addy RC, Thiel M, et al. Behavioral and psychosocial effects of two middle school sexual health education programs at tenth-grade follow up. J Adolesc Health. 2014;54:151–9.
46. Ford K, Sohn W, Lepkowski JM. Ethnicity or race, area characteristics, and sexual partner choice among American adolescents. J Sex Res. 2003;40(2):211–8.
47. Lampis J, Cataudella S, Busonera A, Skowron EA. The role of differentiation of self and dyadic adjustment in predicting codependency. Contemp Fam Ther. 2017;39(1):62–72.
48. Mezzich AC, Tarter RE, Giancola PR, Lu S, Kirisci L, Parks S. Substance use and risky sexual behavior in female adolescents. Drug Alcohol Depend. 1997;44:157–66.

18

Female genital mutilation: current awareness, believes and future intention in rural Egypt

Eman S. Mohammed*, Amany E. Seedhom and Eman M. Mahfouz

Abstract

Background: Female genital cutting, also termed female genital mutilation (FGM), is a damaging practice with no health benefits for girls or women, and is considered to be a violation of children's rights.

Methods: A cross-sectional, community-based study using interview administered questionnaire to explore knowledge and attitude of people living in a rural area in Minia. Systematic random sampling was used to interview 618 males and females above the age of 18 in the period from September to November 2016.

Results: FGM was performed on 76.6% of females, complications occurred in 35.6% of them. Females demonstrated a higher level of knowledge than males. Nearly 56% of respondents believed that this practice should continue. Females were more supportive of the continuation of FGM than men (60.3% vs. 47.9%). The attitude that FGM is a good practice, knowledge level, women's status and religion were significantly associated with women's willingness to subject their daughters to FGM in the future. Attitude was the only significant predictor associated with men's willingness to subject their daughters to FGM.

Conclusion: The strong correlation between social pressure and intentions to carry out FGM means that FGM practice will continue to be embraced among future generations unless policies are put in place to eradicate this practice through empowering females by education and reasonable income.

Keywords: Female genital mutilation, Attitude, Predictors, Rural, Egypt

Plain English summary

Previous research assessed either female or male knowledge or attitude to FGM; this research explores gender perspectives and attitudes. Another important studied point is ability to explore future intention to undertake the practice to their daughters. Involving males in the battle against FGM is essential and necessitate innovative measures. Empowering females through education and reasonable income helps discouraging the practice of FGM.

Background

Female genital cutting, also termed female genital mutilation (FGM), is a damaging practice with no health benefits for girls and women, and is considered to be a violation of children's rights [1]. FGM is primarily widespread in certain high-risk countries including Egypt, and its rate is directly related to women's social status and Gender Equity (GE) [2]. The age of the girls who underwent this procedure usually varies from weeks after birth to puberty [3].

FGM practice is usually driven by religious, social and cultural impetus. Many people believe that religion is the reason behind their practice of FGM. In fact, religious scholars have different views regarding FGM. Some oppose the practice while others endorse it [4]. In some societies people practice FGM because of social pressure. One study has shown to what extent people in Minia governorate might be keen to perform FGM due to their solid belief of its direct relation to modesty and virginity. On other hand, others believe that removing "unclean" parts of the girl's body is essential to maintain femininity [5].

* Correspondence: emansameh7@yahoo.com
Public Health and Preventive Medicine, Faculty of Medicine, Minia University, Minia 1666, Egypt

According to the most recent Egyptian Health Issues Survey (EHIS) (2015), 87% of all Egyptian women, in the ages from 15 to 49 have been subjected to FGM. However, the results also suggested that the rate of the practice has declined among younger women. While the percentage of women subjected to FGM in the age group 25–49 exceeds 87%, the percentage in the age group under 25 does not exceed 70% [6]. It is noteworthy that the FGM rate for women age 15–49 shown in the 2015 EHIS is relatively low (87%) when compared to the 2008 Egyptian Demographic Health Survey (EDHS) in which the rate was as high as 91% [7].

UNICEF (2013) report shows that the level of support for the continuation of FGM among men and women varies widely across countries. In Egypt, the majority of boys and men report that they want FGM to continue. By contrast, more women than men report they would like the practice to halt. This suggests that altering FGM practice should involve not only women, but also entire communities, including men, particularly in settings where men participate in the decision-making process [3]. Therefore, we aimed to investigate the sex-specific intention of parents to continue FMG practice on their daughters. It was also crucial to assess the knowledge and attitudes of women and men in rural Upper Egypt regarding FGM.

Methods

Study design

This community-based cross-sectional study was conducted in a randomly chosen rural area (Nazlet El-falahin), El-Minia governorate between September and November, 2016.

Administrative design

The local municipal of Nazlet El-falahin gave its approval for the authors to obtain demographic data about the village as to the total number of residents, the total number of homes and the total number of women and men above the age of 18.

Sample size

The sample size was calculated using EP Info version 2000 by entering the prevalence of FGM (87%), the number of women and men above the age of 18 years (6253) and the confidence level (99.99%). Accordingly, the minimum required sample size was (600); 400 females and 200 males, which represents 9.6% of the total age-eligible inhabitants.

Therefore, we used a systematic random sampling technique by numbering the houses in the village choosing the first house at random, and then every fifth house to survey an expected number of (644 participants). Data were collected from 618 participants; 418 women and 200 men who agreed to be interviewed and to participate in the study. The remaining women and men declined to participate in the study. The response rates of women and men were 96.7% and 94.3% respectively. Noteworthy, we do not have reproductive data for the 26 (14 female and 12 male) who refused to participate in the study. However, there was no significant difference between those who participated and those who refused to participate as regards the distribution of socio-demographic characteristics such as age, religion, educational level, and marital status.

A pilot study was performed on 60 persons from the same village from an area away from the sampled households to ensure their non-inclusion in the final sample and the questionnaire was further validated through a review panel process where each item was considered for appropriateness. The data for these 60 persons was not included in the study results.

The questionnaires were administered, face to face, by 10 of fourth grade medical students. The medical students had attended one week of training on FGM and social research skills before filling the questionnaires. We did not sample different households for men and women. All eligible men and women who had consented to participate were interviewed. However, in most households, the number of interviewed subjects was not more than three eligible participants. We could not match couples as husbands and wives, because of the possibility that the interviewed males could be brothers, brothers-in-law, or other relatives co-residing with the interviewed women, and vice versa. Eligible men were interviewed by male interviewers, while eligible women were interviewed by female interviewers.

Data collection

The questionnaire was divided into four sections covering the following topics:

1- Personal characteristics and socio-demographic details including gender, age, educational level, religion and marital status.
2- The participants' knowledge about FGM was assessed through questions about its health consequences, reasons given for performing this practice and sources of this knowledge. The total knowledge score for each participant was calculated based on the answers given to each question: "correct answer" was assigned a score of 1; "incorrect/do not know" was assigned a score of 0. Scores less than 50% (less than 5 points) were categorized as "poor knowledge level", and scores between 50 and 100% were categorized as "good knowledge level".

3- Participants' attitude towards the practice of FGM was assessed using questions including: whether it should be considered a good practice, its continuation, husbands' preference for wives subjected to FGM, discrimination against girls who did not undergo FGM, the involvement of men in the debate on FGM, whether it decreased promiscuity and whether this practice can ever be eliminated in Egypt. Participants' attitudes were positive, negative or neutral.

The total attitude score for each participant was calculated based on the answers given to each question: "positive attitude" was assigned a score of 1; "neutral and negative attitude" was assigned a score of 0. Scores less than 50% (less than 4 points) were categorized as "Not in favour of FGM", and scores between 50 and 100% were categorized as "In favour of FGM". The eight questions that determined the attitude constituted of some negative statements, for which the scorings were reversed.

4- *The practice* was also assessed by asking if females were subjected to FGM or not, by whom, whether any complications have occurred (the interviewers mentioned the immediate and long term complications one by one) and whether they would subject their own daughters to this practice in the future.

Table 1 Socio-demographic profile of studied population, rural Minia, Egypt, during September–November 2016

Socio-demographic variables	Frequency	Percentage
Sex		
Male	200	32.4
Female	418	67.6
Age		
Range (mean ± SD)	18–78 (31.8 ± 14.6)	
Educational level		
Illiterate	100	16.2
Read and write	64	10.4
1ry education	52	8.4
2nd education	164	26.5
University	238	38.5
Religion		
Muslims	558	90.3
Christian	60	9.7
Marital status		
Single	252	40.8
Married	342	55.3
Divorced	4	0.6
Widowed	20	3.2
Total	618	100

Statistical analysis

The Statistical Program SPSS for windows version 20 was used in data analysis. Univariate and bivariate analyses with chi square tests were conducted to detect differences in knowledge and attitude between both sexes. For multivariate analyses the dependent variable was women's and men's willingness to subject their daughters to FGM in the future. Risk ratios were estimated by odds ratios (OR) via both binary logistic regression and Generalized Estimating Equations (GEE) analyses. Statistical significance was set at $p < 0.05$.

Results

The study highlighted the key characteristics that either foster or discourage the continuation of the practice. A total of 618 rural dwellers were included in the present study. Respondents' average age was 31.8 ± 14.6 years. About 90% were Muslims, 67.6% were women and 55.3% were married (Table 1).

Correct answers about the reasons of FGM were significantly higher among female than among male participants. The percentage of those who did not consider FGM as a mandatory religious practice was 64.1% of females versus 49% of males, did not consider it a proper protection to virginity (41.6% versus 26%) and did not view it as hygiene for vagina (47.8% versus 32%). All these differences were statistically significant.

Evaluation of rural dwellers' knowledge on FGM-related complications showed that 57.9% of females knew that the practice badly affected girls' health and welfare. Correct answers that FGM causes difficulties during delivery and leaves scars were reported among 25.8% and 53.1% of females respectively compared to 10% and 38% of males respectively ($p < 0.0001$). Nearly half of female participants versus 38% of men were aware of FGM being illegal (Table 2).

Of all participants studied, 37.1% had a poor level of knowledge while 62.9% had a good level of knowledge. Females demonstrated a higher level of knowledge than males ($P = 0.01$). The main source of information was television or radio which are used more often by females compared to males ($p = 0.006$).

Questions which were designed to measure the attitude of rural residents towards the practice of FGM showed that about 56% of rural residents believed that this practice should be continued. Females were more supportive of the continuation of FGM than men (60.3% vs. 47.9%). Also in this study, it was found that 47.3% Muslims versus 30% Christians ($p = 0.01$) believed that FGM is a good practice and should be continued.

Table 2 Knowledge of female genital mutilation among the rural dwellers, rural Minia, Egypt, during September–November 2016

Knowledge	Females no. (%) $n = 418$	Males no. (%) $n = 200$	Total no. (%) $n = 618$	X2 *P* value
Reported answers of rural dwellers about reasons of FGM				
FGM is a mandatory religious practice?				
Incorrect answer/don't know	150 (35.9)	102 (51)	250 (40.8)	14.3
Correct answer	268 (64.1)	98 (49)	366 (59.2)	0.001
FGM is hygienic for vagina				
Incorrect answer/don't know	218 (52.2)	146 (68)	354 (57.3)	14.9
Correct answer	200 (47.8)	64 (32)	264 (42.7)	0.001
FGM protects virginity				
Incorrect answer/don't know	244 (58.4)	148 (74)	392 (99.4)	14.5
Correct answer	174 (41.6)	52 (26)	226 (36.6)	0.001
Reported answers of rural dwellers about consequences on health of FGM				
Bleeding				
Incorrect answer/don't know	184 (44)	78 (39)	262 (42.4)	1.4
Correct answer	234 (56)	122 (61)	356 (57.6)	0.2
Reduction of sexual desire				
Incorrect answer/don't know	214 (51.2)	80 (40)	294 (53.7)	8.8
Correct answer	204 (48.8)	120 (60)	324 (52.4)	0.01
Transmission of infectious diseases				
Incorrect answer/don't know	248 (59.3)	114 (57)	362 (58.6)	0.3
Correct answer	170 (40.7)	86 (43)	256 (41.4)	0.6
Difficulty during delivery				
Incorrect answer/don't know	310 (74.2)	180 (90)	490 (79.3)	21.6
Correct answer	108 (25.8)	20 (10)	128 (20.7)	< 0.0001
Affects health and welfare of women				
Incorrect answer/don't know	176 (42.1)	118 (59)	294 (47.6)	15.5
Correct answer	242 (57.9)	82 (41)	324 (52.4)	< 0.0001
Scar formation				
Incorrect answer/don't know	196 (46.9)	124 (62)	320 (51.8)	12.4
Correct answer	222 (53.1)	76 (38)	298 (48.2)	< 0.0001
There is a law against FGM				
Incorrect answer/don't know	214 (51.2)	124 (62)	338 (54.7)	6.7
Correct answer	204 (48.8)	76 (38)	280 (45.3)	0.03
Knowledge score				
Poor knowledge level	141 (33.7)	88 (44)	229 (37.1)	6.1
Good knowledge level	277 (66.3)	112 (56)	389 (62.9)	0.01
Source of information				
Newspapers	18 (4.3)	4 (2)	22 (3.6)	17.9
TV/radio	202 (48.4)	72 (36)	274 (44.3)	0.006
Social meetings	14 (3.3)	8 (4)	22 (3.6)	
Mosque or church	10 (2.4)	2 (1)	12 (1.9)	
Friends and relatives	140 (33.5)	84 (42)	224 (36.2)	
More than one answer	34 (8.1)	30 (15)	64 (10.4)	

Discrimination against girls who did not undergo FGM was found in 39.8% of rural residents. Discrimination was found to be higher among females than males (41.9% vs. 35.6%) but this difference was statistically not significant (Table 3).

Nearly 49% of the participants considered that men should be involved in the debate on FGM. This opinion was significantly more embraced among males than females (61.9% vs. 43.2%). Also, about 49% of rural residents believed that FGM could be eliminated in Egypt. Males were more supportive of this attitude (56.9% vs. 45.6%).

About 55% of rural residents believed that husbands preferred that their wives be subjected to FGM. Males tended to endorse this attitude more than females (71.4% vs. 46.8%). Nearly 57% of rural residents believed that FGM should be criminalized. This attitude was more supported by females (66% vs. 36.7%). Thirty one percent of rural residents believed that FGM reduced promiscuity. Males were more supportive of this attitude (46.1% vs. 23.8%).

Type I (clitoris or the clitoral hood is cut off) and II (clitoris and inner lips are cut off) FGM were performed on 320 (76.6%) of females. The average age of circumcision was 11.5 ± 2.3 years. The practice was performed by a doctor in only 8.7% of the cases whereas 91.3% of them were by non-medical persons. Complications occurred in 35.6% of females who were subjected to FGM, 97.2% of them have been cut by non-medical persons (Table 4).

Table 5 provided the adjusted OR and 95% CI that quantified the association between the combined effect of independent variables and the outcome variable (women's willingness to subject their daughters to FGM in the future). These estimates were obtained using the logistic regression analysis. Attitude that FGM is a good practice, knowledge level, women's status and religion were significantly associated with women's willingness to subject their daughters to FGM in the future. The results suggest that while education is not significantly associated with women's willingness to subject their daughters to FGM, attitude that FGM is a good practice represented the major cause.

Table 3 Positive and negative attitudes of FGM among male and female rural dwellers, rural Minia, Egypt, during September–November 2016

Attitude	Females no. (%)	Males no. (%)	Total no. (%)	X2 *P* value
FGM is a good practice				
Positive attitude	148 (39.5)	107 (57.8)	225 (45.5)	16.9
Negative attitude	227 (60.5)	78 (42.2)	305 (54.5)	< 0.0001
FGM should continue				
Positive attitude	245 (60.3)	92 (47.9)	337 (56.4)	8.2
Negative attitude	161 (39.7)	100 (52.1)	261 (43.6)	0.004
Uncircumcised girls should be discriminated against				
Positive attitude	170 (41.9)	69 (35.6)	239 (39.8)	2.2
Negative attitude	236 (58.1)	125 (64.4)	361 (60.2)	0.1
FGM can ever be eliminated in Egypt				
Positive attitude	185 (45.6)	111 (56.9)	296 (49.3)	6.8
Negative attitude	221 (54.4)	84 (43.1)	305 (50.7)	0.009
Men should be involved in the debate on FGM				
Positive attitude	176 (43.2)	122 (61.9)	298 (49.3)	18.5
Negative attitude	231 (56.8)	75 (38.1)	306 (50.7)	< 0.0001
Husband prefer wives subjected to FGM				
Positive attitude	191 (46.8)	140 (71.4)	331 (54.8)	32.4
Negative attitude	217 (53.2)	56 (28.6)	273 (45.2)	< 0.0001
Should FGM be criminalized				
Positive attitude	268 (66)	72 (36.7)	340 (56.5)	46.1
Negative attitude	138 (34)	124 (63.3)	262 (43.5)	< 0.0001
FGM decreases promiscuity				
Positive attitude	97 (23.8)	89 (46.1)	186 (31)	30.4
Negative attitude	310 (76.2)	104 (53.9)	414 (69)	< 0.0001

NB Neutral attitude was excluded from both female and male categories

Table 4 Practice of FGM among studied females, rural Minia, Egypt, during September–November 2016

Practice	Yes no. (%)	No no. (%)
Was FGM performed on you?	320 (76.6)	98 (23.4)
Was FGM performed by a doctor?	28 (8.7)	292 (91.3)
Did any complication occurs (as perceived by her)?	114 (35.6)	206 (64.4)
Age at circumcision		
Range	4–17	
(mean ± SD)	11.5 ± 2.3	
Age groups (number of women)	no. circumcised (percentage)	
< 19 (208)	136 (65.4)	
20–24 (58)	46 (79.3)	
25–29 (42)	38 (90.5)	
30–34 (26)	22 (84.6)	
35–39 (24)	22 (91.7)	
40–44 (24)	24 (100)	
45–49 (16)	14 (87.5)	
≥ 50 (20)	18 (90)	
Marital status (number of women)	no. circumcised (percentage)	
Never married (230)	148 (64.3)	
Ever married (188)	172 (91.5)	
Total	418	100

Table 6 showed logistic regression analysis of the independent variables and the outcome variable (men's willingness to subject their daughters to FGM in the future). Attitude that FGM is a good practice was the only significant factor associated with men's willingness to subject their daughters to FGM in the future.

Discussion

Researcher's attention has increasingly been directed towards FGM over the last decades due to its effect on women's health representing a severe violation of a basic human right: bodily integrity [8]. Previous studies have shown that FGM occurred among females in all social strata, uneducated and highly educated, urban and rural residents [9]. Studies on FGM among the general population in Egypt have reported that 87% of Egyptian women have been subjected to FGM [10, 11].

Evaluation of rural residents' knowledge on FGM-related complications showed that 57.9% of females knew that the practice badly affected girls' health and welfare. Similar finding was reported by Moges et al. (2014) in a study conducted to assess knowledge of women towards FGM in Ethiopia [12].

About 55% of rural residents had knowledge that FGM was against the law, which was similar to that of Emam et al. who noticed that despite women's awareness that FGM was illegal, they would still practice it. This showed that the law alone was not sufficient to eradicate this habit, and it seemed that laws forbidding FGM led to changes in the patterns of the practice [13].

Eventually, of all participants studied, 37.1% had a poor level of knowledge and 62.9% had a good level of knowledge. Females demonstrated a higher level of knowledge more than males ($P = 0.01$). This finding was in agreement with Abdel Magied and Makki, 2004 who found that female respondents were far more knowledgeable about the negative consequences of FGM [14].

Our results showed that females were more supportive of the continuation of FGM than men (60.3% vs 47.9%) because females are greatly affected by the culture that supports inequality between men and women. In contrast to this, the study done in Somalia reveals that male respondent (96%) supported the continuation of FGM. This difference may be explained by the fact that the achieved progress towards the abandonment of the practice in Somalia has been known to be very limited due to the unprecedented prevalence of the practice in Somalia [15].

In the current study, 54.8% of rural residents believed that husbands preferred that their wives being subjected to FGM. Males were more supportive of this attitude (71.4% vs. 46.8%). This was not in coherence with Abathun et al. who found that more than half of the studied young boys preferred to marry girls not subjected to FGM. This implies that young boys had

Table 5 Logistic regression of factors independently associated with women's willingness to subject their daughters to FGM in the future, rural Minia, Egypt, during September–November 2016

Risk factors	OR (95% CI)	p
Women status		
No FGM	1.00 (Reference)	0.004[a]
Complicated FGM	0.07 (0.02–0.34)	
Not complicated FGM	1.13 (1.02–1.97)	
Attitude that FGM is a good practice		
No	1.00 (Reference)	0.0001[a]
Yes	2.35 (1.73–8.95)	
Knowledge level about FGM		
Good	1.00 (Reference)	0.001[a]
Poor	1.28 (1.14–1.59)	
Religion		
Christian	1.00 (Reference)	0.03[a]
Muslim	1.02 (0.93–1.25)	
Educational level		
University level	1.00 (Reference)	0.2
Secondary education	0.17 (0.04–0.81)	
Basic education	0.89 (0.1–4. 92)	
Illiterate	1.28 (0.2–3.54)	
Marital status		
Never married	1.00 (Reference)	0.07
Ever married	0.82 (0.4–1.23)	
Age group		
< 25 year	1.00 (Reference)	0.84
> 25 year	1.83 (0.53–4.21)	

Cox & Snell R Square = 0.56
NB dependent variable is women's willingness to subject their daughters to FGM in the future, OR odds ratio, CI confidence interval
[a]Statistically significant

Table 6 Logistic regression of factors independently associated with men's willingness to subject their daughters to FGM in the future, rural Minia, Egypt, during September–November 2016

Risk factors	OR (95% CI)	p
Attitude that FGM is a good practice		
No	1.00 (Reference)	0.0001[a]
Yes	1.63 (1.07–2.89)	
Spouse' status		
No FGM	1.00 (Reference)	0.32
Complicated FGM	1.75 (0.15–20.3)	
Not complicated FGM	8.58 (0.38–196.2)	
Knowledge level about FGM		
Good	1.00 (Reference)	0.82
Poor	1.84 (0.19–3.71)	
Religion		
Christian	1.00 (Reference)	0.87
Muslim	1.25 (0.09–16.9)	
Educational level		
University level	1.00 (Reference)	0.6
Secondary education	0.14 (0.01–1.78)	
Basic education	1.31 (0.17–12.8)	
Illiterate	1.94 (0.11–7.74)	
Marital status		
Never married	1.00 (Reference)	0.9
Ever married	0.78 (0.02–41.3)	
Age group		
< 25 year	1.00 (Reference)	0.2
> 25 year	1.1 (0.003–3.67)	

Cox & Snell R Square = 0.50
NB dependent variable is men's willingness to subject their daughters to FGM in the future, OR odds ratio, CI confidence interval
[a]Statistically significant

unrestrained freedom to obtain knowledge about the harmful effect of FGM on sexuality [16].

The overall prevalence of FGM among female participants in this study is considered to be low when compared with the 2015 DHS data [6]. Yet, as data disaggregated by age, the higher prevalence of FGM is evident for the older age group of females (> 25 years) rather than younger age group. In the current study, more than half of the studied females aged below 25 years; meanwhile, nearly 90% of females in the older age group were found to be subjected to FGM, which is more or less approaching what was reported by the national EHIS, 2015.

By comparing the percentages of those who had reported living with FGM across different age categories in the current study with the respective percentages of the EHIS, 2015, FGM prevalence in our study was slightly lower in the age categories (15–19 years 65.4% vs. 69.6%) and (20–24 years 79.3% vs. 81.6%) and (35–39 years 91.7% vs. 95.4%) and (45–49 years 87.5% vs. 97.1%); but was slightly higher in the age categories (25–29 years 90.5% vs. 89.2%) and (40–44 years 100% vs. 94.9%). Likewise the EHIS, 2015, we found that the highest prevalence of FGM was in the age groups (35–39) and (25–29) years; both came the second and third top percentages in both studies respectively. The percentages of FGM among the never- married females in our study was lower than that among ever-married females (64.3% vs. 91.5%), which are found to be slightly lower than the findings of EHIS, 2015 (67.6% vs. 91.5%) [6].

The practice was performed by a doctor in only 8.7% of the cases while 91.3% of them were by non-medical persons. This result was inconsistent with the finding of Rasheed et al. which was carried out also in Upper Egypt and aimed to estimate the influence of the 2007 criminalization law on the prevalence and yearly incidence of FGM, and it was found that in their vast majority, the procedures were performed by general practitioners. In total, 88.2, 34.3 and 14.9% of nurses, young physicians, and senior physicians, respectively, approved the practice. This difference may be explained by the fact that the study of Rasheed et al. was performed from September 2008 to September 2010, shortly after the criminalization law was enacted in Egypt, so physicians were unaware of the consequences of this criminal action [17].

The logistic regression analysis showed that knowledge, attitude, religion and women's status are significant predictors of future FGM practice among the daughters of females, with attitude that FGM is a good practice representing the major cause. These findings were in agreement with Pashaei et al. who examined the determinants of women's intentions to subject their daughters to FGM, and it was found that attitude was the strongest predictor of perpetuation of FGM [18]. Therefore, intervention programs to decrease FGM might focus primarily on converting women's positive attitude toward FGM into negative attitude, and on alleviating the perceived social pressure to mutilate one's daughter [19].

Men's contribution in the prevention of this harmful practice is indeed needed. The prospects of eliminating FGM will most likely to come to an end if due attention is given to male attitudes [20]. In a rural Upper Egyptian society, like our study focus, where the majority of men lead, and decide for women who to interact with and who to socialize with, it is highly advised that men be included in all efforts to prevent/eliminate FGM adequately [21]. However, researches involving men's future intentions and their influence on the perpetuation of the FGM are limited.

This study found that the attitude was the only significant predictor for men's willingness to subject their daughters to FGM; so we recommend conducting health education sessions to the rural educated men, and consequently they will most likely help to change positive attitudes of none and low educated men in their families towards continuation of FGM. Television and other media have an important role in changing the attitude of rural men and so contribute to discontinuation of FGM.

This study revealed that the participants were trapped in customary traditions, and found out controversy and divergence between the participants' perception of the harmful effects of FGM and their inclination towards maintaining FGM, giving an impetus to advance strong measures against the harmful practice. A proper measure in this regard is the Transtheoretical Model which facilitates the process of intentional behavior change in different community settings.

People can move through a series of stages during behavior modification to reduce resistance, facilitate progress, and prevent relapse of the FGM behavior [22]. The stages include: precontemplation (not ready), contemplation (getting ready), preparation, action and maintenance. As population move from *preparation* to *action*, the gap between sense of self-efficacy and temptation gets closer, and behavior change is achieved. So, to redress these harmful behaviors, people need to become aware of the possibility of change, have a favorable opinion towards change, choose to adopt or reject the change, put change into practice, and reinforce or reject change when faced with conflict or difficulty [22].

Limitations of the study

Some women and men refused to participate in the study. The response rates were 96.7% and 94.3% for women and men respectively. Refusal of participation could be attributed to their sense of shame, or because FGM is an illegal practice. The possibility to recall bias, or reporting bias was another limitation. Despite the fact that accuracy of self-reported data can be compromised by real ignorance about status or purposeful misrepresention of their status, yet, the validity of the results was not affected by this type of bias as it did not exceed 8% in previous studies in Egypt between the reported FGM and actual status. Because circumcision is a sensitive issue, our data collectors were skillful and used appropriate procedures adjusted for participant's response.

Another point worth mentioning is the fact that often more than one participant was recruited from the same household and therefore there is a possibility for violation of the independent observation assumption of logistic regression analysis. We dealt with this issue in several ways, first we checked if the distribution of number of interviewed participants per a household among each group of outcome (willing to subject their daughter to FGM versus not willing to do so, and we found no significant difference in this distribution. Second, we addressed this clustering of the measurements through the empirical variance estimation method (the robust standard error method) by running GEE analysis with robust covariance matrix in SPSS. This GEE analysis yielded more or less similar parameter estimates (OR) as those obtained by the binary logistic regression.

Conclusions and recommendations

Women's knowledge, attitude, religion and status are proved to be significant predictors of the women's future intentions to carry out FGM practice on daughters, thereby, concrete efforts need to be exerted in these specific areas, particularly through securing and realizing quality education to the fullest potential, offering explanatory role by religious leaders that FGM is neither mandated nor recommended by either Islam or Christianity, and approaching females by health education messages in schools, MCH and in any other opportunity of contact.

Female genital mutilation needs to be reframed within the broader issue of gender inequity and inequality which cuts across geography, socioeconomic, religion and education. Promoting gender justice and equality through taking actual steps towards empowering women and improving their position and status by ensuring quality education will enhance decision making capacity and will pave the way towards elimination of the FGM practice.

The findings of the study highlighted the welcoming attitude of men towards the continuity of FGM practice. So sincere scientific efforts of changing men's attitudes are greatly needed through involving them seriously and adequately in all efforts of prevention and elimination of FGM.

It is essential to strengthen and scale up the momentum for change brought about by the recent issuing of a law that banned and criminalized the FGM act, especially in rural areas in Upper Egypt, in order to turn the potentials into actual changes in attitudes and behaviors.

Implications of the study

It's important to train health care providers on how to address the complications of FGM and to make sure that the concerned health services are able to deal with these cases.

Abbreviations

EDHS: Egyptian Demographic Health Survey.; EHIS: Egyptian Health Issues Survey; FGM: Female genital mutilation; GE: Gender Equity

Acknowledgements

The authors would like to offer their sincere thanks to fourth grade medical students for their help in field work. We are grateful for all the women and men of Nazlet El-falahin village, Minia, Egypt, for their participation in the study. Many thanks to Mr. Mohamed S. Mostafa for language revision and for his continuous support.

Authors' contributions

ES had the original idea of the study and had made substantial contributions to conception and design and perform analysis and interpretation of data. AS and EM participate in the result section of the paper and they had been involved in drafting the manuscript or revising it critically for important intellectual content. All authors read and approved the final manuscript.

Competing interests

The authors declare that they have no competing interests.

References

1. Female genital mutilation, fact sheet: World Health Organization; 2013 (http://www.who.int/about/licensing/copyright_form/en/index.html. Accessed 20 Nov 2016).
2. Van Rossem R, Meekers D, Gage AJ. Women's position and attitudes towards female genital mutilation in Egypt: a secondary analysis of the Egypt demographic and health surveys, 1995-2014. BMC Public Health. 2015;15:874. https://doi.org/10.1186/s12889-015-2203-6 https://www.ncbi.nlm.nih.gov/pmc/articles/PMC4566495/. Accessed 15 Nov 2016.
3. United Nations Children's Fund (UNICEF). Female Genital Mutilation/Cutting: A statistical overview and exploration of the dynamics of change. https://www.unicef.org/media/files/UNICEF_FGM_report_July_2013_Hi_res.pdf. Accessed 1 Dec 2016.
4. Jones SD, Ehiri J, Anyanwu E. Female genital mutilation in developing countries: an agenda for public health response. Eur J Obstetr Gynecol Reprod Biol. 2004;116(2):144–51.
5. Yount KM. Symbolic gender politics, religious group identity, and the decline in female genital cutting in Minya, Egypt. Social Forces. 2004;82(3):1063–90.
6. Ministry of Health and Population [Egypt], El-Zanaty and Associates [Egypt], and ICF International. 2015. Egypt Health Issues Survey 2015. Cairo, Egypt and Rockville, Maryland, USA: Ministry of Health and Population and ICF International. https://dhsprogram.com/publications/publication-FR313-DHS-Final-Reports.cfm. Accessed 3 Nov 2016.
7. El-Zanaty F, Way AA. Egypt demographic and health survey. Cairo: Ministry of Health, El-Zanaty and Associates, and Macro International; 2008. (2009)
8. Schroeder P. Female genital mutilation – a form of child abuse. N Engl J Med. 1994;331(11):739–40.
9. Female genital mutilation. Geneva: World Health Organization; 2014 [Updated February 2014]. (http://www.who.int/mediacentre/factsheets/fs241/en/. Accessed 15 Nov 2016).
10. Yount KM. Like mother, like daughter? Female genital cutting in Minia, Egypt. J Health SocBehav. 2002;43:336–58.
11. El-Zanaty FH, Way AA. Egypt interim demographic and health survey, 2003: Ministry of Health and Population; 2004.
12. Moges NA, Mullu G, Gedfew M, Redi M, Molla M, Ayenew S, Fentahun S, Adisie S, Dagnew Z. Knowledge, attitude and practice of women towards female genital mutilation in LejetKebele, Dembecha Woreda, Amhara regional state, northwest, Ethiopia, 2014. J Gynecol Obstetr. 2015;3(2):21–5. https://doi.org/10.11648/j.jgo.20150302.11.
13. Emam E, EL-Maghawri A, Labeeb S. Cultural awareness about female genital mutilation among female employees of Minia University. J Amer Sci. 2011;7(4):611–7.
14. Abdel Magied A, Makki AE. Knowledge and attitudes of Sudanese youth towards female genital mutilation / female circumcision (FGM / FC). Case study: College of Technological Sciences (Tigana). Ahfad J. 2004;21(1):29–40.
15. Gele AA, Bø BP, Sundby J. Have we made progress in Somalia after 30 years of interventions? Attitudes toward female circumcision among people in the Hargeisa district. BMC Res Notes. 2013;6:122.
16. Abathun AD, Gele AA, and Sundby J. Attitude towards the Practice of Female Genital Cutting among School Boys and Girls in Somali and Harari Regions, Eastern Ethiopia. Obstet Gynecol Int. 2017; Article ID 1567368:1–9.
17. Rasheed SM, Abd-Ellah AH, Yousef FM. Female genital mutilation in upper Egypt in the new millennium. Int J Gynaecol Obstet. 2011;114(1):47–50. https://doi.org/10.1016/j.ijgo.2011.02.003 Epub 2011 Apr 21.
18. Pashaei T, Ponnet K, Moeeni M, Khazaee-pool M, Majlessi F. Daughters at risk of female genital mutilation: examining the determinants of Mothers' intentions to allow their daughters to undergo female genital mutilation. PLoS One. 2016;11(3):e0151630. https://doi.org/10.1371/journal.pone.0151630.
19. Saleh Z. Female genital mutilation in Egypt. In: A paper presented to the faculty of University of North Carolina at Chapel Hill; 2013. https://cdr.lib.unc.edu/indexablecontent/uuid:5d857dc2-e79b-4e7a-be49-9b723dde6e24. Accessed 5 Dec 2016.
20. Zelalem B. Male involvement in the practice of female genital mutilation in shone town southern nation nationality regional government, Ethiopia a thesis submitted as partial fulfillment of masters of philosophy in international community health, institute of community medicine, Oslo university 2000–2002; 2002.
21. Shaheen HM, Kasemy ZA, Salah Eldeen FM. The current situation regarding awareness about female genital mutilation among men working in schools of Benha City, Qaluobia governorate. Menoufia Med J. 2017;30(1):23–7.

Maternal socioeconomic factors and the risk of premature birth and low birth weight in Cyprus

Paraskevi Stylianou-Riga[1], Panayiotis Kouis[2*], Paraskevi Kinni[2], Angelos Rigas[3], Thalia Papadouri[1], Panayiotis K. Yiallouros[2] and Mamas Theodorou[4]

Abstract

Background: Prematurity and low birth weight are significant predictors of perinatal morbidity and mortality and are influenced by the overall health and socioeconomic status of the pregnant mother. Although Cyprus is characterized by the highest prematurity rate in Europe (13.1% in 2014), the relationship between maternal health and socioeconomic characteristics with prematurity and low birth weight has never been investigated. We aimed to investigate the association of maternal demographic, clinical and socioeconomic characteristics with premature delivery and low neonatal birth weight in Cyprus.

Methods: In a case-control design, questionnaire data were collected from 348 women who gave birth prematurely (cases) and 349 women who gave birth at term (controls). Information was obtained on gestation duration and birth weight as well as maternal demographic, socioeconomic and clinical profiles, including parameters such as smoking, body mass index, alcohol consumption, presence of gestational diabetes and mental health factors.

Results: Premature delivery was associated with greater maternal age (OR: 1.12, 95% CI: 1.06–1.18), absence of gestational diabetes (OR: 0.53, 95% CI: 0.30–0.97), long working hours (OR: 3.77, 95% CI: 2.08–6.84) and emotional stress (OR: 8.5, 95% CI: 3.03–23.89). Within the cases group, emotional stress was also associated with lower birth-weight (β: -323.68 (95% CI: -570.36, – 77.00).

Conclusions: The findings of this study demonstrate the positive association of maternal psychological factors, working conditions as well as maternal age with prematurity and low birth weight in Cyprus. Additional, prospective, studies are needed in the country to further investigate these associations and inform public health intervention measures.

Keywords: Preterm birth, Low birth weight, Maternal risk factors, Socioeconomic factors

Plain english summary

Prematurity and low birth weight are important determinants of neonatal health and are influenced by the overall health and socioeconomic conditions of the pregnant mother. While prematurity rates vary significantly across the world, Cyprus is characterized by the highest prematurity rate in Europe. However, the factors that are associated with prematurity and low birth weight in Cyprus have never been studied.

This study was designed to understand the influence of demographic, mental health and socioeconomic factors on premature delivery and low birth weight in Cyprus. We identified 348 mothers with premature deliveries at the island's largest maternity unit during a one year period and we also enrolled 349 mothers with term pregnancies as controls. Through the use of a specifically designed questionnaire we obtained data on socioeconomic characteristics from both groups of mothers. Basic information about clinical and demographic characteristics was available from medical charts.

Comparison between mothers with preterm pregnancies and mothers with term pregnancies demonstrated that maternal age at birth, long working hours and emotional

* Correspondence: kouis.panayiotis@ucy.ac.cy
[2]Medical School, University of Cyprus Shakolas Educational Center of Clinical Medicine, Palaios Dromos Lefkosias Lemesou 215/6, 2029 Aglantzia, Nicosia, Cyprus
Full list of author information is available at the end of the article

stress were associated with a higher risk for prematurity while emotional stress was also associated with lower birth weight among premature neonates. Combinations of two or more factors were associated with a sharp increase of prematurity risk, demonstrating a cumulative effect.

Healthcare professionals should take into account the overall socioeconomic status of pregnant women during observation, towards identifying high risk pregnancies for prematurity and implementation of appropriate clinical management. Furthermore, healthcare policy makers should aim for the development of public health intervention measures targeting high risk pregnant women.

Background

Optimal fetal development is widely recognized (World Health Organization – WHO, 2006) as an important factor of infant's survival and subsequent social development. In particular, birth weight, neonatal viability and gestational age, are considered as important health determinants throughout lifetime [1]. Furthermore, the good health and the favorable socioeconomic environment of the pregnant mother are also considered essential prerequisites for the mental and physical well-being of the infant [2].

Preterm labor is the leading cause of perinatal morbidity and mortality in developed countries, where the majority of deaths occur in neonates with a gestational age of less than 32 weeks [3–5]. In recent years, the care provided in Neonate Intensive Care Units (NICU) settings increased the survival of premature infants but at the same time increased duration of hospitalization and costs. As a result, the care of premature neonates currently accounts for a large proportion of the total in-hospital costs worldwide [6]. In total, fifteen million premature births are reported annually worldwide [4] and although the frequency of preterm labor varies considerably between countries, almost 90% of these premature births occur in developing countries in Africa and Asia [7]. In 2014, the rate of preterm births was 10% in the US [8], while in Europe in 2010, preterm birth rates varied markedly from 5 to 10.6% among live births [9]. Cyprus is characterized by the highest premature birth rate in Europe, reaching 10.6% and 13.1% in 2010 and 2014 respectively [10, 11] partly due to increase of multiple pregnancies following in-vitro fertilization [12].

Furthermore, low birth weight (LBW) is associated with increased mortality as well as acute and long-term health problems [13–15]. In Europe the percentage of LBW ranged between 4 and 9% in 2010 [10]. LBW infants also face significant neurodevelopmental problems, whereas in adulthood they are at higher risk to develop type 2 diabetes mellitus, hypertension and coronary artery disease [16].

Several risk factors have been found to be associated with premature birth and LBW, including maternal age, ethnicity, lifestyle maternal characteristics such as smoking and alcohol consumption, education level, working conditions, access to obstetric observation, diabetes mellitus, mental stress and depression, body mass index (BMI) before pregnancy and additional weight-gain during pregnancy [5]. Despite the increasing incidence of premature births in Cyprus, there is lack of knowledge regarding the prevalent maternal risk factors for premature birth and LBW, which is a necessary prerequisite for development of prevention strategies by the national health system and awareness initiatives among the public and health professionals. We aimed to assess the relation of demographic and maternal socioeconomic and lifestyle characteristics with the risk of premature birth among Cypriot pregnant women and investigate the contribution of the same characteristics to LBW risk among premature infants.

Methods

Study population

The source population were all mothers that gave birth between March 2015 and April 2016 at "Archbishop Makarios III" hospital in Nicosia, Cyprus. "Archibishop Makarios III" hospital is the main tertiary maternal and pediatric hospital in Cyprus which hosts the only tertiary NICU on the island. Mothers who gave birth to premature neonates (gestation < 37 weeks) were included in the study as cases and mothers that gave birth to term neonates (gestation > 37 weeks) were included in the study as controls. Data collection commenced in March 2015 and was completed in April 2016. Mothers with multiple pregnancies or mothers that underwent infertility treatment as well as mothers of stillborn neonates and mothers of neonates with chromosomal abnormalities were excluded from the study. Sample size calculation was performed using OpenEpi [17] assuming a 1:1 ratio of cases to controls, 95% confidence level, 80% power and a least extreme Odds Ratio (OR) to be detected equal to 1.55. The calculated sample size was 333 cases and 333 controls. All participants provided written informed consent and the study protocol was approved by the Cyprus National Bioethics Committee (EEBK ΕΠ 2015.01.25) and the Cyprus Ministry of Health (Protocol approval: 0282/2015).

Data collection and data processing

Information on duration of gestation period and birth weight was obtained from hospital records while all other information was collected through a structured self-administered questionnaire. The questionnaire (Additional file 1) was adopted from similar previous studies [18, 19] and consisted of questions on basic demographic (age, ethnicity) and socioeconomic factors such as marital status, socioeconomic status (income, education level, profession, working conditions (manual labour, standing, > 8 h shifts). Data on anthropometric indices and other potential maternal risk factors such as gestational diabetes, stress, depression, antidepressants consumption, alcohol consumption, and smoking before and during pregnancy were also obtained through the questionnaire and the responses were crosschecked with available information in the mothers' medical records. Anthropometric and clinical parameters such as weight, height, gestational diabetes and depression were derived from clinical assessments while experience of emotional stress and use of antidepressants or anxiolytics during pregnancy were obtained from self-assessment by the participants using binary (YES or NO) questions. Composite scores for variables describing working conditions and socioeconomic deprivation were developed with individual factors carrying the same weight.

Statistical analysis

All variables used in the analysis were checked for normality with the use of histograms. Summary statistics for participant characteristics were calculated separately for cases and controls and categorical variables are reported as absolute and relative (%) frequencies, while continuous variables are reported as mean estimates and standard deviation. In unadjusted analyses, differences in participant characteristics between cases and controls were investigated using chi square test in the case of categorical variables and independent *t*-test in the case of continuous variables. A multivariate logistic regression including all variables that were found to be significantly associated with prematurity ($p_{value} < 0.10$) in the unadjusted analysis was used in order to calculate the OR and 95% Confidence Intervals (95% CI) for pre-term birth.

Among cases, the relationship between different characteristics and gestational age as well as birth weight were examined using the Pearson correlation coefficient and adjusted analyses were performed using a multivariate linear regression model. The linear regression models included all variables that were significantly correlated with birth weight ($p_{value} < 0.10$).

To further illuminate the role of clustering of risk factors for prematurity, a cumulative individual risk score was calculated for each mother by summing the values (0 for negative or 1 for positive) of each significant risk factor. Lastly, to demonstrate the extent to which different significant risk factors overlap, a Venn diagram was produced using Venny software [20]. The OR of combinations of risk factors with significant overlap was calculated using binary logistic regression.

For the multivariate logistic, binary logistic and linear regressions a two tailed *p*-value < 0.05 was applied to demonstrate statistical significance. All statistical analyses were performed using STATA (Version 12, StataCorp, College Station, TX).

Results

A total of 697 mothers were included in the study (348 cases and 349 controls). Only one mother did not complete the questionnaire resulting in a final response rate of 99.8% for cases and 100% for controls. Cases were older than controls (30.7, 95% CI: 19.4–41.9 vs 28.8, 95% CI: 18.8–38.7, $p_{value} < 0.001$) and more frequently reported practicing a manual labour profession (33.3% vs 19.8%, $p_{value} = 0.001$) or working >8 h per day (34.9% vs 11.6%, $p_{value} < 0.001$). Birth weight was significantly lower in cases (mean: 2173 g, 95% CI: 829–3277 among cases Vs mean: 3225 g, 95% CI: 2433–4148 among controls, $p_{value} < 0.001$). The distribution of birth weight in the two groups according to the WHO categorisation is displayed in Fig. 1.

Table 1 presents basic demographic and clinical characteristics of cases and controls. Between the two

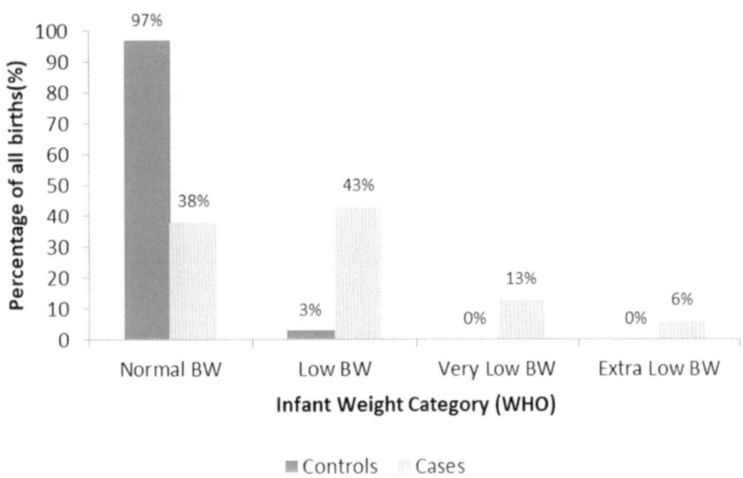

Fig. 1 Distribution of infant weight in births from cases and controls. Distribution of infant weight (according to WHO categorization) among births from cases (preterm pregnancies) and controls (term pregnancies). BW: Birth Weight

Table 1 Distribution of demographic characteristics and maternal risk factors for prematurity among mothers with term (controls) and mother with pre-term deliveries (cases)

Maternal characteristic	Controls *N* (%)	Cases *N* (%)	Statistical Significance†
Demographic			
Age at childbirth[a]	28.8 (18.8–38.7)	30.7 (19.4–41.9)	< 0.001‡
Family status			
Married	339/341 (98.3%)	319/341 (93.6%)	
Divorced	0/341 (0%)	4/341 (1.2%)	0.001
Single	4/341 (1.2%)	18/341 (5.28%)	P_{trend}: < 0.001
Education level			
Primary	35/343 (10.2%)	36/341 (10.6%)	
Secondary	107/343 (31.2%)	110/341 (32.3%)	
Post-secondary	70/343 (20.4%)	73/341 (21.4%)	0.02
Tertiary	116/343 (33.8%)	87/341 (25.5%)	
Post-graduate	15/343 (4.4%)	35/341 (10.3%)	P_{trend}: 0.85
Working Conditions			
Unemployed	77/307 (25.1%)	89/320 (27.8%)	0.44
Partner unemployed	64/338 (18.9%)`	54/321 (16.8%)	0.48
Manual labour	46/232 (19.8%)	76/228 (33.3%)	0.001
Prolonged standing at work	103/232(44.4%)	112/229 (48.9%)	0.33
Working > 8 h per day	27/232 (11.6%)	80/229 (34.9%)	< 0.001
Life-Style			
Smoking before pregnancy	92/340 (27.1%)	97/339 (28.6%)	0.65
Smoking during pregnancy	35/341 (10.3%)	38/339 (11.2%)	0.69
Clinical			
Additional weight gain during pregnancy[a]	12.23 (0.3–23.7)	10.96 (3–24)	0.003‡
Body mass index			
BMI < 20	56/334 (16.8%)	65/279 (23.3%)	
20 < BMI < 25	166/334 (49.7%)	132/279 (47.3%)	
25 < BMI < 30	66/334 (19.8%)	55/279 (19.7%)	0.23
30 < BMI < 35	31/334 (9.3%)	19/279 (6.8%)	
BMI > 35	15/334 (4.5%)	8/279 (2.9%)	P_{trend}: 0.04
Gestational diabetes	74/341 (21.7%)	44/338 (13.0%)	0.003
Clinically diagnosed depression	5/339 (1.5%)	12/339 (3.5%)	0.09
Stress during gestation	12/341 (3.5%)	64/337 (19.0%)	< 0.001

[a]Mean and 95% Confidence Interval
†Independent Sample T test ‡ Pearson Chi Square

groups, there were statistically significant differences in the distributions of maternal age, family status, manual labour, long working hours, additional weight gain during pregnancy, pre-gestation BMI, gestational diabetes, depression and stress during pregnancy. Multivariate analysis demonstrated that significant maternal risk factors for prematurity were age (OR: 1.12,95% CI: 1.06–1.18, $p_{value} < 0.001$), gestational diabetes (OR: 0.53,95% CI: 0.30–0.97, $p_{value} = 0.038$), stress (OR: 8.5, 95% CI: 3.03–23.89, $p_{value} < 0.001$) and long working hours (OR: 3.77, 95% CI: 2.08–6.84, $p_{value} < 0.001$). The results of multivariate analysis for prematurity are summarized in Table 2.

Among the significant maternal risk factors for prematurity, clustering of two or more factors was associated with a sharp increase of prematurity risk as displayed in Table 3. Compared to baseline (no risk factor), the OR for the presence of any one risk factor was 2.37 (95% CI: 1.69–3.32, $p_{value} < 0.001$), the OR for the presence of any two risk factors was 6.13 (95% CI: 3.48–10.80, $p_{value} < 0.001$) and the OR for the presence for any three risk factors was 25.70 (95% CI: 3.31–199.70, $p_{value} = 0.002$). Trend

Table 2 Association between maternal risk factors and prematurity in multivariate analysis

Risk Factor	Contrast	Odds Ratio (95% CI)	*P*-value
Age at child birth	Continuous	1.12 (1.06, 1.18)	< 0.001
Pre-gestation BMI	Continuous	0.96 (0.92, 1.01)	0.11
Gestational diabetes	Categorical	0.53 (0.30, 0.97)	0.04
Depression	Categorical	1.38 (0.25, 7.61)	0.71
Stress	Categorical	8.5 (3.03, 23.89)	< 0.001
Family status	Categorical	1.11 (0.57, 2.15)	0.77
Manual labour	Categorical	1.54 (0.90, 2.65)	0.11
Long working hours	Categorical	3.77 (2.08, 6.84)	< 0.001

test calculation was statistically significant (p_{value} for trend< 0.001). Figure 2, presents the different combinations of significant maternal risk factors in a 3-way Venn diagram. The most frequent combination was advanced maternal age and long working hours (OR: 5.17, 95% CI: 2.60–10.30, $p_{\text{value}} < 0.001$) followed by the combination of advanced maternal age and stress (OR: 9.89, 95% CI:3.66–26.72, $p_{\text{value}} < 0.001$).

Multivariate analysis within the group of preterm infants, demonstrated that stress was the only parameter that was significantly associated with birth weight (β: -323.68, 95% CI: -570.36, -77.00, $p_{\text{value}} = 0.010$). The remaining parameters were not found to significant predictors of birth weight among preterm infants. Table 4 summarizes the results of multivariate analyses for gestational age and infant birth weight within the cases.

Discussion

This is the first study conducted in Cyprus, which investigates socioeconomic risk factors for spontaneous premature labor and low birth weight. Our results indicate that advanced maternal age during childbirth, maternal stress and working conditions, are important predictors for preterm delivery and low birth weight.

During the past three decades, an increase in the average childbearing age has been observed among women in high income countries. In the European Union, the average childbearing age was 29.8 years in 2009, compared to 29.3 in 2003 [21] while a similar trend was observed in Australia [22], Canada [23] and the United Kingdom [24, 25]. In 2016, the mean age of mothers at the first childbirth varied between the European Union Member States. The lowest mean age for the first childbirth was recorded in Bulgaria (26.0 years), followed by Romania (26.4), Latvia (26.8), Slovakia (27.0), Poland (27.2) and Lithuania (27.3). In contrast, the mother's age for the first childbirth was above 30 in Italy (31.0 years), Spain (30.8), Luxembourg (30.5), Greece (30.3) and Ireland (30.1) [26]. In Cyprus, the average childbearing age has increased from 28 to 30.2 years between 1995 and 2015 [23]. Our results are in line with previous findings demonstrating that advanced childbearing age, is a risk factor for premature birth, low birth weight and for adverse pregnancy outcomes such as fetal distress and emergency caesarean section [22, 27, 28]. The increased risk is partly explained by the co-existence of conditions such as diabetes and hypertension [22] and the natural ageing of reproductive tissues which may result in reduced fetal intake of necessary nutrients for intrauterine growth [29].

Table 3 Combined score and associated risk for prematurity

Risk Score[a]	Total Number	Controls (*N* = 343)	Cases (*N* = 342)	OR (95% CI)	*P*-value
0	259	172	87	–	–
1	330	150	180	2.37 (1.69–3.32)	< 0.001
2	82	20	62	6.13 (3.48–10.80)	< 0.001
3	14	1	13	25.70 (3.31–199.70)	0.002

[a]The cumulative individual risk score for each mother was calculated as the sum of values (0 for negative or 1 for positive) for each significant risk factor (long working hours, stress and maternal age). Maternal age was classified as 1 for values ≥30 years old and as 0 for values < 30 years old (30 years was the median value for mother age at childbirth in our dataset)

Unfavorable working conditions, characterised by manual labour and long working hours in particular, were associated with preterm birth among Cypriot women in this study. Previous findings have also demonstrated a positive association of physical exertion related work, long hours and/or shift work with poor pregnancy outcomes [30, 31]. These effects can be attributed to muscles physical stress at work and increased release of catecholamines and arteriol constriction, which causes redistribution of blood flow in the pregnant woman and reduced blood flow to the placenta, as well as hormonal disturbances and nutritional deficits that can also adversely affect fetal growth [32]. Overall, although there is considerable inhomogeneity in the employment settings among the published studies that explore the relationship between working conditions and pregnancy outcomes [33], it is now well documented that long working hours constitute a significant risk factor for premature birth and low birth weight [34, 35].

Maternal stress during pregnancy was also a statistically significant predictor in the occurrence of both preterm birth and low birth weight in our study. Despite the heterogeneity of previous studies' design and approaches to measuring stress, published literature indicates a strong association between stress during pregnancy and risks for premature birth and low birth weight [36, 37]. In a recent Swedish study more than 50% of pregnant women reporting stress during pregnancy experienced a premature labor [37], while other studies besides preterm birth associated stress with low birth weight and low head circumference [38, 39]. As a consequence, it is necessary for pregnant women to be monitored regularly to detect development

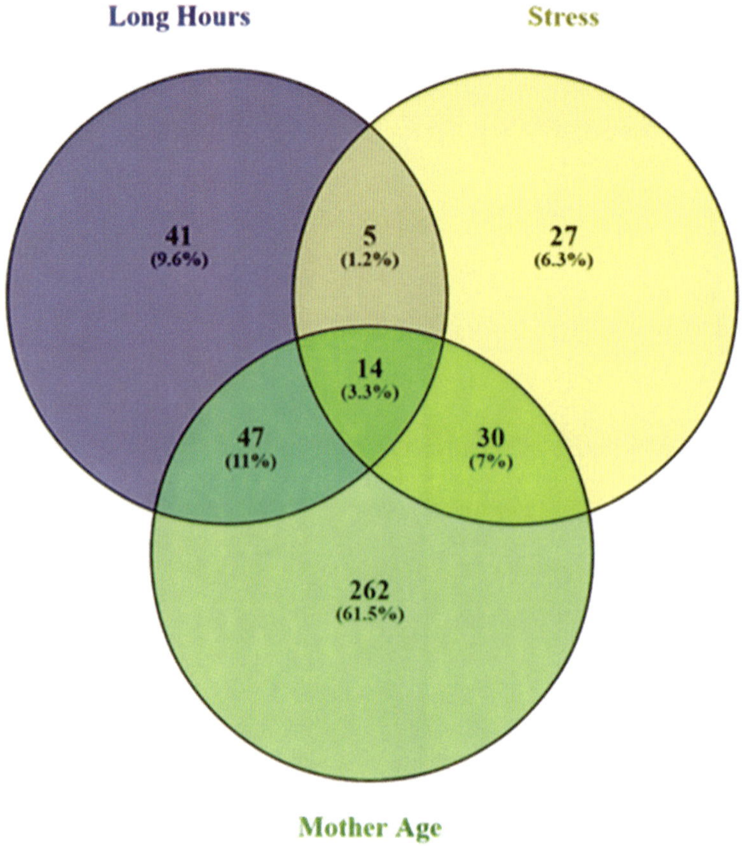

Fig. 2 Overlap of significant risk factors for prematurity. Overlap of risk factors that were found to be significant predictors of prematurity (stress, long working hours, mother age > 30 years)

of stress and other psychological problems [40]. According to the guidelines of the American College of Obstetricians and Gynaecologists, it is recommended that pregnant women are screened at least once every trimester during pregnancy for their psychological condition, irrespectively of the social and educational level, race and ethnicity, and referred for specialised treatment if applicable [40, 41].

In general, gestational diabetes mellitus has been found to be associated with medically indicated premature labor and lower gestational age [42, 43]. However, in our study, we found that the frequency of gestational diabetes was lower in mothers who had premature birth compared to controls. Similar negative associations between pregnancy outcomes and gestational diabetes have been also reported by few recent studies [44, 45]. These discrepancies can be attributed to the possibility of good glycemic control of women with gestational diabetes in these studies through good obstetric monitoring, balanced diet and insulin treatment, factors which have not been specifically assessed in our study [46, 47]. A recent study demonstrated that although presence of uncontrolled gestational diabetes and obesity during pregnancy is associated with negative prognosis, their effects can be counterbalanced by the application of glycaemic control combined with controlled weight gain [48]. Furthermore, comparison with previous studies is inherently difficult as the effect of gestational diabetes on perinatal outcomes is influenced by racial factors [49], the different diagnostic criteria for gestational diabetes that are used in each country, the heterogeneity of study populations and differences in the detection programs that are applied in each country, which

Table 4 Association between maternal risk factors and birth weight within premature infants group

Risk Factor	Contrast	Coefficient (95% CI)	*P*-value
Age at child birth	Continuous	−16.00 (−33.52, 1.54)	0.07
Pre-gestation BMI	Continuous	13.37 (−8.43, 35.16)	0.23
Gestational diabetes	Categorical	201.13 (−69.37, 471.64)	0.14
Depression	Categorical	−34.81 (− 647.09, 577.46)	0.91
Stress	Categorical	−323.68 (−570.36, −77.00)	0.01
Family status	Categorical	145.16 (−66.15, 356.46)	0.18
Manual labour	Categorical	− 154.636 (− 362.05, 52.77)	0.14
Long working hours	Categorical	123.25 (−80.72, 327.22)	0.24

eventually result in a wide range of gestational diabetes frequency from less than 1% to above 10% across the world [46].

This study benefited largely by including data from consecutive births in Cyprus, accurate assessment of study outcomes, a very high response rate and a questionnaire that captured responses on a wide array of socioeconomic factors. However, our study has several limitations, primarily originating from its retrospective nature which precluded the acquisition of participants' detailed clinical data such as obstetric complications [50, 51], use of corticosteroids [52] and other medications that may affect occurrence of premature birth [28] and the type and quality of the provided obstetric care [53]. Like any questionnaire study, this study might have been influenced by subjectivity and recall bias, although factors like family status, working conditions and smoking habits during pregnancy are usually easily recollected characteristics by mothers. Furthermore, assessment of factors, such as emotional stress with the use of a one-time questionnaire during the postpartum period that was not specifically designed to address psychological parameters, might have also introduced some bias in our results [54]. Future studies, need to further explore the findings of the present study in the Cyprus population with a prospective study design and the use of validated instruments for measurement of mental health attributes [55–57]. Furthermore, our study excluded women with multiple pregnancies or infertile women who underwent infertility treatment. As a result, the generalizability of our findings is limited to women with singleton pregnancies following natural conception.

Conclusions

In summary, stress, prolonged working hours and advanced maternal age at childbirth, are associated with increased odds of preterm delivery and low birth weight in Cyprus, while the combination of adverse socioeconomic risk factors appears to have a cumulative effect on the odds of prematurity. Further, prospective, studies should further investigate risk factors for adverse pregnancy outcomes and eventually inform local public health authorities towards the development of evidence-based management protocols to limit premature births and subsequent neonatal complications and related healthcare costs.

Abbreviations

BMI: Body Mass Index; CI: Confidence Intervals; LBW: Low Birth Weight; NICU: Neonatal Intensive Care Unit; OR: Odds Ratio; WHO: World Health Organisation

Acknowledgements

We would like to thank the study participants and the nursing staff of "Archbishop Makarios III" hospital for their cooperation.

Authors' contributions

PSR conceived the hypothesis for this manuscript. PSR and TP collected patient data and performed the field work of the study. PK and PK performed the statistical analysis under the guidance of PKY. AR and PKY contributed to the interpretation of the findings. MT contributed towards the study design, supervised collection of data and contributed to the interpretation of the findings. All authors assisted in the interpretation of findings and critically revised the manuscript. All authors have read and approved the final version of the manuscript.

Competing interests

The authors declare that they have no competing interests

Author details

[1]Neonatal Intensive Care Unit, "Archbishop Makarios III" Hospital, Nicosia, Cyprus. [2]Medical School, University of Cyprus Shakolas Educational Center of Clinical Medicine, Palaios Dromos Lefkosias Lemesou 215/6, 2029 Aglantzia, Nicosia, Cyprus. [3]Apollonion Hospital, Nicosia, Cyprus. [4]Faculty of Economics and Management, Open University of Cyprus, Nicosia, Cyprus.

References

1. Barker DJ, Eriksson JG, Forsén T, Osmond C. Fetal origins of adult disease: strength of effects and biological basis. Int J Epidemiol. 2002;31(6):1235–9.
2. World Health Organisation, Promoting optimal fetal development: report of a technical consultation, 2006 [http://apps.who.int/iris/handle/10665/43409].
3. Offiah I, O'Donoghue K, Kenny L. Clinical risk factors for preterm birth. In: Preterm Birth-Mother and Child. InTech; 2012.
4. Blencowe H, Cousens S, Chou D, Oestergaard M, Say L, Moller A, Kinney M, Lawn J. Born too soon: the global epidemiology of 15 million preterm births. Reprod Health. 2013;10(1):S2.
5. Goldenberg RL, Culhane JF, Iams JD, Romero R. Epidemiology and causes of preterm birth. Lancet. 2008;371(9606):75–84.
6. Comert S, Agzikuru T, Akin Y, Telatar B, Tan PD, Ergen SG, Dervisoglu P. The cost analysis of preterm infants from a NICU of a state Hospital in Istanbul. Iran J Pediatr. 2012;22(2):185–90.
7. Beck S, Wojdyla D, Say L, Betran AP, Merialdi M, Requejo JH, Rubens C, Menon R, Van Look PF: The worldwide incidence of preterm birth: a systematic review of maternal mortality and morbidity. Bull World Health Organ 2010, 88:31–38.
8. Center for Disease Control and Prevention, Preterm Birth, 2018, [https://www.cdc.gov/reproductivehealth/maternalinfanthealth/pretermbirth.htm].
9. Delnord M, Blondel B, Zeitlin J. What contributes to disparities in the preterm birth rate in European countries? Curr Opin Obstet Gynecol. 2015; 27(2):133–42.
10. Macfarlane A, Dattani N: European Perinatal Health Report Health and care of pregnant women and babies in Europe in 2010.
11. Cyprus Health Monitoring Unit, Perinatal health indicators for the year 2014, 2014, [https://www.moh.gov.cy/Moh/MOH.nsf/All/8DC461429CBC4DE7C22579CE002EF07D?OpenDocument].
12. Zeitlin J, Szamotulska K, Drewniak N, Mohangoo A, Chalmers J, Sakkeus L, Irgens L, Gatt M, Gissler M, Blondel B. Preterm birth time trends in Europe: a study of 19 countries. BJOG Int J Obstet Gynaecol. 2013;120(11):1356–65.
13. Shah MK, Gee RE, Theall KP. Partner support and impact on birth outcomes among teen pregnancies in the United States. J Pediatr Adolesc Gynecol. 2014;27(1):14–9.
14. Lawn JE, Cousens S, Zupan J. Lancet neonatal survival steering team: 4 million neonatal deaths: when? Where? Why? Lancet. 2005;365(9462):891–900.
15. OECD/WHO, Health at a Glance Asia/Pacific 2012, OECD Publishing [https://www.oecd-ilibrary.org/social-issues-migration-health/health-at-a-glance-asia-pacific-2012_9789264183902-en].
16. Bian Y, Zhang Z, Liu Q, Wu D, Wang S. Maternal risk factors for low birth weight for term births in a developed region in China: a hospital-based study of 55,633 pregnancies. J Biomed Res. 2013;27(1):14–22.

17. Sullivan KM, Dean A, Soe MM. On academics: OpenEpi: a web-based epidemiologic and statistical calculator for public health. Public Health Rep. 2009;124(3):471–4.
18. Sebayang SK, Dibley MJ, Kelly PJ, Shankar AV, Shankar AH, SUMMIT Study Group. Determinants of low birthweight, small-for-gestational-age and preterm birth in Lombok, Indonesia: analyses of the birthweight cohort of the SUMMIT trial. Tropical Med Int Health. 2012;17(8):938–50.
19. Alijahan R, Hazrati S, Mirzarahimi M, Pourfarzi F, Ahmadi Hadi P. Prevalence and risk factors associated with preterm birth in Ardabil. Iran Iran J Reprod Med. 2014;12(1):47–56.
20. Heberle H, Meirelles GV, da Silva FR, Telles GP, Minghim R: InteractiVenn: a web-based tool for the analysis of sets through Venn diagrams. BMC Bioinformatics 2015, 16(1):169.
21. Kenny LC, Lavender T, McNamee R, O'Neill SM, Mills T, Khashan AS. Advanced maternal age and adverse pregnancy outcome: evidence from a large contemporary cohort. PLoS One. 2013;8(2):e56583.
22. Ludford I, Scheil W, Tucker G, Grivell R. Pregnancy outcomes for nulliparous women of advanced maternal age in South Australia, 1998–2008. Aust N Z J Obstet Gynaecol. 2012;52(3):235–41.
23. Adema W, del Carmen Huerta M, Panzera A, Thevenon O, Pearson M. The OECD family database: developing a cross-national tool for assessing family policies and outcomes. Child Indic Res. 2009;2(4):437.
24. Eurostat, LUCAS micro data 2015 [http://ec.europa.eu/eurostat/web/lucas/data/primary-data/2015].
25. Public Health England, United Kingdom National Statistics, [https://www.ons.gov.uk/peoplepopulationandcommunity/birthsdeathsandmarriages/livebirths/bulletins/birthsbyparentscharacteristicsinenglandandwales/2016].
26. Eurostat, Births and fertility in 2016, 2018, [http://ec.europa.eu/eurostat/documents/2995521/8774296/3-28032018-AP-EN.pdf].
27. Khoshnood B, De Vigan C, Vodovar V, Goujard J, Lhomme A, Bonnet D, Goffinet F. Trends in prenatal diagnosis, pregnancy termination, and perinatal mortality of newborns with congenital heart disease in France, 1983-2000: a population-based evaluation. Pediatrics. 2005;115(1):95–101.
28. Fuchs F, Monet B, Ducruet T, Chaillet N, Audibert F. Effect of maternal age on the risk of preterm birth: a large cohort study. PLoS One. 2018; 13(1):e0191002.
29. Aras RY. Is maternal age risk factor for low birth weight? Archives of Medicine and Health Sciences. 2013;1(1):33.
30. Mozurkewich EL, Luke B, Avni M, Wolf FM. Working conditions and adverse pregnancy outcome: a meta-analysis. Obstet Gynecol. 2000;95(4):623–35.
31. Bonzini M, Coggon D, Palmer KT. Risk of prematurity, low birthweight and pre-eclampsia in relation to working hours and physical activities: a systematic review. Occup Environ Med. 2007;64(4):228–43.
32. Mahmoodi Z, Karimlou M, Sajjadi H, Dejman M, Vameghi M, Dolatian M, Mahmoodi A. Association of maternal working condition with low birth weight: the social determinants of health approach. Annals of medical and health sciences research. 2015;5(6):385–91.
33. Saurel-Cubizolles MJ, Zeitlin J, Lelong N, Papiernik E, Di Renzo GC, Breart G. Europop group: employment, working conditions, and preterm birth: results from the Europop case-control survey. J Epidemiol Community Health. 2004;58(5):395–401.
34. Niedhammer I, O'Mahony D, Daly S, Morrison J, Kelleher C. Occupational predictors of pregnancy outcomes in Irish working women in the Lifeways cohort. BJOG Int J Obstet Gynaecol. 2009;116(7):943–52.
35. Van Melick M, van Beukering M, Mol B, Frings-Dresen M, Hulshof C: Shift work, long working hours and preterm birth: a systematic review and meta-analysis. Int Arch Occup Environ Health 2014, 87(8):835–849.
36. Wadhwa PD, Entringer S, Buss C, Lu MC. The contribution of maternal stress to preterm birth: issues and considerations. Clin Perinatol. 2011;38(3):351–84.
37. Lilliecreutz C, Larén J, Sydsjö G, Josefsson A. Effect of maternal stress during pregnancy on the risk for preterm birth. BMC pregnancy and childbirth. 2016;16(1):5.
38. Su Q, Zhang H, Zhang Y, Zhang H, Ding D, Zeng J, Zhu Z, Li H. Maternal stress in gestation: birth outcomes and stress-related hormone response of the neonates. Pediatrics & Neonatology. 2015;56(6):376 81.
39. Henrichs J, Schenk J, Roza S, Van den Berg M, Schmidt H, Steegers E, Hofman A, Jaddoe V, Verhulst FC, Tiemeier H. Maternal psychological distress and fetal growth trajectories: the generation R study. Psychol Med. 2010;40(4):633–43.
40. American College of Obstetricians and Gynecologists. Psychosocial risk factors: perinatal screening and intervention. ACOG Committee opinion number 343. ObstetrGynecol. 2006;108:469–77.
41. Jomeen J. The importance of assessing psychological status during pregnancy, childbirth and the postnatal period as a multidimensional construct: a literature review. Clin Eff Nurs. 2004;8(3–4):143–55.
42. Gasim T. Gestational diabetes mellitus: maternal and perinatal outcomes in 220 saudi women. Oman Med J. 2012;27(2):140–4.
43. Köck K, Köck F, Klein K, Bancher-Todesca D, Helmer H. Diabetes mellitus and the risk of preterm birth with regard to the risk of spontaneous preterm birth. J Matern Fetal Neonatal Med. 2010;23(9):1004–8.
44. Mahalakshmi MM, Bhavadharini B, Maheswari K, Anjana RM, Jebarani S, Ninov L, Kayal A, Malanda B, Belton A, Uma R, Mohan V, Unnikrishnan R. Current practices in the diagnosis and management of gestational diabetes mellitus in India (WINGS-5). Indian J Endocrinol Metab. 2016;20(3):364–8.
45. Aviram A, Guy L, Ashwal E, Hiersch L, Yogev Y, Hadar E. Pregnancy outcome in pregnancies complicated with gestational diabetes mellitus and late preterm birth. Diabetes Res Clin Pract. 2016;113:198–203.
46. Xiong X, Saunders L, Wang F, Demianczuk N. Gestational diabetes mellitus: prevalence, risk factors, maternal and infant outcomes. Int J Gynecol Obstet. 2001;75(3):221–8.
47. Au CPY, Raynes-Greenow CH, Turner RM, Carberry AE, Jeffery HE. Antenatal management of gestational diabetes mellitus can improve neonatal outcomes. Midwifery. 2016;34:66–71.
48. Benhalima K; Robyns K, Van Crombrugge P, Deprez N, Seynhave B, Devlieger R, Verhaeghe J, Mathieu C, Nobels F: Differences in pregnancy outcomes and characteristics between insulin-and diet-treated women with gestational diabetes. BMC pregnancy and childbirth 2015, 15(1):271.
49. Silva JK, Kaholokula JK, Ratner R, Mau M. Ethnic differences in perinatal outcome of gestational diabetes mellitus. Diabetes Care. 2006;29(9):2058–63.
50. Zhang Y, Liu X, Gao S, Wang J, Gu Y, Zhang J, Zhou X, Li Q. Risk factors for preterm birth in five maternal and child health hospitals in Beijing. PLoS One. 2012;7(12):e52780.
51. Temu TB, Masenga G, Obure J, Mosha D, Mahande MJ. Maternal and obstetric risk factors associated with preterm delivery at a referral hospital in northern-eastern Tanzania. Asian Pacific Journal of Reproduction. 2016;5(5):365–70.
52. Bonanno C, Wapner RJ. Antenatal corticosteroids in the management of preterm birth: are we back where we started? Obstet Gynecol Clin N Am. 2012;39(1):47–63.
53. Beeckman K, Louckx F, Downe S, Putman K. The relationship between antenatal care and preterm birth: the importance of content of care. The European Journal of Public Health. 2012;23(3):366–71.
54. Witt WP, Litzelman K, Cheng ER, Wakeel F, Barker ES. Measuring stress before and during pregnancy: a review of population-based studies of obstetric outcomes. Matern Child Health J. 2014;18(1):52–63.
55. Cohen S, Kamarck T, Mermelstein R. A global measure of perceived stress. J Health Soc Behav. 1983;24(4):385–96.
56. Gunning M, Denison F, Stockley C, Ho S, Sandhu H, Reynolds R. Assessing maternal anxiety in pregnancy with the state-trait anxiety inventory (STAI): issues of validity, location and participation. Journal of Reproductive and Infant Psychology. 2010;28(3):266–73.
57. Sidebottom AC, Harrison PA, Godecker A, Kim H. Validation of the patient health questionnaire (PHQ)-9 for prenatal depression screening. Archives of women's mental health. 2012;15(5):367–74.

Condom use at last sex by young men in Ethiopia: the effect of descriptive and injunctive norms

Aparna Jain[1*], Elizabeth Tobey[1], Hussein Ismail[2] and Annabel Erulkar[2]

Abstract

Background: Condoms are an important prevention method in the transmission of HIV and sexually transmitted infections as well as unintended pregnancy. Individual-level factors associated with condom use include family support and connection, strong relationships with teachers and other students, discussions about sexuality with friends and peers, higher perceived economic status, and higher levels of education. Little, however, is known about the influence of social norms on condom use among young men in Ethiopia. This study examines the effect of descriptive and injunctive norms on condoms use at last sex using the theory of normative social behavior.

Methods: A cross-sectional survey was implemented with 15-24 year old male youth in five Ethiopian regions in 2016. The analytic sample was limited to sexually active single young men ($n = 260$). Descriptive statistics, bivariate and multivariate logistic regressions were conducted. An interaction term was included in the multivariate model to assess whether injunctive norms moderate the relationship between descriptive norms and condom use.

Results: The descriptive norm of knowing a friend who had ever used condoms significantly increased respondents' likelihood of using condoms at last sex. The injunctive norm of being worried about what people would think if they learned that the respondent needed condoms significantly decreased their likelihood to use condoms. The injunctive norm did not moderate the relationship between descriptive norms and condom use. Young men who lived closer to a youth friendly service (YFS) site were significantly more likely to have used condoms at last sex compared to those who lived further away from a YFS site.

Conclusions: Social norms play an important role in decision-making to use condoms among single young men in Ethiopia. The interplay between injunctive and descriptive norms is less straightforward and likely varies by individual. Interventions need to focus on shifting community-level norms to be more accepting of sexually active, single young men's use of condoms and need to be a part of a larger effort to delay sexual debut, decrease sexual violence, and increase gender equity in relationships.

Keywords: Social norms, Condom use, Theory of normative social behavior, Young men, Ethiopia

Plain English summary

Condoms are an important tool to prevent the spread of HIV, sexually transmitted infections, and unwanted pregnancies. Research conducted in Ethiopia and elsewhere has shown various factors that influence young men's use of condoms. One important but understudied factor is the effect of social norms on condom use. This study assessed how social norms influenced whether young men in Ethiopia used condoms the last time they had sex by applying the theory of social normative behavior. Results showed that social norms do affect condom use: young men who knew of friends who had used condoms were more likely to have used condoms at last sex, and young men who were not worried about what people would think of them if they found out they needed condoms were more likely to have used condoms as well. Interventions should look to change community norms by increasing the acceptance of condom use among young men who are sexually active and not married, and this should be a

* Correspondence: apjain@popcouncil.org
[1]Population Council, 4301 Connecticut Avenue NW, Suite 280, Washington DC 20008, USA
Full list of author information is available at the end of the article

part of a larger effort to delay the age of first sex, reduce sexual violence, and promote health masculinities and gender equity.

Background

Eastern and Southern Africa have the highest HIV prevalence rates among young people aged 15–24 in the world with 3.4% of young women and 1.6% of young men living with HIV in 2016 [1]. Though Ethiopia has a relatively low HIV prevalence rate for this region, at 0.4% of young women and 0.5% of young men (UNAIDS 2017) [1], it has the second-highest population in Africa (after Nigeria) at 105 million people in mid-2017 [2]. This large population translates to a high burden of people living with HIV across Ethiopia: in 2016, there were 87,000 young people living with HIV and 8700 new cases among young people across the country [1].

In 2015, the World Health Organization, UNAIDS, and UNFPA issued a position statement encouraging the promotion of condoms to young people, among other populations, as a critical intervention for preventing the spread of HIV, sexually transmitted infections (STIs), and unintended pregnancies [3]. Condom use is also an important indicator for assessing never-married young men's access to family planning and reproductive health (FP/RH) services. Among Ethiopian men aged 25–49, the median age at first marriage is 23.7 and the median age at first sex is 21.2, 2.5 years before marriage [4]. Furthermore, of the 13.8% of never-married men have who had sexual intercourse in the past 12 months with a person who was neither their wife nor a partner who lived with them, only slightly more than half (53.9%) reported using a condom during last sex with such a partner [4].

Several studies have assessed individual-level factors associated with condom use among young men in Ethiopia. Factors that have shown to support the use of condoms include family support and connection, strong relationships with teachers and other students, discussions about sexuality with friends and peers, higher perceived economic status, and higher levels of education [5–7]. Risk factors associated with non-use of condoms or other risky sexual behaviors include low involvement in religious activities, high levels of alcohol consumption, and poor knowledge of HIV/AIDS [5, 8]. Thus, there is a need to focus on increasing use of condoms among young men, for the prevention of HIV, STIs, and unintended pregnancy. There is also a need for interventions to focus on the contextual factors surrounding pre-marital sex by addressing violence in early sexual encounters, and gender equity.

Evidence on the role of social norms in young men's decision making to use condoms is mixed. A study of young adults in rural Ethiopia found that social norms influenced intention to use condoms but not reported use of condoms [9]. In four studies in South Africa, Tanzania, Uganda and Swaziland, where norms were measured by different statements, social norms were shown to influence male and female adolescents' use of condoms [10–13]. However, a study of adolescents in rural Tanzania that examined the role of social norms through statements including the following: "I agree with the opinion of my friends that I should use condoms when having sex" found that norms did not directly predict condom use [14]. These results are inconclusive and do not capture the full range of social norms that can influence behavior.

Theory of normative social behavior

The theory of normative social behavior (TNSB) [15] is a framework used to explain how social norms influence behavior. TNSB distinguishes between two types of social norms: descriptive norms, which are individuals' perceptions about the prevalence of a behavior [16], and injunctive norms, which are perceived social pressures to conform [17, 18]. Injunctive norms influence behavior because failure to conform carries the threat of social sanctions [15]. TNSB holds that both descriptive and injunctive norms directly affect behavior, but that the relationship between descriptive norms and behavior is moderated by injunctive norms, among other factors [15]. This theory has been tested for various health behaviors, including contraceptive use [19], alcohol consumption [20], handwashing [21], and physical activity [22].

The purpose of this study is to explore the role of social norms, both descriptive and injunctive, on condoms use at last sex, and to determine whether injunctive norms moderate the relationship between descriptive norms and condom use among young men in Ethiopia.

Methods

Data

A cross-sectional household survey of 15–24-year-old males living in rural and peri-urban Ethiopia was conducted in Amhara, Benishangul-Gumuz, Oromia, Southern Nations, Nationalities, and Peoples' Region (SNNP), and Tigray regions from January to July 2016. The sampling strategy was designed to measure the effect of distance to a youth friendly service (YFS) health center on utilization of a range of health services. Of 247 eligible YFS sites identified in these regions by the Regional Health Bureaus, 5% were randomly selected for inclusion and the number of sites in each region was determined by probability proportional to size. A total of 14 YFS sites were selected from five regions. One non-YFS health center was randomly selected from each region for comparison.

A stratified, two-stage cluster design was employed where enumeration areas (EAs) were the sampling unit for stage one and selected within 5 km of YFS site, within 5 km of a non-YFS site, and within 5-10 km of a YFS site. Households comprised the second stage and approximately 37 households with eligible respondents were randomly selected per EA, and one respondent per household was selected using a Kish grid [23]. A more detailed description of the sampling strategy is available in the study report [24]. The total number of males interviewed was 1244.

The questionnaires included modules on background characteristics; household characteristics; social cohesion and autonomy; puberty, family planning, and sexual activity; and facility visits for condoms, sexually transmitted infections, HIV, and basic health services. The questionnaires were translated into Amharic, Afan Oromo, and Tigrigna.

Sample population

The sample was limited to 15–24 year old never-married young men who had ever had sexual intercourse. Young men who were married/in-union were excluded from the analysis because they reported low condom use at last sex (1.3%) because they were trying to get pregnant, were in a steady/committed relationship, or because of religious prohibition.

Measures

The dependent variable is condom use at last sex measured by responses to the question "Did you use a condom the last time you had sexual intercourse?". Though this measure does not capture consistent condom use, it is advantageous as it minimizes recall bias by only asking about one recent incidence of sex [25]. Respondents who used a condom at last sex were coded as 1 and those who did not use a condom were coded as 0.

Descriptive norms were measured by asking respondents whether they knew of any friend who had ever used a condom. Respondents who knew of a friend who had ever used condoms were coded as 1 and those who did not know of a friend or were unsure were coded as 0.

Injunctive norms were measured by the following attitudinal statement: "I would be worried about what people in my community would say about me if they found out I needed condoms." This statement was measured on a four-point Likert scale ranging from strongly agree to strongly disagree. The responses were combined to form a dichotomized variable of agree or worry coded as 0 and disagree or not worried coded as 1.

Additional independent variables included in the model were: respondent's age; education; religion; wealth quintile; ownership of personal savings to assess financial autonomy; living with both parents; chewing khat, drinking alcohol, or smoking cigarettes in the past month; distance living away from a YFS facility to assess physical access and presence of age-appropriate services; age at first sex; and whether the respondent had gone for HIV testing or counseling in the last 6 months.

Analysis

Descriptive statistics were calculated for respondent characteristics, dependent and independent variables. Bivariate analyses of condom use at last sex were conducted using Pearson's chi-squared tests and t-tests for significance. Multivariate logistic regression models were used and were adjusted by variables that were statistically significant in the bivariate analysis or were theoretically important. Akaike's Information Criterion (AIC) was employed to compare relative quality and fit of several models, and the model with the lowest AIC was chosen. The final model was run with and without an interaction term to assess the moderating effect of injunctive norms on descriptive norms. The likelihood-ratio test was used to determine if inclusion of the interaction term improved model fit. Lastly, the Hosmer-Lemeshow test was applied to the final model to assess model fit to the data. All analyses were conducted using Stata v15.

Results

Table 1 shows characteristics of sexually active single young men aged 15–24 ($n = 260$). Three out of five (60%) respondents were aged 20–24 years and the median age at first sex was 17 years. Most respondents were out of school at the time of the survey (70%), were living with both parents (64%), and did not have their own savings (72%). Approximately half were Orthodox Christian (49%) and the remaining half were Muslim (41%) or Protestant (10%). Over one-third (37%) of respondents lived within 5 km of a YFS site while 38% lived within 5-10 km, and the remaining quarter (25%) lived within 5 km of a non-YFS site. Respondents were of all wealth quintiles, though the greatest proportion was in the lowest wealth quintile (27%).

Slightly more than half of the sample had either chewed khat, drank alcohol, and/or smoked cigarettes (51%) in the past month. Most respondents had not gone for HIV testing or counseling in the last 6 months (90%), while virtually all respondents knew of HIV (99.6%) and knew that HIV can be transmitted by unprotected sex (96%). Fifty-seven percent of respondents knew of a friend who had ever used a condom (descriptive norm) and 63% agreed that they would be worried about what people in their community would say if they found out the respondent needed condoms (injunctive norm). Two-thirds (66%) of the respondents had ever used condoms and 56% of the sample used a condom at last sex.

Table 2 presents the results of the bivariate analyses for condom use at last sex. Young men who had attended secondary education or higher were significantly more likely to report condom use at last sex (65%) than those had never attended or only attended primary school (49%). Young men who lived < 5 km

Table 1 Respondent Characteristics ($n = 260$)

	Percent	Number
Age		
15–19	40.8	106
20–24	59.2	154
Age at first sex (median, range)	17.0	(10–23)
School status		
In school	30.4	79
Out of school	69.6	181
Education[a]		
Never attended school	4.6	12
Primary	55.0	143
Secondary/technical/vocational/higher	40.0	104
Living with both mother and father		
No	35.8	93
Yes	64.2	167
Has own savings		
No	71.5	186
Yes	28.5	74
Religion		
Muslim	41.2	107
Orthodox Christian	48.8	127
Protestant	10.0	26
Region		
SNNP	24.2	63
Tigray	21.2	55
Amhara/Benishangul-Gumuz	17.3	45
Oromia	37.3	97
Proximity to health facility/YFS		
< 5 km from YFS	36.5	95
5-10 km from YFS	38.5	100
< 5 km from non-YFS	25.0	65
Wealth quintile		
Lowest	26.5	69
Lower	14.2	37
Middle	19.2	50
Higher	20.4	53
Highest	19.6	51
Chewed khat, drank alcohol, smoked cigarettes in past month		
Did not do any behavior	49.2	128
Did one or more behaviors	50.8	132
Has ever heard of HIV		
No	0.4	1
Yes	99.6	259
Knows HIV can be transmitted via unprotected sex[a]		
No	3.5	9
Yes	96.2	250
Has gone for HIV testing or counseling in last 6 months		
No	89.2	232
Yes	10.8	28
Descriptive norm: Knows a friend who has ever used condoms		
No/don't know	43.5	113
Yes	56.5	147
Injunctive norm: "I would be worried about what people in my community would say if they found out I needed condoms"		
Disagree	37.3	97
Agree	62.7	163
Ever used of condoms		
No	33.8	88
Yes	66.2	172
Condom use at last sex		
No	44.2	115
Yes	55.8	145

[a]Percent and number do not add to 100% or 260 due to missing values

from a YFS site were significantly more likely to have used a condom at last sex (65%) compared to those who lived < 5 km from a non-YFS (55%) and those who lived 5-10 km away from a YFS site (47%). Young men living in higher wealth quintiles were more likely than those in lower wealth quintiles to report condom use at last sex, with a range from 67% in the highest wealth quintile to 41% in the lowest.

In terms of norms, condom use at last sex was significantly associated with both descriptive and injunctive norms. Among those who knew of a friend who had ever used a condom (descriptive norm), 67% used a condom at last sex, compared to 41% of those who did not know of a friend who had used condoms. Condom use at last sex was significantly higher among young men who disagreed with the measure of injunctive norm: those who disagreed (that is, would not worried about what people would say if they found out the respondent needed condoms) were significantly more likely to have used condoms at last sex (65%) than those who agreed (50%).

A t-test was conducted to determine if mean age at first sex differed for those who used condoms at last sex and those who did not. The mean age was 17.2 for both populations, and the difference was not significant (data not shown). Since nearly all respondents reported HIV awareness and knowledge that unprotected sex can transmit HIV, these two measures were excluded from bivariate and multivariate analysis.

Table 2 Bivariate analysis of condom use at last sex ($n = 260$)

	Condom use at last sex (%)
Age	
15–19	59.4
20–24	53.2
School status	
In school	60.8
Out of school	53.6
Education	
Never attended school/Primary	49.0
Secondary/technical/vocational/higher	65.4*
Living with both mother and father	
No	58.1
Yes	54.5
Has own savings	
No	52.2
Yes	64.9
Religion	
Orthodox	50.4
Muslim	61.7
Protestant	57.7
Region	
Oromia	53.6
Tigray	50.9
Amhara/Benishangul-Gumuz	53.3
SNNP	65.1
Proximity to health facility/YFS	
< 5 km from YFS	65.3*
5-10 km from YFS	47.0
< 5 km from non-YFS	55.4
Wealth quintile	
Lowest	40.6
Lower	54.1
Middle	52.0
Higher	69.8
Highest	66.7**
Chewed khat, drank alcohol, smoked cigarettes in past month	
Did not do any behavior	58.6
Did one or more behaviors	53.0
Has gone for HIV testing or counseling in last 6 months	
No	54.7
Yes	64.3
Descriptive norm: Knows a friend who has ever used condoms	
No/don't know	40.7
Yes	67.3**
Injunctive norm: "I would be worried about what people in my community would say if they found out I needed condoms"	
Disagree	64.9
Agree	50.3*

* *p*-value ≤0.05; ** *p*-value ≤0.01

Table 3 presents the adjusted odds ratios (AORs) of the effect of descriptive and injunctive norms on condom use at last sex, adjusting for respondent characteristics, distance to a YFS facility, and use of khat, alcohol, or cigarettes. Though theoretically relevant and shown elsewhere as significant predictors to condom use at last sex, we removed five variables from the multivariate model because these measures were not significant in the bivariate analysis, and to ensure a stronger fit of the data: age at first sex, school status, living with mother and father, has own savings, and used HIV testing or counseling in the past 6 months.

The likelihood-ratio test was used to test the difference between the model with the interaction term of injunctive and descriptive norms and the model without the interaction. The test was borderline significant with a *p*-value of 0.0952. The final model presented in Table 3 includes the interaction term.

Among respondents who agreed with the injunctive norm statement (would be worried about what people in their community would say if they found out they needed condoms), those who knew of a friend who had ever used condoms were 4.7 times (95% CI: 2.26–9.95) more likely to use condoms at last sex than those who did not have a friend who had used condoms. Furthermore, among respondents who did not know of a friend who had ever used a condom, those who disagreed with the injunctive norm statement (or would not be worried) were 3.4 times (95% CI: 1.38–8.35) more likely to have used a condom at last sex compared to those who agreed with the statement. The interaction term of descriptive norm × injunctive norm was not statistically significant, and no synergistic effect of condom use at last sex was observed.

Respondents who lived 5-10 km away from a YFS facility were significantly less likely to have used a condom at last sex compared to those who lived within 5 km of a YFS site (AOR = 0.46, 95% CI: 0.23–0.92). There was no significant difference in the odds of condom use at last sex for those who lived within 5 km from a non-YFS site compared to those who lived within 5 km from a YFS site. No significant difference was observed among those who lived 5-10 km from YFS to those who lived < 5 km from non-YFS in condom use at last sex (data not shown). Those who lived in the higher wealth quintile were

Table 3 Adjusted odds ratios of condom use at last sex ($n = 260$)

	AOR	95% CI
Age		
15–19	ref	
20–24	0.61	(0.33–1.12)
Education		
Never attended school/Primary	ref	
Secondary/technical/vocational/higher	1.84	(0.99–3.42)
Religion		
Orthodox Christian	ref	
Muslim	2.07	(0.96–4.45)
Protestant	1.63	(0.51–5.23)
Region		
Oromia	ref	
Tigray	1.12	(0.46–2.71)
Amhara/Benshangul-Gumuz	1.07	(0.44–2.63)
SNNP	1.67	(0.72–3.87)
Proximity to health facility/YFS		
< 5 km from YFS	ref	
5-10 km from YFS	0.46*	(0.23–0.92)
< 5 km from non-YFS	0.47	(0.22–1.05)
Wealth quintile		
Lowest	ref	
Lower	2.31	(0.87–6.14)
Middle	1.64	(0.70–3.85)
Higher	3.10*	(1.24–7.73)
Highest	1.99	(0.79–4.99)
Chewed khat, drank alcohol, smoked cigarettes in past month		
Did not do any behavior	ref	
Did one or more behaviors	0.88	(0.45–1.70)
Descriptive Norm: Knows a friend who has ever used condoms		
Yes	4.74**	(2.26–9.95)
Injunctive norm: "I would be worried about what people in my community would say if they found out I needed condoms"		
Disagree	3.39**	(1.38–8.35)
Descriptive norm × Injunctive norm		
Descriptive Norm: Yes × Injunctive Norm: Disagree	0.37	(0.12–1.19)

* *p*-value ≤0.05; ** *p*-value ≤0.01

significantly more likely to have used a condom at last sex than those in the lowest quintile (AOR = 3.10, 95% CI: 1.24–7.73).

The Hosmer-Lemeshow goodness-of-fit test demonstrated that the model fits the data reasonably well ($p = 0.601$).

Discussion

The purpose of this study was to assess the role of social norms in condom use at last sex among sexually active single young men in Ethiopia. Using the TNSB, the study looked at how perceptions of friends' use of condoms (descriptive norm) and worry of what community members would say if they learned that the respondent needed condoms (injunctive norm) influenced condom use at last sex. This study also explored whether the injunctive norm moderated the relationship between the descriptive norm and condom use. The results show that, in the context of never-married, sexually active young men in Ethiopia, while descriptive and injunctive norms individually influence condom use at last sex, injunctive norms do not moderate the relationship between descriptive norms and condom use.

A study of contraceptive use using the TNSB framework in India also found that injunctive norms do not have a strong moderating effect on the relationship between descriptive norms and behavior [19]. Condom use, like contraceptive use, is a semi-private behavior in that it generally occurs between partners with limited public knowledge of the behavior. The lack of moderation may have occurred because private behaviors are not observed by others and are thus not subjected to the same levels of public scrutiny or stigma as public behaviors. In addition, the lack of moderation on condom use suggests that descriptive and injunctive norms may function differently for individuals and their interaction is more complex.

The study results are important for the Ethiopian government to reach its ambitious goals related to HIV knowledge, condom use and HIV testing and counseling by 2020 [26]. Different programmatic strategies with young men need to be tested and evaluated. For instance, the Ethiopian government is exploring the inclusion of FP/RH and HIV education in school-based programming [26]. In our sample, the vast majority (95%) had attended at least primary school, though only 40% went on to secondary school. Using primary schools as a space where age-appropriate information can be shared about FP/RH and HIV at earlier ages may provide young men with the knowledge and tools that they need to make better and safer decisions around condom use in the future.

The study results also showed that respondents who are worried and concerned about how they would be perceived if others in their community learned that they needed condoms suggest that even in a place like Ethiopia, where condoms are relatively ubiquitous, fear of how one who uses condoms is perceived can weigh heavily on adopting protective behaviors. As has been shown with programs to delay girls' marriage [27, 28], the Ethiopian government may consider holding community conversations to engage young men and their parents to begin addressing social norms that restrict adolescents from using condoms, especially in rural areas where traditional notions forbidding pre-marital sex exist.

The study showed that unmarried young men who know of a friend who has used condoms are more likely to use condoms themselves suggests that communication and sharing of information within social and peer networks is important in changing behaviors. Condom use is by and large a private behavior that is not explicitly known or seen by others. Knowledge of a friend's use of condoms would likely occur in discussions and so if young men brag to their friends about sex [29, 30], then perhaps the narrative around sexual discourse has changed to also include condom use. A study in Ethiopia showed that discussions about sexuality with friends had a positive association with condom use, though "discussions of sexuality" was not well defined [6]. Condom use may be also considered a sign of autonomy or increased status, where young men can obtain condoms without shame. The government may consider creating young mens' groups to engage unmarried young men in a range of health and relationship issues, including the importance of condoms use, and to provide referrals to facilities for HIV counseling and testing.

The study also showed that respondents who lived closer to a YFS facility were significantly more likely to use condoms at last sex compared to those who lived further away from a YFS facility, and marginally more likely than those who lived close to a non-YFS facility. This finding suggests that proximity to a facility, especially one that has received programmatic interventions to increase its youth friendliness, is important to young men's use of condoms at last sex. Ethiopia is scaling YFS sites across the country, and this may additionally contribute to increased condom use among young men. The results of this study suggest that increasing YFS, however, is not sufficient to increase condom use - social norms also must be addressed.

Interventions aimed at increasing condom use and addressing social norms should also focus on greater contextual factors in Ethiopia. Because early sexual encounters in Ethiopia are often in the context of force or coercion [6, 31, 32], interventions should consider the role of gender-based violence and inequitable gender norms in condom use. For young women and girls in Ethiopia, the formation of girls' groups and community conversations about child marriage were shown to be effective not only in raising the age at marriage [27, 28], but also in increasing FP/RH knowledge and voluntary contraceptive use [27]. Adaptations of these interventions may include forming young men's groups and convening community conversations to engage young men, their parents, and community leaders to begin shifting social norms that inhibit condom use and address gender norms, raise the age of sexual debut, and decrease gender-based violence among young people in Ethiopia.

Further research is necessary especially on positive deviants, that is the young men who did use condoms at last sex, to understand the pathways that lead to them to this decision including where they first heard about condoms, how they learned to use them or where to get them, negotiating with their partner, among many other issues.

Examining the factors associated with condom use at last sex among young males is paramount, as there is evidence to suggest that decision-making on condom use rests predominantly with males [6]. Efforts to examine and increase condom use must therefore include and target boys and young men, as the present study has, and empower them to access and use condoms. However, social change is also critical to enable inclusion of girls and young women in the discourse around condoms, so that condom decision-making becomes more equitable between partners.

Study limitation

A limitation of this study is the lack of temporality. Because this is a cross-sectional survey, it is not certain that knowledge of friend's use of condoms influenced condom use at last sex or whether use of condoms at last sex influenced the respondent to discuss condoms with their friends. Either way, communication around condom use with friends and peers appears to be important.

Conclusions

This study examined condom use at last sex among single young men in rural Ethiopia through the theory of normative social behavior to assess the relationship of descriptive and injunctive norms on behavior. More than half of single young men used condoms at last sex. Those who knew of a friend who had used condoms (descriptive norm), and who were not worried about what members of their community would say if they found out they needed condoms (injunctive norms) were more likely to use condoms at last sex, though there was no moderating effect of injunctive norms. Young men who lived close to a YFS site were also more likely to use condoms at last sex. The results of this study suggest that social change is needed to improve access to and use of condoms at last sex in Ethiopia.

Abbreviations

AIC: Akaike's information criterion; AIDS: Acquired immune deficiency syndrome; AOR: Adjusted odds ratio; CI: Confidence interval; FP/RH: Family planning and reproductive health; HIV: Human immunodeficiency virus; SNNP: Southern Nations, Nationalities, and Peoples' Region; STI: Sexually transmitted infection; TNSB: Theory of normative social behavior; UNAIDS: Joint United Nations Programme on HIV and AIDS; UNFPA: United Nations Population Fund; USAID: United States Agency for International Development; WHO: World Health Organization; YFS: Youth friendly services

Acknowledgements

We thank Lemi Negeri who served as a research coordinaor during this study. We also thank the research assistants and drivers who collected the data in Ethiopia. We sincerely thank our colleagues Mihira Karra, Erika Martin, and Erika Houghtaling of USAID for their feedback on the manuscript. The manuscript benefitted from feedback received at the IUSSP conference held in Cape Town, South Africa, in November 2017, where it was presented as an oral presentation. Finally, we are grateful to the youth who participated in the study and shared their time and experiences.

Funding

The Evidence Project is made possible by the generous support of the American people through the United States Agency for International Development (USAID) under the terms of cooperative agreement no. AIDOAA-A-13-00087. The contents of this manuscript are the sole responsibility of the Evidence Project and Population Council and do not necessarily reflect the views of USAID or the United States Government.

Authors' contributions

AJ was the Principal Investigator for the study, conceptualized the article, carried out analyses and contributed to writing of all sections of the manuscript. ET carried out analyses and contributed to writing of all sections. HI was Co-Principal Investigator on the study. HI and AE contributed to study conceptualization and data collection and provided substantive comments to the manuscript. All authors read multiple drafts and approved the final manuscript.

Competing interests

The authors declare that they have no competing interests.

Author details

[1]Population Council, 4301 Connecticut Avenue NW, Suite 280, Washington DC 20008, USA. [2]Population Council, Heritage Plaza, 4th floor, Bole Medhaneialem Road, Addis Ababa, Ethiopia.

References

1. UNAIDS: AIDSinfo. http://aidsinfo.unaids.org (2017). Accessed 26 Oct 2017.
2. Population Reference Bureau. 2017 World population data sheet. Washington, DC: Population Reference Bureau; 2017.
3. UNAIDS. UNFPA, WHO and UNAIDS: Position statement on condoms and the prevention of HIV, other sexually transmitted infections and unintended pregnancy.(2015) http://www.unaids.org/en/resources/presscentre/featurestories/2015/july/20150702_condcon_prevention. Accessed 26 Oct 2017.
4. Central Statistical Agency (CSA) [Ethiopia] and ICF. Ethiopia Demographic and Health Survey 2016. Addis Ababa, Ethiopia, and Rockville, Maryland: CSA and ICF; 2016.
5. Abebe M, Tsion A, Netsanet F. Living with parents and risky sexual behaviors among preparatory school students in Jimma zone, south West Ethiopia. Afr Health Sci. 2013;13(2):498–506.
6. Bogale A, Seme A. Premarital sexual practices and its predictors among in-school youths of shendi town, west Gojjam zone, North Western Ethiopia. Reprod Health. 2014;11:49.
7. Maria W. Sexual behaviour, knowledge and awareness of related reproductive health issues among single youth in Ethiopia. Afr J Reprod Health. 2007;11(1):14–21.
8. Kassa G, Degu G, Yitayew M, Misganaw W, Muche M, Demelash T, Mesele M, Ayehu M. Risky sexual behaviors and associated factors among Jiga high school and preparatory school students, Amhara region, Ethiopia. Int Sch Res Notices. 2016;2016:1–7. https://doi.org/10.1155/2016/4315729.
9. Molla M, Nordrehaug Åstrøm A, Brehane Y. Applicability of the theory of planned behavior to intended and self-reported condom use in a rural Ethiopian population. AIDS Care. 2007;19(3):425–31.
10. Bryan A, Kagee A, Broaddus M. Condom use among south African adolescents: developing and testing theoretical models of intentions and behavior. AIDS Behav. 2006;10(4):387–97.
11. Eggers S, Aarø L, Bos A, Mathews C, Kaaya S, Onya H, de Vries H. Sociocognitive predictors of condom use and intentions among adolescents in three sub-Saharan sites. Arch Sex Behav. 2015;45(2):353–65.
12. Sacolo H, Chung M, Chu H, Liao Y, Chen C, Ou K, Chang L, Chou K. High risk sexual behaviors for HIV among the in-school youth in Swaziland: a structural equation modeling approach. PLoS One. 2013;8(7):e67289.
13. Rijsdijk L, Bos A, Lie R, Ruiter R, Leerlooijer J, Kok G. Correlates of delayed sexual intercourse and condom use among adolescents in Uganda: a cross-sectional study. BMC Public Health. 2012;12:817.
14. Kalolo A, Kibusi S. The influence of perceived behaviour control, attitude and empowerment on reported condom use and intention to use condoms among adolescents in rural Tanzania. Reprod Health. 2015;12(1):105.
15. Rimal R, Real K. How behaviors are influenced by perceived norms: a test of the theory of normative social behavior. Commun Res. 2005;32(3):389–414.

16. Cialdini R, Reno R, Kallgren C. A focus theory of normative conduct: recycling the concept of norms to reduce littering in public places. J Pers Soc Psychol. 1990;58(6):1015–26.
17. Rimal R, Real K. Understanding the influence of perceived norms on behaviors. Commun Theor. 2003;13(2):184–203.
18. Lapinski M, Rimal R. An explication of social norms. Commun Theor. 2005; 15(2):127–47.
19. Rimal R, Sripad P, Speizer I, Calhoun L. Interpersonal communication as an agent of normative influence: a mixed method study among the urban poor in India. Reprod Health. 2015;12:71.
20. Jang S, Rimal R, Cho N. Normative influences and alcohol consumption: the role of drinking refusal self-efficacy. Health Commun. 2013;28(5):443–51.
21. Lapinski M, Anderson J, Shugart A, Todd E. Social influence in child care centers: a test of the theory of normative social behavior. Health Commun. 2014;29(3):219–32.
22. Priebe CS, Spink KS. When in Rome: descriptive norms and physical activity. Psychol Sport Exerc. 2011;12(2):93–8.
23. Kish L. A procedure for objective respondent selection within the household. J Am Stat Assoc. 1949;44(247):380–7.
24. Jain A, Ismail H, Tobey E, Erulkar A. Understanding adolescent and youth sexual and reproductive health-seeking behaviors in Ethiopia: implications for youth friendly service programming. Washington, DC: Population Council; 2017.
25. MEASURE Evaluation. Condom use at last high-risk sex. In: Family planning and reproductive health indicators database; 2017. https://www.measureevaluation.org/prh/rh_indicators/womens-health/stis-hiv-aids/condom-use-at-last-high-risk-sex. Accessed 26 Oct. 2017.
26. Ministry of Health of Ethiopia. National adolescent and youth health strategy (2016–2020). Addis Ababa: Federal Democratic Republic of Ethiopia; 2017.
27. Erulkar A, Muthengi E. Evaluation of Berhane Hewan: a program to delay child marriage in rural Ethiopia. Int Perspect Sex Reprod Health. 2009;35(1):6–14.
28. Erulkar A, Medhin G, Weissman E. The impact and cost of child marriage prevention in three African settings. Addis Ababa. New York: Population Council; 2017.
29. Selikow T, Ahmed N, Flisher A, Mathews C, Mukoma W. I am not "umqwayito": a qualitative study of peer pressure and sexual risk behavior among young adolescents in Cape Town, South Africa. Scand J Public Healt. 2009;37(Suppl 2):107–12.
30. Izugbara C. Notions of sex, sexuality and relationships among adolescent boys in rural southeastern Nigeria. Sex Educ. 2004;4(1):63–79.
31. Annabel Erulkar, Abebaw Ferede, (2009) Social Exclusion and Early or Unwanted Sexual Initiation Among Poor Urban Females in Ethiopia. International Perspectives on Sexual and Reproductive Health. 35(04):186–93.
32. Lelissa G, Yusuf L. A Cross Sectional Study on Prevalence of Gender Based Violence in Three High Schools, Addis Ababa, Ethiopia. Ethiop J Reprod Health.

A survival analysis of the timing of onset of childbearing among young females in Nigeria: are predictors the same across regions?

Michael O N Kunnuji[1*], Idongesit Eshiet[1] and Chinyere C P Nnorom[2]

Abstract

Background: Early childbearing comes at high health costs to girls, the children they bear, their future life chances and the larger society. Nationally representative data suggest variation in onset of childbearing across regions and states of the country. Yet, there is need for strong evidence on how background characteristics explain time to first birth among young females across regions in Nigeria.

Methods: We analysed the 2013 DHS dataset using Kaplan Meier and Cox Regression. The outcome variable is age at onset of childbearing with location (rural/urban), education, religion, wealth index, region and having ever married/cohabited as covariates. Models were computed for national level analysis and the six regions of the country.

Results: The effect of marriage/cohabitation on time to first birth is strong and universal across the regions. Ever married girls had higher adjusted hazard ratios for starting childbearing than single girls, ranging from 5.35 in the South South to 44.62 in the North West ($p < 0.001$ in all models). Education also has significant effect on time to first birth across regions. The significance of state of residence, wealth, and religion varies across regions.

Conclusion: We conclude that the combinations of factors that explain onset of childbearing vary across regions. Therefore, context specific factors should be considered in program designs aimed at achieving a significant reduction in early childbearing and similar problems in Nigeria.

Keywords: Adolescent childbearing, Regional variation in Nigeria, Early marriage and cohabitation, Reproductive health, Survival analysis, Wealth

Plain English summary

When compared to adolescents within the age group of 10 and 19 years in other countries of the world, a large proportion of adolescents in Nigeria give birth to babies. The problem with adolescents giving birth is that the experience of childbearing often results in ill health for the adolescents and their babies. In addition, it affects the future of these adolescents and their babies. The adolescent mothers are often not able to continue with their education, or to acquire any meaningful training that will allow them get good jobs later in life. Previous research on the health of people in Nigeria tells us that in Nigeria, girls in certain regions, especially the northern zones are more likely to start having children than those from the southern zones, but we are yet to know whether the factors that predispose adolescents to childbearing are the same across regions. We used survival analysis to show the factors that determine how much time it takes adolescents in different regions to begin childbearing. At the national level, empirical evidence suggest that the predictors of the timing of onset of childbearing include being ever married/having ever lived with a man as if married, the zone in which an adolescent is located, how rich or poor an adolescent is, literacy and education. In the different regions, we still found that being ever married/having ever lived with a man as if married is a constant predictor of onset of childbearing. Other factors

* Correspondence: michaelkunnuji@gmail.com
[1]Department of Sociology, University of Lagos, Lagos, Nigeria
Full list of author information is available at the end of the article

such as state of residence, how rich or poor one is, religion and education can also help us understand the onset of childbearing in some of the regions. We conclude that the combination of factors that explain onset of childbearing vary across regions and context specific factors should be considered in program designs aimed at achieving a significant reduction in early childbearing among young people.

Background

Nigeria, the most populous country in Africa with a 2017 population of 191 million has an adolescent birth rate of 122 births per 1000 women ages 15 to 19 years [1]. About 74% of adolescent girls who give birth in the country do so at home [2] and they are exposed to many child delivery-related complications [3, 4] and poor birth outcomes [5]. Early childbearing is also a risk factor for cervical cancer [6]. In addition, research shows that early childbearing, typically before the age of 16 years, is associated with an increased risk of maternal anemia, infections, eclampsia and preeclampsia, emergency cesarean delivery, postpartum depression and inadequate breastfeeding initiation [7]. Studies further show that infants of teenage mothers are more likely to be premature and have a low birth weight [8], and are at an increased risk for respiratory distress syndrome and autism later in life [7].

Apart from these reproductive health implications, early childbearing comes at high socio-economic cost to girls and the society at large. It is associated with low educational attainment [8–10], high likelihood of staying unmarried [9, 11], marital instability, overall poor socio-economic status and welfare dependency in adult life [9–11] and lower levels of children's education [8]. Also, it leads to stigma with psychological effects such as shame and guilt [12]. In terms of longevity, teenage mothers have lower life expectancy when compared with non-teen mothers [8]. By implication, early childbearing has negative implications for girls, their children and the society at large.

A number of studies have explored probable determinants of early childbearing, often implicating social and environmental factors. For instance, some studies show that girls living in underserved or high-poverty communities are at a high risk of beginning childbearing early [11–13] or teenage pregnancy (whether they carry the pregnancy to term or not) [14]. Early childbearing is also associated with low educational aspiration, dropping out of school and having friends, majority of whom have experienced pregnancy or are teenage mothers [11, 15] or having older sexually active siblings/pregnant or parenting sisters or having suffered sexual abuse [16]. The diversity of Nigeria which we present in the paragraph that follows explains why it is important to explore the predictors of time to first birth differently for different regions of the country.

The Nigerian population is made up of about 374 ethnic groups [2] which are politically organised into 36 states. The 36 states are often clustered into six regions/regions – North Central, North East and North West, South East, South South and South West [2] each composed of contiguous states with approximately similar ethnic groups. The North West region is home to the Hausa and Fulani Ethnic groups. In the North East region, the Kanuri, Hausa and Fulani are the majority ethnic groups but the zone is also inhabited by several smaller ethnic groups. The North Central zone is inhabited by several of Nigeria's minority groups such as the Nupe, Tiv, Idoma and Gbagi. The majority ethnic group in the South West is the Yoruba while the Igbo are the majority ethnic group in the South East. The South South is occupied by minority ethnic groups such as the Edo, Urhobo, Itsekiri, Izon, Ibibio/Efik etc. [17]. The people in the North West and North East zones are mainly Muslims while those in the South South and South East are mainly Christians. The South West and North Central zones have mixed populations of Christians and Muslims. Generally, development indicators are better in the southern regions than the northern regions. For example, mean years of schooling are higher in the southern regions than the northern regions. On the other hand, gender inequality index is highest in the North West, followed by the North East and the North Central. Similarly, poverty is higher in the three northern regions than in any of the southern regions [18].

A recent study explained regional variation in adolescent childbearing with a model for each of the regions in Nigeria [19] focusing on first births in adolescence, as well as long after adolescence among adults in Nigeria. Consequently, the analysis includes young people and adults up to the age of 49 years. In addition, the study fails to include entry into marital union/cohabitation which is a potential predictor of onset of childbearing [20–22] and (dis)continuation of education [23, 24]. By implication, understanding adolescent childbearing requires controlling the confounding effect of entry into marriage/cohabitation. The current study of adolescents and young people includes entry into marriage or cohabitation as a covariate in explaining the onset of childbearing, contrary to the technique adopted by the mentioned previous study.

Prevalence of adolescent childbearing varies significantly across Nigeria's regions, suggesting that region is a predictor of age at first birth [2]. Apart from region, our preliminary unadjusted national level analysis shows that factors such as living in a rural community, having little or no education, being a Muslim, and not having access to wealth also contribute to the explanation of early childbearing. Although region is a strong predictor of variance, young girls within the same region also have varied chances of becoming mothers. We ask, therefore: In the different regions of the country, what are the significant background predictors of time to first birth? Our study set out to answer this question. The danger in relying on a single explanatory model in the explanation of onset of childbearing in Nigeria is that predictive factors may differ across regions and sub-national differences may be subsumed in a national level analysis. Consequently, interventions designed on this limited understanding of the sexuality of young people across regions may fail simply because they are not context specific.

Explaining variation in time to first birth across regions in Nigeria

A theory for regional variance in the persistence of traditional norms and resistance to international norms is found in the explanation that socio-cultural context and degree of conservatism due to religious beliefs are an important factor [25, 26]. Certain religious teachings hold the view that menarche signifies that a girl is ripe for motherhood. For instance, child-marriage is common in the Hausa-Fulani dominated Northwestern region of Nigeria where Islam is used to justify the prescription that the girl child should be married off before or at menarche to prevent premarital sex and out-of-wedlock births [27, 28]. Behind the veil of religion, however, the tradition of polygyny and poverty are major factors associated with child marriage [27, 29]. Girls married off or made to live with men under such circumstances are exposed to sex, pregnancy and childbearing. One can therefore hypothesize that entry into marriage/cohabitation will be a universal predictor of onset of childbearing.

Location may also explain time to first birth as spelt out in the metropocentric explanation [30]. The explanation holds that communities within major cities in Nigeria are better served by government in terms of provision of infrastructure and services than communities in the periphery of the state. This argument applies to access to education and reproductive health information and services which are potential predictors of reproductive health behaviour. In contexts where the theory holds, living in a rural community may reduce time to first birth as access to campaigns on the negative implications of early childbearing and access to reproductive health information and services may be limited. Against the backdrop of these explanations, we seek to identify specific predictors of time to first birth in each of the regions of Nigeria. These explanations draw from the ecological and contextual frameworks which recognise macro level factors that set the contexts that influence community, family, school and peer factors which in turn influence entry into marital unions and onset of childbearing among young females [31–33]. Ecological and contextual frameworks emphasise conceptual issues relating to the context in which reproductive health behaviour takes place and enhance the effectiveness of research and innovations on the subject matter. In the context of this study, the framework helps us explore the influence of contextual factors such as location, education, religion and entry into marital unions on the onset of childbearing.

Methods

This study employs the 2013 Nigeria Demographic and Health Survey which is a nationally representative study that administered a structured questionnaire to 17,359 men and 38,948 women (15–49 years) across the 36 states and Federal Capital Territory of Nigeria. The survey covers a wide range of topics, including fertility, entry into marital union, reproductive health, domestic violence etc. We extracted the data for all the young females (15–24 years), a total of 14,619 respondents included in the study for the purpose of this analysis. Details about the DHS sampling techniques and sample size are available at http://www.dhsprogram.com/. The Nigeria DHS research protocol complies with the WHO ethical and safety recommendations and the National Health Research Ethics Committee guidelines. We did not gather primary data for the study, so we did not require any further ethical approval outside the approval obtained by the National Population Commission and ICF International.

This is a time-to-event analysis which models time (in years) until the event of first childbirth [34, 35]. We used the Kaplan-Meier test to estimate mean ages at first birth for different categories of young females. Kaplan-Meier survival estimate is mathematically denoted by

$$S(t_j) = S(t_{j-1})\left(1 - \frac{d_j}{n_j}\right).$$

The computation represents the cumulative probability of not having started childbearing at a given time t_j, where n_j is the number of young females yet to begin childbearing just before t_j and d_j the number of first childbirths at t_j. We present estimated mean ages for categories of young females and use the Log Rank test to compare means for significant difference. Survival functions for background characteristics are presented in charts.

We used the Cox proportional hazards models to estimate the probability that an individual will have first childbirth around a particular point in time. The model is written as

$$h(t) = h_0(t) \times \exp\{b_1 x_1 + b_2 x_2 + \ldots + b_p x_p\}.$$

Adjusted hazard ratios comparing young females of different categories with reference groups are presented and flagged where they are statistically different from the reference categories in seven models, the first for the entire national sample of young females and one for each of the six regions. Age at first child birth was used as the Time variable while having had a child is the event of interest. Covariates included in the analysis are place of residence (rural/urban), highest educational qualification, religion, being ever married/having ever cohabited, wealth index and state. In the national level analysis, region was used instead of state. All the covariates are categorical and the first category was used as the reference category in all the models.

Results

The background characteristics of the study participants are presented in Table 1. As the table shows, about 60% of the respondents were drawn from the rural parts of Nigeria, 54% of them had secondary education (about 12 years of formal education) and 56% were single/never married. The table further shows that 36% of them had begun having children.

Estimated mean ages at first birth

The results presented in Table 2 show that the Kaplan-Meier estimated mean age at first birth is higher in urban areas than rural areas (21.83 vs 19.67), and among single/never married young females than those who had ever married/cohabited (23.35 vs 18.33). The results further reveal that the mean age at first birth increases with education and wealth index. For the different regions, the estimated mean ages at first birth range from 18.81 years in the North West to 22.29 years in the South East. The Cox regression model shows that only education, wealth index, having ever married/cohabited, and region are significant predictors of time to first birth at the national level when background characteristics are adjusted for as shown by the adjusted hazard ratios in Table 2.

The North East, North West and South South have significantly higher adjusted hazard ratios (1.24, 1.21 and 1.45, $p < 0.001$) than the North Central region as shown in Table 2. The South West also has a marginally higher adjusted hazard ratio (1.14, $p < 0.05$). Figure 1 further shows the variableness of the proportion of young females who have begun childbearing across the states of the federation. The proportion is least in Osun state (13.2%) and highest in Jigawa state (66.3%). In the whole of Nigeria, 36.4% have begun childbearing. The highest proportions

Table 1 Background characteristics of respondents by region

	North Central	North East	North West	South East	South South	South West	Nigeria
	$N = 2432$ (%)	$N = 2531$ (%)	$N = 3580$ (%)	$N = 1647$ (%)	$N = 2439$ (%)	$N = 1990$ (%)	$N = 14,619$ (%)
Location							
Urban	823 (33.8)	660 (26.1)	935 (26.1)	1115 (67.7)	844 (34.6)	1454 (73.1)	5831 (39.9)
Rural	1609 (66.2)	1871 (73.9)	2645 (73.9)	532 (32.3)	1595 (65.4)	536 (26.9)	8788 (60.1)
Education							
No education	410 (16.9)	1260 (49.8)	2225 (62.2)	11 (0.7)	28 (1.1)	91 (4.6)	4025 (27.5)
Primary	382 (15.7)	377 (14.9)	444 (12.4)	166 (10.1)	335 (13.7)	154 (7.7)	1858 (12.7)
Secondary	1464 (60.2)	810 (32.0)	849 (23.7)	1347 (81.8)	1928 (79.0)	1511 (75.9)	7909 (54.1)
Higher	176 (7.2)	84 (3.3)	62 (1.7)	123 (7.5)	148 (6.1)	234 (11.8)	827 (5.7)
Religion							
Catholics	312 (13.1)	83 (3.3)	80 (2.3)	801 (48.8)	239 (9.9)	87 (4.4)	1602 (11.1)
Other Christians	1004 (42.1)	454 (18.1)	160 (4.5)	836 (50.9)	2138 (88.3)	1289 (65.2)	5881 (40.7)
Muslims	1070 (44.8)	1978 (78.6)	3287 (93.2)	4 (0.2)	44 (1.8)	600 (30.4)	6983 (48.3)
Wealth quintile							
Poorest	176 (7.2)	782 (30.9)	1122 (31.3)	72 (4.4)	13 (0.5)	25 (1.3)	2190 (15.0)
Poorer	437 (18.0)	731 (28.9)	1117 (31.2)	236 (14.3)	237 (9.7)	143 (7.2)	2901 (19.8)
Middle	780 (32.1)	466 (18.4)	607 (17.0)	427 (25.9)	665 (27.3)	303 (15.2)	3248 (22.2)
Richer	550 (22.6)	332 (13.1)	456 (12.7)	507 (30.8)	854 (35.0)	659 (33.1)	3358 (23.0)
Richest	489 (20.1)	220 (8.7)	278 (7.8)	405 (24.6)	670 (27.5)	860 (43.2)	2922 (20.0)
Ever/never married							
Single never married	1504 (61.8)	920 (36.3)	995 (27.8)	1348 (81.8)	1873 (76.8)	1546 (77.7)	8186 (56.0)
Ever married/cohabited	928 (38.2)	1611 (63.7)	2585 (72.2)	299 (18.2)	566 (23.2)	444 (22.3)	6433 (44.0)
Has begun childbearing							
No	1664 (68.4)	1288 (50.9)	1715 (47.9)	1322 (80.3)	1764 (72.3)	1543 (77.5)	9296 (63.6)
Yes	768 (31.6)	1243 (49.1)	1865 (52.1)	325 (19.7)	675 (27.7)	447 (22.5)	5323 (36.4)

Table 2 Summary of Kaplan-Meier survival tests & Adjusted hazard ratios for age at first birth

	Event	Summary of Kaplan-Meier tests	Adjusted Hazard ratios
	Began childbearing (%)	Estimated mean age (in years) at first birth (95% CI)	HR (95% CI)
Location			
Urban (RC)	1395 (23.9)	21.83 (21.73–21.92)	
Rural	3928 (44.7)	19.67 (19.58–19.75)	1.06 (0.98–1.14)
Log Rank (Mantel-Cox) Chi-square		991.03 ($p < 0.001$)	
Education			
No education (RC)	2539 (63.1)	18.03 (17.93–18.14)	
Primary	907 (48.8)	19.16 (18.98–19.34)	0.96 (0.88–1.05)
Secondary	1772 (22.4)	21.71 (21.63–21.79)	0.70 (0.64–0.77)***
Higher	105 (12.7)	23.38 (23.26–23.50)	0.36 (0.29–0.45)***
Log Rank (Mantel-Cox) Chi-square		3703.39 ($p < 0.001$)	
Religion			
Catholics (RC)	367 (22.9)	21.94 (21.77–22.12)	
Other Christians	1503 (25.6)	21.63 (21.53–21.72)	1.06 (0.94–1.19)
Muslims	3383 (48.4)	19.30 (19.20–19.39)	0.98 (0.86–1.13)
Log Rank (Mantel-Cox) Chi-square		1371.861 ($p < 0.001$)	
Wealth quintile			
Poorest (RC)	1260 (57.5)	18.16 (18.00–18.32)	
Poorer	1429 (49.3)	19.17 (19.02–19.32)	0.89 (0.83–0.96)**
Middle	1169 (36.0)	20.50 (20.36–20.64)	0.86 (0.79–0.94)**
Richer	964 (28.7)	21.38 (21.26–21.51)	0.72 (0.65–0.81)***
Richest	501 (17.1)	22.53 (22.42–22.64)	0.56 (0.49–0.64)***
Log Rank (Mantel-Cox) Chi-square		2199 ($p < 0.001$)	
Ever/never married			
Single never married	450 (5.5)	23.35 (23.29–23.41)	
Ever married/cohabited	4873 (75.8)	18.33 (18.25–18.40)	10.60 (9.56–11.75)***
Log Rank (Mantel-Cox) Chi-square		5813.19 ($p < 0.001$)	
Region			
North Central	768 (31.6)	21.11 (20.96–21.27)	
North East	1243 (49.1)	19.26 (19.10–19.42)	1.24 (1.12–1.37)***
North West	1865 (52.1)	18.81 (18.68–18.95)	1.21 (1.10–1.33)***
South East	325 (19.7)	22.29 (22.14–22.45)	1.02 (0.88–1.17)
South South	675 (27.7)	21.36 (21.21–21.52)	1.45 (1.29–1.62)***
South West	447 (22.5)	21.96 (21.80–22.11)	1.14 (1.01–1.29)*
Log Rank (Mantel-Cox) Chi-square		1777.26 ($p < 0.001$)	

* $p < 0.05$, ** $p < 0.01$, *** $p < 0.001$
HR Hazard ratio, *RC* Reference Category, *CI* Confidence Interval

of young females who have begun childbearing are found in the North East and North West states of Jigawa, Katsina, Bauchi, Zamfara and Gombe.

Figure 2 shows the survival functions for wealth index, region, location, education, religion and marital status. The charts suggest that having ever married/cohabited, education and wealth have the most effect on time to first birth.

Regional variation in predictors of time to first birth

Predictors of time to first birth vary across regions. In the North Central region, young females with secondary education have a lower hazard ratio for beginning childbearing (0.75, $p < 0.01$) compared to those with no formal education in Table 3. Girls in the Richer and Richest quintiles also have lower hazard ratios for beginning childbearing (0.66, $p < 0.05$; 0.51, $p < 0.01$). Ever married/

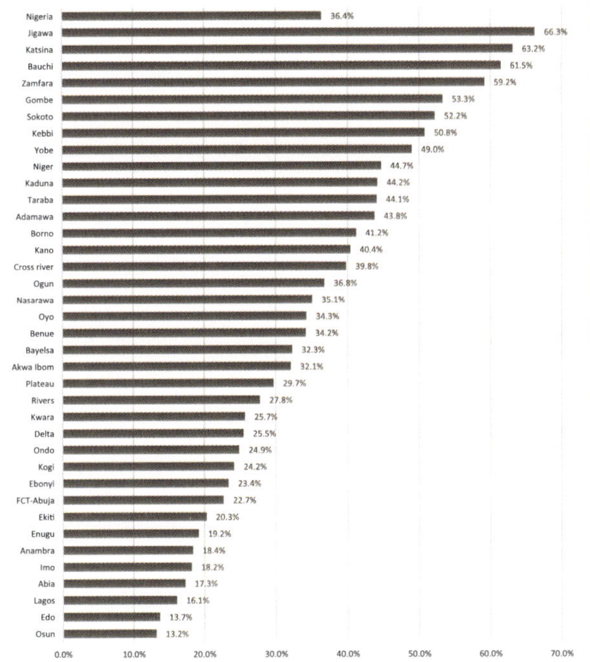

Fig. 1 Proportions of young females (15–24 years) who have begun childbearing by state

cohabited girls have a hazard ratio 20.37 times that of single/never married girls. The analysis also shows that states are significantly different within the region. In the North East, having a secondary or higher education reduces the likelihood of beginning to have children at any given time within the first 24 years of life. The effect of wealth is, however, marginal and inconsistent. The hazard ratio for ever married/cohabited girls is 11.31 times higher than the hazard ratio for single girls ($p < 0.001$). States within the region also have varying effects on time to first childbirth. In the North West, education, wealth and religion have significant effect on time to first child birth. Lower hazard ratios were found for girls with secondary (0.63, $p < 0.001$) and higher education (0.41, $p < 0.05$). Girls from higher wealth quintiles also had lower adjusted hazard ratios when compared with girls in the Poorest quintile. Ever married/cohabited girls have an adjusted hazard ratio that is 44.62 times that of never married girls.

In the South East region, lower hazard ratios are associated with higher wealth. Having higher education also significantly affects time to first birth, with an adjusted hazard ratio of 0.26 ($p < 0.05$). The adjusted hazard ratio for ever married/cohabited young females is 10.55 times that of single/never married girls. No state has an adjusted hazard ratio different from the reference state. In the South South on the other hand, all the states have significantly higher adjusted hazard ratios for beginning childbearing when compared to the reference state (Edo) and girls with higher education have a significantly lower adjusted hazard ratio (0.30, $p < 0.01$) than girls with no formal education. Having ever married/cohabited has the strongest effect on time to first birth, with an adjusted hazard ratio of 5.35 ($p < 0.001$). In the South West, having a higher education significantly increases time to first birth in comparison with girls with no formal education ($p < 0.01$). Ever married/cohabited girls have an adjusted hazard ratio of 12.66 ($p < 0.001$).

Discussion

Having ever married/cohabited is a universal and strong predictor of time to first birth across all six regions of the country. This confirms findings from earlier studies that living in marital unions or cohabiting exposes girls

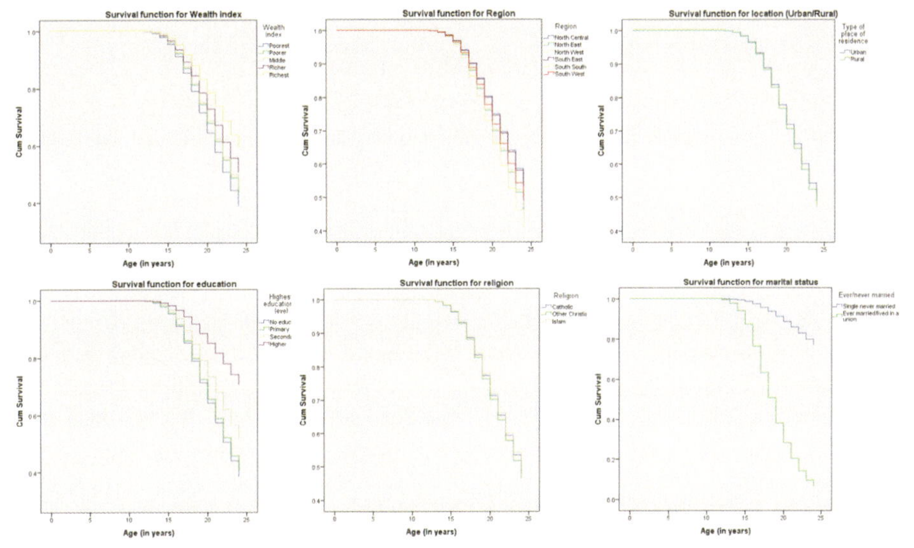

Fig. 2 Survival functions for background characteristics

Table 3 Adjusted hazard ratios for age at first birth by region

	North Central HR (95% CI)	North East HR (95% CI)	North West HR (95% CI)	South East HR (95% CI)	South South HR (95% CI)	South West HR (95% CI)
Location						
Urban (RC)						
Rural	0.97 (0.78–1.20)	1.00(0.84–1.21)	0.97 (0.82–1.15)	1.25 (0.96–1.63)	1.01 (0.83–1.23)	1.10 (0.84–1.44)
Education						
No education (RC)						
Primary	0.99 (0.79–1.24)	0.89 (0.75–1.06)	0.96 (0.83–1.12)	1.22 (0.43–3.49)	1.17 (0.69–1.97)	1.16 (0.78–1.72)
Secondary	0.75 (0.60–0.93)**	0.67 (0.55–0.81)***	0.63 (0.52–0.77)***	0.91 (0.333–2.53)	0.85 (0.51–1.42)	0.84 (0.57–1.24)
Higher	0.68 (0.42–1.11)	0.27 (0.14–0.51)***	0.41 (0.20–0.86)*	0.26 (0.72–0.92)*	0.30 (0.14–0.62)**	0.46 (0.28–0.77)**
Religion						
Catholics (RC)						
Other Christians	1.14 (0.88–1.48)	0.94 (0.63–1.40)	0.34 (0.21–0.55)***	0.99 (0.78–1.25)	1.46 (1.08–1.96)*	1.25 (0.73–2.12)
Muslims	1.06 (0.78–1.43)	0.89 (0.60–1.32)	0.38 (0.26–0.57)***	0.87 (0.32–2.42)	1.36 (0.70–2.63)	1.11 (0.63–1.94)
Wealth quintile						
Poorest (RC)						
Poorer	0.99 (0.74–1.32)	0.96 (0.83–1.10)	0.86 (0.78–0.96)**	0.54 (0.33–0.90)*	0.76 (0.24–2.43)	0.47 (0.25–0.89)*
Middle	0.91 (0.68–1.22)	0.82 (0.68–0.99)*	0.77 (0.666–0.89)**	0.75 (0.46–1.22)	0.75 (0.24–2.37)	0.64 (0.34–1.23)
Richer	0.66 (0.47–0.92)*	0.81 (0.64–1.03)	0.82 (0.65–1.04)	0.53 (0.33–0.87)*	0.55 (0.18–1.75)	0.53 (0.27–1.03)
Richest	0.51 (0.34–0.77)**	0.69 (0.48–0.99)*	0.69 (0.50–0.97)*	0.47 (0.27–0.80)**	0.37 (0.12–1.20)	0.44 (0.21–0.90)
Ever/never married						
Single never married						
Ever married/ cohabited	20.37 (14.69–28.25)***	11.31 (8.35–15.31)***	44.62 (25.06–79.46)***	10.55 (8.08–13.757)***	5.35 (4.53–6.32)***	12.66 (9.57–16.75)***
State[a]						
Reference state						
State 2	0.84 (0.61–1.15)	1.02 (0.82–1.28)	1.13 (0.95–1.35)	0.90 (0.63–1.29)	1.92 (1.37–2.68)***	0.80 (0.56–1.15)
State 3	0.73 (0.56–0.95)*	1.27 (1.02–1.58)*	1.18 (0.99–1.40)	1.32 (0.91–1.90)	2.05 (1.50–2.81)***	1.00 (0.69–1.45)
State 4	0.66 (0.49–0.89)**	1.16 (0.95–1.42)	1.11 (0.93–1.31)	0.89 (0.57–1.39)	1.46 (1.04–2.03)*	1.15 (0.82–1.61)
State 5	0.85 (0.6–1.17)	1.41 (1.17–1.69)***	0.94 (0.79–1.11)	0.94 (0.63–1.40)	2.26 (1.68–3.05)***	0.94 (0.65–1.36)
State 6	0.83 (0.62–1.10)	1.37 (1.10–1.71)**	1.26 (1.03–1.53)*		1.48 (1.08–2.02)*	1.17 (0.83–1.65)
State 7	0.75 (0.57–0.98)*		0.93 (0.77–1.11)			

HR Hazard Ratio, *RC* Reference Category, *CI* Confidence Interval
* $p < 0.05$, ** $p < 0.01$, *** $p < 0.001$
[a] North Central states: Ref state – Niger, State 2 – FCT, State 3 – Nasarawa, State 4 – Plateau, State 5 – Benue, State 6 – Kogi, State 7 – Kwara
North East states: Ref state – Yobe, State 2 – Borno, State 3 – Adamawa, State 4 – Gombe, State 5 – Bauchi, State 6 – Taraba
North West states: Ref state – Sokoto, State 2 – Zamfara, State 3 – Katsina, State 4 – Jigawa, State 5 – Kano, State 6 – Kaduna, State 7 – Kebbi
South East states: Ref state – Anambra, State 2 – Enugu, State 3 – Ebonyi, State 4 – Abia, State 5 – Imo
South South states: Ref state – Edo, State 2 – Cross River, State 3 – Akwa Ibom, State 4 – Rivers, State 5 – Bayelsa, State 6 – Delta
South West states: Ref state – Oyo, State 2 – Osun, State 3 – Ekiti, State 4 – Ondo, State 5 – Lagos, State 6 – Ogun

to pregnancy and childbearing [20–22, 36–38]. A major implication of this finding is that all interventions that seek to reduce early childbearing among adolescents need to also seek to stop the practice of child marriage and cohabitation. It also stresses the need for the adoption and implementation of the Child Rights Act/Law across states in Nigeria. The law prohibits any form of marriage or cohabitation with persons under the age of 18 years. Implementing this law will protect children who are below the age of consent from adults who wish to 'marry' them or cohabit with them.

The second most import factor in time to first birth is education. In all three northern regions, having secondary education has a significant effect on time to first birth while in the southern regions, only higher education significantly affects time to first birth. This supports earlier studies that associate early onset of childbearing with poor education [11, 15, 39] even though it does not address the problem of temporal sequence as we are not able to determine whether low educational aspiration drives adolescent childbearing or vice versa. The current study shows that even when marriage or cohabitation is held constant, education continues to have a significant effect on time to first birth. There is need, therefore, for the full implementation of the universal basic education policy that requires that the first 9 years of education be free and compulsory for all in Nigeria. The implementation of this policy has the potential of increasing reproductive health knowledge and outcomes.

Wealth also has significant influence on time to first birth in all but one of the six regions, albeit, with some inconsistency in some regions. Generally speaking, however, the likelihood of starting to have children is lower for all the four top quintiles than for the Poorest quintile in all the regions even though the result is not significant in some cases. This finding is in agreement with earlier studies [39]. One possible explanation for the role of wealth in time to first birth is that poverty reduces access to sexual and reproductive health knowledge and services [40] which may in turn predict adolescent childbearing. In addition, females from poor households may be involved in relationships with older, richer men for survival [41]. The implication of this finding for programming is that an ecological approach to the problem of early childbearing is required. The provision of sexual and reproductive health information and services should be reinforced with better economic conditions that reduce the lure of relationships with older, richer men.

Generally, young females in the northern states begin to have children earlier. This supports the position in the literature [25, 26]. It is, however, interesting to note that state of residence is also a source of variation in time to first birth in contexts that are assumed to be largely homogeneous. Only the South East and South West regions have states that are homogeneous in respect to time to first birth among young females. In the other regions, we observed state level variations, contrary to the assumption that regions approximate socio-cultural clusters with a measure of internal homogeneity. We argue that variation in sub-national political administration makes a difference in time to first birth. This shows the need for a study to document the effect of state level administration on youth sexual and reproductive health in general, and exposure to pregnancy and childbearing in particular. Such context-specific study will focus on what state governments are doing differently in terms of policy adoption and implementation, state level laws, and the activities of non-government organizations and how these affect the onset of childbearing among young people. The South South represents a classic case of variation with all the states having adjusted hazard ratios that differ significantly from the reference state (Edo). This region requires a state level analysis.

Limitations of the study

The survey is based on self reports which may be inaccurate due to poor recall of events. The choice of covariates in the analysis is also limited to background characteristics. There is the possibility, however, that other variables not included in the analysis significantly affect time to first birth. This study is also limited in scope. For instance, it is desirable to have state-level analyses but this is outside the scope of this study.

Conclusion

The negative health implications of early onset of childbearing stress the importance of evidence-based interventions. Interventions that will yield positive results need to target adolescents at high risk of early marriage, and those living in extreme poverty. While in-school adolescents may have access to some sexuality education, those not registered in schools may be left out and may have limited access to reproductive health information and services. Interventions should therefore seek to address the specific needs of out-of-school girls. Such interventions must also be multi-level in nature, in order to address contextual factors that reinforce the belief in marrying girls off early at the community and national levels. In addition, the most hit states identified in this study should be prioritized in programming. While it may be convenient for governments and non-governmental organizations to pilot their interventions in cities, addressing the problem of adolescent childbearing and similar problems may be more successful if the worst hit states are prioritized.

The concentration of strong non-governmental organizations in cities like Lagos, Abuja, Kano, Calabar and Port Harcourt often gives those cities too much attention at the expense of many less developed states. In the North West for instance, the proportion of young females who have begun childbearing is lowest in Kano state which has a greater likelihood than any of the other states to attract intervention programs because of its relative cosmopolitan nature and population. Yet, Jigawa, Katsina, Bauchi, Zamfara and Kebbi states require greater attention, especially those households living in extreme poverty in these states. The findings of this study also have wider implications within the Nigerian context. Addressing similar reproductive health problems such as youth uptake of human immune-deficiency virus testing and unsafe sex also require an approach that prioritizes the worst hit states of the country, and the poorest of the poor in such states.

Abbreviations

CI: Confidence interval; HR: Hazard ratio; RC: Reference category

Acknowledgements

The authors wish to thank the Demographic and Health Surveys Program for providing access to the dataset.

Funding
The study did not benefit from any funding. The University of Lagos, however, provided a travel grant which made it possible for the initial draft to be presented at an international conference.

Authors' contributions
MK conceived of the study, obtained permission to use the data, analysed the data and drafted the manuscript; IE participated in the interpretation of the data and in critically revising the manuscript; CN participated in the interpretation of the data, in critically revising the statistical analysis and in revising the manuscript. All authors read and approved the final manuscript.

Competing interests
The authors declare that they have no competing interests.

Author details
[1]Department of Sociology, University of Lagos, Lagos, Nigeria. [2]Department of Sociology/Psychology/Criminology & Security Studies, Faculty of Management & Social Sciences, Alex Ekwueme Federal University Ndufu-Alike Ikwo (AE-FUNAI), Abakaliki, Ebonyi State, Nigeria.

References
1. Population Reference Bureau. 2017 world population data sheet. Washington, DC: Population Reference Bureau; 2017.
2. National Population Commission (NPC) [Nigeria] & ICF International. Nigeria Demographic and Health Survey 2013. Rockville: NPC and ICF International; 2014.
3. Tuladhar H, Khanal R, Kayastha S, Shrestha P, Giri A. Complication of home delivery: Our experience at Nepal Medical College Teaching Hospital. Nepal Med Coll J. 2009;11(3):164–9.
4. Tabatabaie MG, Moudi Z, Vedadhir A. Home birth and barriers to referring women with obstetric complications to hospitals: a mixed-methods study in Zahedan, southeastern Iran. Reprod Health. 2012;9:5. https://doi.org/10.1186/1742-4755-9-5.
5. Phipps MG, Sowers M. Defining early adolescent childbearing. Am J Public Health. 2002;92(1):125–8.
6. El-Moselhy EA, Borg HM, Atlam SA. Cervical Cancer: sociodemographic and clinical risk factors among adult Egyptian females. Adv Oncol Res Treat. 2016;1(1):106.
7. Jeha D, Usta I, Ghulmiyyah L, Nassar A. A review of the risks and consequences of adolescent pregnancy. J Neonatal-Perinatal Med. 2015;8:1–8.
8. Karra M, Lee M. Human capital consequences of teenage childbearing in South Africa, research brief. Washington, DC: Population Reference Bureau; 2012.
9. Otterblad OP, Bengt H, Gunilla RW, Sven C. Teenage childbearing and long-term socioeconomic consequences: a case study in Sweden. Fam Plan Perspect. 2001;33(2):70–4.
10. Oyefara JL. Socio-economic consequences of adolescent childbearing in Osun state, Nigeria. KASBIT Bus J. 2009;2(1 & 2):1–18.
11. Rowlands S. Social predictors of repeat adolescent pregnancy and focused strategies. Best Pract Res Clin Obstet Gynaecol. 2010;24(5):605–16.
12. Chambers BD, Erausquin JT. The promise of intersectional stigma to understand the complexities of adolescent pregnancy and motherhood. J Child Adolesc Behav. 2015;3(5):249. https://doi.org/10.4172/2375-4494.1000249.
13. Harding DJ. Counterfactual models of neighbourhood effects: the effect of neighbourhood poverty on dropping out and teenage pregnancy. Am J Sociol. 2003;109(3):676–719.
14. Amoran OE. A comparative analysis of predictors of teenage pregnancy and its prevention in a rural town in Western Nigeria. Int J Equity Health. 2012;11:37.
15. Raneri LG, Wiemann CM. Social ecological predictors of repeat adolescent pregnancy. Perspect Sex Reprod Health. 2007;39(1):39–47. https://doi.org/10.1363/3903907.
16. Millner BC, Benson B, Galbraith KA. Family relationships and adolescent pregnancy risk: a research synthesis. Dev Rev. 2001;21:1–38.
17. Harper Collins. Social studies atlas for Nigeria. Hong Kong: HaperCollins Publishers; 2009.
18. United Nations Development Program. National human development report 2015: human security and human development in Nigeria. New York: UNDP; 2015.
19. Adebowale AS, Fagbamigbe AF, Adebayo AM. Regional differences in adolescent childbearing in Nigeria. J Popul Soc Stud. 2016;24(2):101–16.
20. Holland JA. Love, marriage, then the baby carriage? Marriage timing ad childbearing in Sweden. Demogr Res. 2013;29:275–306.
21. Goli S, Rammohan A, Singh D. The effect of early marriages and early childbearing on women's nutritional status in India. Matern Child Health J. 2015;19(8):1864–80.
22. Manning WD, Cohen JA. Teenage cohabitation, marriage, and childbearing. Popul Res Policy Rev. 2015;34(2):161–77.
23. Okereke CI, Uwakwe JO, Nwamuo P. Education an antidote against early marriage for the girl-child. J Educ Soc Res. 2013;3(5):73–8.
24. Kyari GV, Ayodele J. The socio-economic effect of early marriage in North Western Nigeria. Mediterr J Soc Sci. 2014;3(5):73–8.
25. Rosen J. Advocating for Adolescent Reproductive Health: Addressing Cultural Sensitivities. InFocus, November. 2000. On the web at: http://www2.pathfinder.org/pf/pubs/focus/IN%20FOCUS/nov_2000.htm.
26. Rosen JE, Murray NJ, Moreland S. Sexuality education in schools: The international experience and implications for Nigeria: Policy working paper series 12. Abuja: USAID; 2004.
27. United Nations Children's Fund. Early marriage: child spouses. Innocenti digest, no. 7. Florence: UNICEF; 2001.
28. Fayokun KO. Legality of child marriage in Nigeria and inhibitions against realisation of education rights. US-China Educ Rev. 2015;5(7):460–70.
29. Walker J. Mapping early marriage in West Africa: a scan of trends, interventions, what works, best practices and the way forward. Lagos: Ford Foundation; 2013.
30. Kunnuji MON. Spatial variations in access to improved sanitation and water in Lagos state. J Water Sanit Hyg Dev. 2014;4(4):612–9.
31. Aarø LF, Mathews C, Kaaya S, Katahoire AR, Onya H, Abraham C, et al. Promoting sexual and reproductive health among adolescents in southern and eastern Africa (PREPARE): project design and conceptual framework. BMC Public Health. 2014;14:54. http://www.biomedcentral.com/1471-2458/14/54.
32. Blum RB, Astone NM, Decker MR, Mouili C. A conceptual framework for early adolescence: a platform for research. Int J Adolesc Med Health. 2014;26(3):321–31.
33. Price NL, Hawkins K. A conceptual framework for the social analysis of reproductive health. J Health Popul Nutri. 2007;25(1):24–36.
34. Clark TG, Bradburn MJ, Love SB, Altman DG. Survival analysis part I: basic concepts and first analyses. Br J Cancer. 2003;89:232–8.
35. Thomas L, Reyes EM. Tutorial: survival estimation for cox regression models with time-varying coefficients using SAS and R. J Stat Softw. 2014;61:1–23.
36. Bongaarts J, Frank O, Lesthaeghe R. The proximate determinants of fertility in sub-Saharan Africa. Popul Dev Rev. 1984;10(3):511–37.
37. Alemayehu T, Haider J, Habte D. Determinants of adolescent fertility in Ethiopia. Ethiop J Health Dev. 2010;24(1):30–8.
38. Baizan P, Aassve A, Billari FC. Cohabitation, marriage, first birth: The interrelationship of family formation events in Spain. Rostock: MPIDR Working Paper, WP 2001–036; 2001.
39. Nahar MZ, Zahangir MS. Patterns and determinants of age at first birth in Bangladesh. Turk J Popul Stud. 2013;35:63–77.
40. Casey EA, Lindhorst TP. Toward a multi-level, ecological approach to the primary prevention of sexual assault: prevention in peer and community contexts. Trauma Violence Abuse. 2009;10:91–114.
41. Kunnuji MON. Basic deprivation and involvement in risky sexual behaviour among out-of-school young people in a Lagos slum. Cult Health Sex. 2014. https://doi.org/10.1080/13691058.2014.894206.

"In the hospital, there will be nobody to pamper me": a qualitative assessment on barriers to facility-based delivery in post-Ebola Sierra Leone

Stefanie Theuring[1*], Alimamy Philip Koroma[2] and Gundel Harms[1]

Abstract

Background: Sierra Leone has one of the highest maternal mortality rates in the world. Encouraging the use of skilled birth attendance in health facilities is an important step in the endeavor to increase the number of safe deliveries. However, public trust in health facilities has been greatly damaged during the Ebola epidemic outbreak in Sierra Leone in 2014/2015, and little is known about external and intrinsic barriers to facility-based delivery (FBD) in the country since the end of the Ebola epidemic.

Methods: We conducted a qualitative study on FBD in Princess Christian Maternity Hospital, Freetown, which is the national referral maternity hospital in Sierra Leone. We performed six focus group discussions with providers, pregnant women and recent mothers surrounding experiences, attitudes and behaviors regarding FBD and potential barriers. Discussions were tape recorded, transcribed and evaluated through content analysis.

Results: Women in our study were overall technically aware of the higher safety linked with FBD, but this often diverged from their individual desire to deliver in a supportive and trusted social and traditional environment. Close relatives and community members seemed to be highly influencial regarding birth practices. Many women associated FBD with negative staff attitudes and an undefined fear. Logistic issues regarding transportation problems or late referral from smaller health centers were identified as frequent barriers to FBD.

Conclusions: More supportive staff attitudes and acceptance of an accompanying person throughout delivery could be promising approaches to increase women's confidence in FBDs. However, these approaches also imply revising health systems structures, like staff working conditions that are conducive for a friendly atmosphere, sufficient space in delivery wards allowing the women to bring a birth companion, or like the establishment of a reliable peripheral ambulance system to ensure transportation and fast referral.

Keywords: Maternal mortality, Facility-based delivery, Post-Ebola, Qualitative study, Sierra Leone

Plain English summary

Background: Sierra Leone is one of the countries in the world where most women die when giving birth. Assistance of skilled health workers in health facilities increases safety for mothers. However, after many people died in hospitals in Sierra Leone during the Ebola outbreak in 2014/2015, trust in health facilities decreased. Although the Ebola outbreak ended, there might still be barriers to facility-based delivery (FBD).

Methods: Our aim was to find out what people think of FBD in Freetown, Sierra Leone. We conducted six group discussions in Princess Christian Maternity Hospital with staff, pregnant women and recent mothers on experiences, attitudes and behaviors regarding FBD and potential barriers.

Results: Women in our study were overall aware of FBD being safer than home deliveries. At the same time, they often expressed a desire to deliver in a familiar

* Correspondence: stefanie.theuring@charite.de
[1]Institute of Tropical Medicine and International Health, Charité-Universitätsmedizin, Augustenburger Platz 1, 13353 Berlin, Germany
Full list of author information is available at the end of the article

social and traditional environment. Close relatives and community members often influenced where and how women want to deliver. Many women feared that staff might treat them badly in hospitals and that they might die there. Transportation to hospital from home or from other health centers was named as a problem.

Conclusions: Women might be convinced to use FBD if staff would treat them in a more supportive way and if they could bring a trusted person to stay with them during delivery. This means that hospitals need to improve some conditions, like motivating the staff or offering an ambulance system to ensure transportation even from far away.

Background

Sierra Leone is not only one of the poorest countries in the world; it is also one of the most dangerous countries when it comes to delivering a baby, with a maternal mortality rate of 1360/100.000 births as of 2015. [1] Despite strong efforts to improve health services´ accessibility and availability, e.g. by establishing a peripheral health unit network or reducing financial barriers by introducing the Free Healthcare Initiative for pregnant and lactating women in 2010 [2, 3] immense gaps in the country's health system in terms of quality of care and patient safety remain a problem. Furthermore, the largely inadequate obstetric care offered by an already weak health system in Sierra Leone has been further compromised during the Ebola epidemic with approximately 10 000 cases between 2014 and 2015, forcing many hospitals to close down or reduce their activity to prevent Ebola transmission or because of staff shortages. [3, 4] Many women in the Ebola outbreak-affected countries including Liberia, Sierra Leone and Guinea are likely to have died due to the reduced access to appropriate care during childbirth, and many more to have lost their trust in the reliability and safety of health services during the virus outbreak [3]. While before 2014, facility-based deliveries (FBD) in Liberia were rising up to an all-time high, after the Ebola epidemic, FBDs decreased by up to almost 80%. [5] In Sierra Leone, before 2014, only about half of deliveries were facility-based [6]. A report assessing changes in health services utilization in the early phase of the Ebola outbreak showed that service uptake was seriously compromised with a one-third decline in facility-based deliveries already by September 2014, mostly as a result of women's fear and lack of confidence in health services [7, 8]. Since the Ebola outbreak ended, there is uncertainty whether the public trust in health institutions has been restored, and to date, research regarding the ongoing potential intrinsic and extrinsic barriers to FBD is scarce in this post-outbreak population. This study aimed at capturing the current situation regarding attitudes of patients and providers on FBD in Freetown, Sierra Leone.

Methods

We conducted a cross-sectional qualitative assessment based on six Focus Group Discussions (FGDs) to identify common attitudes, perceptions and behaviors with respect to FBDs, with the goal to design further formative research to increase institutional delivery rates. Our study was located in Princess Christian Maternity Hospital (PCMH) in Freetown, Western Area of Sierra Leone. PCMH is the national referral maternity hospital in the country, with a capacity of about 140 beds and approximately 5700 deliveries in 2016. PCMH is the only facility providing Comprehensive Emergency Obstetric and Neonatal Services in the Western Area, comprising of about 1.5 million inhabitants. [9]

Study procedures

Within PCMH, we conducted two FGDs with health care providers, two FGDs with pregnant women from the ANC ward, and two FGDs with mothers who were waiting for hospital discharge after delivery. This mixture of groups was supposed to offer insight into a wide range of perspectives from different positions. FGD participants were recruited purposively; recruitment criteria included belonging to one of the three target groups, the person not being involved in any medical procedure at the time of recruitment, and willingness to participate. An information sheet on study participation was read out to all participants, and they gave written informed consent by signature or fingerprint. We recruited five to seven participants for each FGD, based on the assumption that a rather small group size can create an encouraging atmosphere for each individual to engage in the discussion [10]. The number of FGDs was subject to data saturation, which was achieved after six groups as we observed reiterating discussion contents and no new information being brought up within those target groups. A local study nurse moderated the FGDs in English and Krio, using a previously prepared discussion guide. The discussion guide comprised questions surrounding general attitudes towards home delivery, institutional delivery, traditional birth attendants (TBAs), perception of barriers to facility-based deliveries, and own experiences with delivery (patients, as well as providers who had previously given birth) or working at the delivery ward (staff). The discussion sessions were located in a privacy-offering counselling room of PCMH and lasted for about 60 min each, a time seeming appropriate for within-group data saturation. For women who spoke in Krio, the study nurse translated questions to Krio and answers to English immediately. Statements of FGD participants were subject to probing and respondent validation. Discussions were audio-taped; in addition, an observing person took notes. This was supposed to support data interpretation, e.g. to capture group dynamics or for the case of affirmation of a statement through body language. We asked each of the participants to fill in a form for basic demographic information before the discussions started. The participants received a refreshment and a small financial compensation for their time spent. The six FGDs were conducted in October 2017.

Analysis

We performed a both tape-based and note-based constant comparison analysis of the data, with an abridged, partly (for key statements) verbatim transcription of audiotapes by one researcher. The data went through a three-step process of inductive coding performed by one researcher (the first author), including initial open coding, axial coding, i.e. grouping and linking identified codes within categories, and selective coding, i.e. deriving themes from the identified categories. [10] The coding procedure involved iterative reading of transcripts and notes combined with writing analytic memos to reflect on the emerging concepts. The content analysis was performed manually.

Results

Thirty-five women took part in our six focus groups; 13 providers and 22 patients. The average age in the provider groups consisting of female nurse/midwives was 43 years, the majority of providers were Christian (9/11; 2 missing data), the minority Muslim (2/11).

Among the patient groups, the average age was 26 years ($n = 19$, 3 missing data). Three quarters of clients were Muslim (15/20, 2 missing data) and one quarter was Christian (5/20). The majority was married (14/17, 5 missing data). Average travel time to the hospital among the patients was 70 min ($n = 16$, 6 missing data). As their occupation, most patients stated they were students or petty traders. Among the participants from the group of recent mothers, the majority had been referred to PCMH for some pregnancy or birth complication.

General views on FBD

The common understanding among all participants, both patients and providers, was that FBD would generally provide best medical care and least health risk for mother and baby.

> *"I think it will be safer for me to deliver in the hospital."* (Pregnant woman, FGD3)

> *"If you come to the hospital, they will know how your baby is, they will know what to do. They will do a scan."* (Pregnant woman, FGD3)

> *"In case of any problem or complication, specialists are available who can help."* (Pregnant woman, FGD3)

> *"I think that is the right way, to deliver in the hospital, because there you can get best medical care."* (Pregnant woman, FGD4)

> *"Home delivery is very risky. (If not going to a health facility), you end up losing the baby and even your own life."* (Recent mother, FGD6)

> *"If you go to the central hospital, and you are delaying and you cannot push, we have a mechanism, the vacuum; we will use it to lift this baby from you. We have so many facilities. (...) If the baby is not responding well, we have a good resuscitation center."* (Health provider, FGD1)

However, contradicting to the positive attitudes participants were describing, at the same time they expressed a general concept of fear, wariness and mistrust regarding health facilities. Most women reporting FBD experiences mentioned an initial fear of going to hospital for delivery, especially for surgery. Reasons remained opaque, but it was vaguely implied that fear was justified. It appeared as if going to the hospital was widely equated with having to die there.

> *"I was frightened, because I never wanted to go to that theater again."* (Recent mother, FGD6)

> *"They told me I am going to need an operation, I feared. (...) I put everything to god."* (Recent mother, FGD6)

> *"Why are women afraid of the hospital? (...) They have their reasons."* (Recent mother, FGD6)

> *"Some women don't want to be referred to hospital. They think it's the end of their lives."* (Recent mother, FGD5)

> *"When Ebola was there, women would not come to hospital, because they said if you come, you will be infected, you will die. Because so many people had Ebola. They are afraid of this."* (Health provider, FGD2)

> *"Most of the (women) will always say, when you go to PCMH to deliver, you die."* (Health provider, FGD1)

> *"Some of the women will tell them (smaller health centers), please don't refer me, I don't want to go to PCMH, I don't want to die."* (Health provider, FGD1)

Attitudes and behavior of delivery staff

Women who had experienced FBD confirmed predominantly positive experiences, having perceived staff as encouraging and supportive.

"They took good care of me, they talked to me, advised me and encouraged me." (Recent mother, FGD6)

"I was giving the nurses a hell of a time. (...) The nurse that night, I congratulate her. She went up and down. Four doctors I think she called for me." (Recent mother, FGD6)

"They are gentle (...) I would still come to this hospital" (Recent mother, FGD5)

"I like the way they took care of me. Staff encouraged me when I was crying, as I was a (primipara), so they encouraged me a lot." (Pregnant woman, FGD3)

"They only gave the best care to me. They were so close and monitoring everything. They encouraged me so much." (Pregnant woman, FGD4)

However, women also reported a number of negative experiences, including communication problems, being neglected by hospital staff, or certain undesirable health workers practices during delivery, like lithotomy position.

"There was a very long delay. (...) I told (the nurse) to do something. She insisted on what she thinks was best. (...) I was admitted on Monday, I went into labor on Tuesday, but C/S was only done on Saturday. (...) (The baby) was alive when I was admitted, but she was born dead." (Recent mother, FGD5)

"I went to a health center closeby; I was thinking that the nurses were very wicked. They just placed me here, nobody talked to me, nobody looked at me, for about ten hours." (Health provider, FGD2)

"I was in pain, I wanted to go to the toilet. Nobody came to me to help, so I myself went to the toilet, and I felt something was coming out, I called the nurses: `come, look at my baby!` I said, `you people are sitting there, talking, talking, talking, and I delivered my baby by myself.´ They were sitting outside the room; after the examination, they just forgot about me." (Health provider, FGD2)

"Some of the nurses we talk to...there's so many attitudes when you are in labor. You may have some kind of behavior that the nurses will not like. But they have to be patient because we are in labor. Their boss should tell them to be patient with us." (Pregnant woman, FGD3)

"The majority of us don't know how to deliver in a bed. We are not used to that. We prefer to deliver on the ground, that is better for us. (...) When you go to the hospital, the nurses will just leave you on the bed. (...) I would like to deliver on the floor. The bed is too high, and we are in a form of fearness." (Pregnant woman, FGD 3)

"All they wanted to do was a vaginal examination. I refused vaginal examination. The area was already sore." (Health provider, FGD2)

The problem of negative staff attitudes possibly deterring women from approaching PCMH was particularly expressed by the providers themselves, who argued that a lack of motivation in underpaid and overworked nurses and midwives would substantially contribute to unfavorable working attitudes of staff.

"It is the attitude of health workers that is not correct. Some of the women will say, ´I don't want to go to this facility to deliver because the nurses don't treat me fair, when I go they shout at me.´ (...) The nurses are stressed." (Health provider, FGD1)

"The salary is very low. It is not encouraging. (...) So we are short of staff. This is the reason why most of us will get annoyed with the patients. (...) I perform three deliveries and I am overworked. I'm stressed with my empty pockets. And when you come around with your own problem, you don't want the problem of others, it just gets me mad." (Health provider, FGD1)

"There is a shortage of health workers. We are dealing with so many patients. So some women may even refuse to come another time, because they say `if I go there, I will stay a long time`. The work is too much for us and there is no motivation. We are working for 24 hours, covering three shifts sometimes. That may lead you to maybe talk a bit hard to the patients." (Health provider, FGD2)

Inhibiting staff attitudes also appeared in the context of the consistently mentioned problem of late referral from smaller health centers to hospitals in emergency cases. Hospital staff described health workers of smaller health centers as often ignoring their limits or overestimating their skills, and thereby causing a delay in referring the patient to hospital.

"The health workers there will be on their limit, but they don't want the community to see: this health worker doesn't know her job. (...) If you check our (PCMH) maternal mortality, you will see that most of the (referred) cases come in as `death on arrival´. (...) So now as a midwife or nurse (...) when you see that

this particular case, you should not handle it, you should refer earlier." (Health provider, FGD1)

"This (late arrival in hospital) can be the fault of colleagues. Sometimes they hold on to these patients for quite long beyond their limits. By the time they refer the patients, by the time they get here if the distance is too long, they come here already obstructed." (Health provider, FGD2)

Role of trusted person/TBAs

As a logical addition to perceived negative attitudes and communication problems with hospital staff, women repeatedly articulated their desire to have a person of trust around when it comes to delivery, like a relative or a TBA. Since delivering woman are usually not allowed to bring an accompanying person into the delivery ward, they fear being unattended and left alone. This imagination causes discomfort and hesitance to choose FBD in many pregnant women despite their knowledge that it is the safer option.

"I will be more comfortable to deliver at home. I am afraid that in latency phase, they will admit you and leave you alone. I am afraid to be alone, I want to deliver at home so I can be with the same midwife." (Pregnant woman, FGD3)

"I am not certain where to deliver, I am having fear. I will have someone at home to pamper me, in the hospital, there will be nobody to pamper me." (Pregnant woman, FGD3)

"(Pregnant women) believe in what older women are telling them, giving them information, helping them at home." (Pregnant woman, FGD4)

"People believe they should deliver at home rather than in hospital, because their grandparents have done it, their great-grandparents were doing it, so they prefer to do it." (Health provider, FGD1)

The large influence of women's trusted social environment also caused delay in hospital referral in some cases where an emergency occurred. When asked why they did not approach the hospital immediately when noticing danger signs, women referred to trusted people in their family/community who advised them, often based on wrong concepts of the symptoms.

"Elder people are experienced. This was my first own pregnancy, so I don´ t have any idea about that. So I took the idea of them. (...) They gave treatments to me." (Recent mother, FGD5)

"I had swollen feet. (My people) said that maybe it is because it is a male child. One day a nurse was passing by. She said: this is a danger sign, go to hospital on Monday. Unfortunately, I was convulsed before Monday. (...) I was having the idea that my feet were swollen because I was having a male child." (Recent mother, FGD5)

From the close social environment, especially husbands seemed to be highly influential on the place of delivery. Reports on partner support with respect to FBD were divergent, including both encouraging and inhibiting attitudes. However, participants described women as generally not authorized for such decision-making without the partner and having to wait for his approval, even in emergency cases.

"My husband also advised me to go to the hospital. Going to the hospital is the best thing." (Pregnant woman, FGD4)

"I asked him why his wife doesn't deliver in hospital; he told me categorically that whenever his wives, because he has several wives, come to the hospital to deliver, they will advise them on family planning. (...) He believes when you advise his wives (on family planning), they will go out with another man." (Health Provider, FGD1)

"The women don't have a right to their own opinion. (...) The nurse will tell them ´I have to refer you to another level, where they will continue your treatment`, the woman will say `I want to wait until my husband comes`. (...) The women don't have a right to make their own decision." (Health provider, FGD1)

"They said she was waiting for the husband. (...) Just as I'm telling you about this knowledge that you should go earlier and save your own life, not your husband's life, but your own life! She will prefer sitting at home waiting for him." (Health provider, FGD1)

TBAs were characterized to have an important role as trusted and respected persons, often with a family bond, whom many women prefer to FBD because of tradition and belief.

"TBAs are in the community, they are very close to the patients. Sometimes these TBAs are women's mothers, or mothers-in-law. So they are trusting them more than the nurses in the hospital." (Health provider, FGD1)

"TBAs, the women know them for a long time, so they think they will be handled with care and treated

better. (...) Also, some of them are their relatives, so they trust in them more than in nurses." (Health provider, FGD2)

"They are the people that are respected in the community. Most of the nurses, they are just young girls. TBAs, maybe she is my mothers or grandmothers age, so they are most trusted." (Health provider, FGD2)

At the same time, participants discussed that TBAs are often lacking medical competencies, and they described the resulting skepticism. Officially, TBAs have no permission to perform deliveries under threat of penalty charge, but recent efforts strived for integrating TBAs into the formal health system. Discussants however agreed that women would never reveal to a health facility if they had been with a TBA, so no one would know or charge a fine.

"TBAs are not trained to a level to attend to complications" (Health provider, FGD2)

"I do not trust them 100% (...) For them, they don't know how to do. They just say the baby is fine." (Pregnant woman, FGD3)

"I am not comfortable with the TBAs because they don't know where the baby lays and how to handle complications." (Pregnant woman, FGD3)

"It was decided to let TBAs join our health workers in the hospital setting. (...) They sent out a call to the TBAs: the greater the number of patients you bring to the hospital (for delivery), the higher they pay you. (...) So the TBA will encourage women to come to the hospital." (Health provider, FGD2)

Travel distance/transportation

Participants frequently expressed long travel distance to PCMH as an important obstacle. It was stated that many women have no means of transportation, especially when labor starts during the night. The failure to approach a health facility for delivery was also perceived as a consequence of poverty and the inability to pay for transportation. Oftentimes, TBAs remain the only accessible option of any skilled attendance in the absence of transportation to a health facility.

"Most pregnant women do not come to the hospital because of transport, because they are living at a distance." (Pregnant woman, FGD4)

"At longer distance, pregnant women will not have transport. Poverty plays a big role to get to the hospital." (Pregnant woman, FGD4)

"Patients go home first to raise money. They are coming here, they don't know anybody, for transport, for food, they need money to take care of themselves. These are very poor patients. Even the blood transfusions have to be paid." (Health provider, FGD2)

"There are places that are not motorable and are far away from any health center. So most of these people now will prefer to go to the TBA." (Health provider, FGD1)

In some cases, PCMH staff had contributed to the transportation barrier to FBD by sending a delivering woman back home because she was not far enough progressed in labor. Staying closer to the hospital around the due date was discussed as an option.

"I came in labor, but it was the latency phase, they returned me back home. Then later, labor progressed in the middle of the night, so I was unable to come back to the hospital, because I was living out of Freetown. (...) I went to a retired midwife and delivered at home because of the distance." (Pregnant woman, FGD3)

"If I lived far off, I would think about a relative that stays very close to the health facility, so about one or two weeks before my delivery time, I go closer to the health center and stay with my sister who is already there. So by the time of contractions, I don't need to delay by getting to the health facility (...) It would ease so many problems." (Health provider, FGD2)

"In PCMH, there is a waiting room. But sometimes the patients refuse to stay, because if they have their farm work to do, they will not leave it there, so they refuse to stay. Also this waiting area is only for women with high risk pregnancy, so the others have to go home." (Health provider, FGD2)

The participants did not consider the ambulance system as helpful to facilitate transportation because of lack of sufficient ambulance cars. Even if women have a possibility to go to PCMH by car, public transport or ambulance, they mentioned that heavy traffic in Freetown would not permit easy access to the hospital.

"Ambulance is there, but there is no fuel, the relatives need to provide fuel, and they don't have the money. Also, the ambulances only cover the district

headquarters. They are not in the villages." (Health provider, FGD2)

"That is another problem. Most of the times these (smaller) health centers don't have an ambulance. So the time they will call for an ambulance, you think of the traffic, you think of the poor road network, the condition of the patient should have gone worse. Most of these patients are dead on arrival" (Health provider, FGD1)

Discussion

This qualitative assessment aimed at reflecting patients´ and providers´ current frames of mind regarding institutional delivery in a setting characterized by extreme poverty, high maternal mortality and ongoing recovery from a major health system collapse during the Ebola outbreak. We observed heterogeneous perspectives on FBD, and identified several intrinsic as well as extrinsic barriers, which were largely concurring with outcomes from a recent systematic review of qualitative evidence on facilitators and barriers to FBD in low- and middle income countries [11].

Overall, study participants expressed a general agreement on health facilities being the safest and most reasonable option for delivering a baby. This confirms earlier findings from Tanzania, where women were highly knowledgeable about the fact that complications during delivery are best manageable at health facilities [12]. Bohren et al. likewise endorsed that health facilities were usually perceived as providing high quality care [11].

At the same time, and somewhat contradictory, the strong perception of advantages of FBD stood alongside a frequently expressed fear of hospital admission and preference for home delivery. This discrepancy, largely acting between the poles of rationality and emotionality, represents a major intrinsic conflict in the context of FBD. The underlying scheme is also transferable to what Bohren et al. have described as an "intersection of traditionalism and modernity" [11]. While "modernity" equates to decision-making in favor of high-standard medical care and obstetric technologies based on the rationale that this will result in increased safety and survival, the "traditionalism" aspect is strongly linked to the influence of a woman's social and cultural environment and the desire to be accompanied and emotionally supported by a trusted person. An event like the Ebola outbreak is likely to increase emotions like fear and mistrust in authorities, and thereby counteracts allegedly rational arguments for institutionalized health care, as also suggested in a systematic review on effects of Ebola on health care utilization [4]. Other studies corroborate the general relevance of our finding that familiar support and care during home delivery might outweigh reasoning for FBD for many women [13, 14].

This is even more the case when women were having bad experiences with inattentive, careless or even rude health staff at the hospital. Unfavorable attitudes of staff were subject to a number of studies in the context of FBD [15–17], and are a constant emerging theme when describing experiences with FBD, ranging from verbal abuse and ignorance to even physical abuse like slapping. A recent study from rural Sierra Leone observed that poor women were particularly prone to unsupportive staff attitudes, with health facilities structurally reflecting social power imbalances within a society [2]. Oyerinde et al. [16] argued that humanized care based on women's dignity during delivery is one of the major determinants of patient satisfaction with maternity services and vital for the public perception of FBD, while a study in Benin concluded that it could even positively influence the progress of birth, like less need of medication [18]. Several studies confirm our finding that patients and especially providers accuse the health system to be responsible for overloaded staff and unbearable working conditions, resulting in a climate of demotivation, frustration and harshness [15]. In any case, respectful and attentive staff attitudes are crucial when aiming at building confidence among delivering women in an institutional environment where they do not know anyone and are in a state of fear. To compete with the trusted social environment of a woman during home delivery, health service implementers need to recognize the pertinence of this topic, and consequently address unfavorable working conditions of staff as well as increase their social and communicative skills in stressful situations. The option of allowing an accompanying person into delivery wards to support a woman throughout the process of giving birth, as it has been practiced in European countries for several generations, could be a worthwhile consideration to improve FBD attractiveness [15, 19, 20]. Continuous emotional support and advocacy may result in increased feeling of control and competence in the delivering woman, with multiple potential benefits. As a Cochrane trial review on the topic showed, one-to-one birth companionship of any person, including unskilled family members, was not only associated with fewer negative views on delivery of the women, but also with improved birth outcomes, like more spontaneous deliveries and less pain medication. [20] In many resource-poor health settings including PCMH, allowing additional persons´ presence in delivery wards is challenging because of restricted space conditions. However, given the importance of this theme and the simplicity of this no-cost measure, health decision makers should take into serious account how this could be realized and included into health policies.

Long distance to the hospital and lack or unaffordability of transportation was among the strongest extrinsic barriers women mentioned for FBD. Poor geographic access and prohibitive costs of transportation are a key barrier for seeking institutional, particularly emergency obstetric care in the sub-Saharan African Region and have been recognized as such for a long time. [2, 11–13, 21, 22] Yet, to date, little innovative thought has been conceded to the question of how delivering women in these resource-poor and often secluded settings can reach a health facility at the right time [23]. As it stands, ambulance systems are not a reliable nor affordable option in our Sierra Leonean setting as well as in many similar other ones. Recent research on a free ambulance system in Ethiopia has shown that its uptake halved pregnancy-related mortality in the related districts, strongly suggesting that this could be a highly valuable strategy if further pursued [23]. Ways to establish free, continuously and widely available ambulance systems covering remote areas should be included as a priority issue into health strategic plans with the goal of reducing maternal mortality.

Limitations

This is one of the first studies after the 2014–2015 Ebola outbreak that looks into perspectives on FBD in Sierra Leone. A limitation of our study is the restriction to participant recruitment from only one health facility, PCMH. Further assessments should involve different facility types including private clinics and peripheral health units, and should also be conducted in other parts of the country including non-urban settings, to be able to generalize our results. Also, we cannot entirely exclude response bias given the FGDs were conducted within the hospital setting; however, all participants were assured that nothing they would discuss would be later attributed to them personally, and our findings generally suggest that there was no shyness among participants to express critical opinions. Logistic constraints of the study setting did not allow for conducting FGDs with home-delivering women directly in their communities or with other influential groups including TBAs and elderly people, nor for comparing experiences of PCMH clients to women having delivered in a facility allowing birth companions in the delivery ward. These aspects could have broadened our spectrum of findings, and further research in this regard would certainly be valuable.

Conclusion

In conclusion, women in our study setting were aware of the higher maternal and newborn safety linked with FBD, but this often diverged from their individual desire to deliver in a supportive and trusted social and traditional environment. In this desire, they seem to be highly susceptible to the influence of close resource persons like husbands or elder family members. Logistic issues with long travel distances and late referral from smaller health centers appeared as another frequent problem for FBDs. Accommodating delivering women's emotional state of insecurity and fear by more supportive staff attitudes and the possibility of an accompanying person at her side throughout the process of giving birth could be promising approaches to increase confidence in health institutions. However, these approaches also imply revising health systems structures, like working conditions of hospital staff conducive for a friendly atmosphere, like sufficient space in delivery wards allowing the women to bring a birth companion, or like the establishment of a reliable peripheral ambulance system. In Sierra Leone, where more women die during childbirth than in virtually any other country, it should be a primary goal of health policy makers to mitigate the barriers to FBD in every possible way, and further implementation research assessing effectiveness of the different approaches would be highly desirable for the future.

Acknowledgements
Many thanks are owed to Ms. Margaret T. Sesay, the study nurse in PCMH conducting the FGDs, and to all the study participants in PCMH, Freetown.

Funding
This study was conducted with support of the ESTHER-clinic partnership program of the German Agency for International Cooperation (GIZ) and the Federal Ministry for Economic Cooperation and Development, who had no influence on the design of the study, on collection, analysis, and interpretation of data, and on writing the manuscript.

Authors' contributions
ST contributed to this research by designing the study, participating as an observer in FGDs, transcribing audio tapes, analyzing the data and writing the manuscript. APK contributed by designing and planning the study and preparing data collection. GH contributed by designing and planning the study. All authors read and approved the final manuscript.

Competing interests
The authors declare that they have no competing interests.

Author details
[1]Institute of Tropical Medicine and International Health, Charité-Universitätsmedizin, Augustenburger Platz 1, 13353 Berlin, Germany.
[2]Department of Obstetrics and Gynecology, Princess Christian Maternity Hospital, Freetown, Sierra Leone.

References

1. WHO, UNICEF. UNFPA, World Bank Group, and United Nations population division, maternal mortality estimation inter-agency group. Maternal mortality in. 1990-2015;2015 http://www.who.int/gho/maternal_health/countries/sle.pdf. Accessed April 18, 2018.
2. Treacy L, Bolkan HA, Sagbakken M. Distance, accessibility and costs. Decision- making during childbirth in rural Sierra Leone: a qualitative study. PLoS One. 2018;13(2):e0188280. https://doi.org/10.1371/journal.pone.0188280.
3. Orya E, Adaji S, Pyone T, Wurie H, van den Broek N, Theobald S. Strengthening close to community provision of maternal health services in fragile settings: an exploration of the changing roles of TBAs in Sierra Leone and Somaliland. BMC Health Serv Res. 2017;17:460.
4. Brolin Ribacke KJ, Nordenstedt H, Höijer J, Molnes R, Froseth TW, et al. The impact of the West Africa Ebola outbreak on obstetric health Care in Sierra Leone. PLoS One. 2016;11(2):e0150080. https://doi.org/10.1371/journal.pone.0150080.
5. Lori JR, Rominski PJE, Munro ML, Williams G, Bell SA, et al. A case series study on the effect of Ebola on facility-based deliveries in rural Liberia. BMC Pregnancy Childb. 2015;15:254. https://doi.org/10.1186/s12884-015-0694-x.
6. Statistics Sierra Leone and ICF International. Sierra Leone Demographic and Health Survey. In: Key findings. Rockville, Maryland, USA: Statistics Sierra Leone and ICF International; 2013. p. 2014. https://dhsprogram.com/pubs/pdf/SR215/SR215.pdf. Accessed April 18, 2018.
7. UNICEF. Sierra Leone Health Facility Survey. Assessing the impact of the EVD outbreak on health systems in Sierra Leone. 2014:2014 https://www.unicef.org/emergencies/ebola/files/SL_Health_Facility_Survey_2014Dec3.pdf. Accessed April 17, 2018.
8. VSO International. Exploring the impact of the Ebola outbreak on routine maternal health services in Sierra Leone. 2015. https://www.vsointernational.org/file/554/download?token=74820Ho8. Accessed April 17, 2018.
9. Princess Christian Maternity Hospital. 2016 annual report of PCMH activities. Freetown, 2017.
10. Onwuegbuzie AJ, Dickinson WB, Leech NL, Zoran AG. A qualitative framework for collecting and analyzing data in focus group research. Int J Qual Meth. 2009;8(3).
11. Bohren MA, Hunter EC, Munthe-Kaas HM, Souza JP, Vogel JP Gülmezoglu M. Facilitators and barriers to facility-based delivery in low- and middle-income countries: a qualitative evidence synthesis. Reprod Health. 2014;11:71.
12. Women´s Dignity, Care International Tanzania. We have no choice. Facility-based childbirth: The perceptions and experiences of Tanzanian women, health workers, and traditional birth attendants. Dar es Salaam, Tanzania: Women´s Dignity and Care International; 2008.
13. Wilunda C, Scanagatta C, Putoro G, Takahashi R, Montalbetti F, Segafredo G, Betran AP. Barriers to institutional childbirth in Rumbek North County, South Sudan: a qualitative study. PLoS One. 2016;11(12):e0168083. https://doi.org/10.1371/journal.pone.0168083.
14. Shiferaf S, Spigt M, Godefrooij M, Melkamu TM. Why do women prefer home births in Ethiopia? BMC Pregnancy Childb. 2013;13(5) https://doi.org/10.1186/1471-2393-13-5.
15. Bohren MA, Vogel JP, Tuncalp Ö, Fawole B, Titiloye MA, Olutayo AO. Mistreatment of women during childbirth in Abuja. Nigeria: a qualitative study on perceptions and experiences of women and healthcare providers Rep Health. 2017;14:9. https://doi.org/10.1186/s12978-016-0265-22017.
16. Oyerinde K, Harding Y, Amara P, Garbrah-Aidoo N, Kanu R, Oulare M, et al. A qualitative evaluation of the choice of traditional birth attendants for maternity care in 2008 Sierra Leone: implications for universal skilled attendance at delivery. Matern Child Health J. 2013;17:862–8. https://doi.org/10.1007/s10995-012-1061-4.
17. D'Ambruoso L, Abbey M, Hussein J. Please understand when I cry out in pain: women's accounts of maternity services during labour and delivery in Ghana. BMC Public Health. 2005;5:140. https://doi.org/10.1186/1471-2458-5-140.
18. Fujita N, Perrin XR, Vodounon JA, Gozo MK, Matsumoto Y, Uchida S, Sugiura Y. Humanised care and a change in practice in a hospital in Benin. Midwifery. 2011;28(4):421–8.
19. Gebrehiwot T, Goicolea I, Edin K, San Sebastian M. Making pragmatic choices: women's experiences of delivery care in northern Ethiopia. BMC Pregnancy Childb. 2012;12:113. https://doi.org/10.1186/1471-2393-12-113.
20. Hodnett ED, Gates S, Hofmeyr GJ, Sakala C. Continuous support for women during childbirth. Cochrane Database Syst Rev. 2013;7 CD003766.
21. Gabrysch S, Cousens S, Cox J, Campbell OMR. The influence of distance and level of care on Deliveryin rural Zambia: a study of linked National Data in a geographic information system. PLoS Med. 2011;8(1): e1000394). https://doi.org/10.1371/journal.pmed.1000394.
22. Panciera R, Khan A, Rizvi SJR, Ahmed S, Ahmed T, Islam R, Adam AM. The influence of travel time on emergency obstetric care seeking behavior in the urban poor of Bangladesh: a GIS study. BMC Pregnancy Childb. 2016;16:240. https://doi.org/10.1186/s12884-016-1032-7.
23. Godefay H, Kinsman J, Admasu K, Byass P. Can innovative ambulance transport avert pregnancy–related deaths? One–year operational assessment in Ethiopia. J Glob Health. 2016;6(1). https://doi.org/10.7189/jogh.06.010410.

Trends in repeated pregnancy among adolescents in the Philippines from 1993 to 2013

Joemer C. Maravilla[1,2*], Kim S. Betts[1,2] and Rosa Alati[1,2,3]

Abstract

Objective: The extent of repeated pregnancy (RP) and repeated birth (RB) among adolescents aged 15–19 is still unknown in the Philippines despite the health and socio-economic consequences. This study aims to investigate the RP and RB prevalence trends in the Philippines from 1993 to 2013.

Methods: A total of 7091 women aged 15–24 who experienced at least one pregnancy were captured in the Philippine demographic health surveys from 1993 to 2013. Annual RP and RB prevalence per age group in three and five categories were calculated and stratified by region, type of residence and wealth index. Cochran–Armitage tests and multivariate logistic regression were applied to determine trend estimates.

Results: Compared to women aged 19–21 years and 22–24 years, for which decreasing patterns were found, RP ([Adjusted Odds ratio (AOR =0.96; 95%Confidence interval (CI) =0.82–1.11) and RB (AOR = 0.90; CI = 0.73–1.10) trends among 15–18 year olds showed negligible reduction over the 20 years. From a baseline prevalence of 20.39% in 1993, the prevalence of RP among adolescents had only reduced to 18.06% by 2013. Moreover, the prevalence of RB showed a negligible decline from 8.49% in 1993 to 7.80% in 2013. Although RP and RB prevalence were generally found more elevated in poorer communities, no differences in trends were noted across wealth quintiles.

Conclusion: For two decades, the Philippines has shown a constant and considerably high RP prevalence. Further investigation, not only in the Philippines but also in other developing countries, is necessary to enable development of secondary prevention programs.

Plain English summary

Despite high and stable levels of adolescent fertility in the Philippines, no specific research has been conducted to specifically measure the trend and magnitude of repeated adolescent pregnancy, which is defined as an adolescent who has had at least two pregnancies. Repeated pregnancy, therefore needs to be investigated as it reflects not only the reproductive health of adolescent mothers but also disparities in service delivery of health, education and welfare support to adolescents after their first pregnancy.

We used the Philippine Demographic and Health Surveys to sample 7091 women aged 15–24 who experienced at least one pregnancy. Annual RP and RB prevalence per age group in three and five categories were calculated and stratified by region, type of residence and wealth quintile. Trends were statistically analysed using Cochran–Armitage tests and multivariate logistic regression.

While a decline was observed in 19–21 and 22–24 year olds, we found a constant prevalence of one in every five in 15–18 years old from 1993 to 2013. This trend was evident across all regions, types of residence and socio-economic status. Our analysis also found that those from the poorest wealth quintile demonstrated a heightened risk of repeated pregnancy compared to other quintiles. The non-decreasing prevalence trend of repeated pregnancy among adolescents indicated the need for secondary prevention programs particularly for the poorest households. Epidemiological investigations are also necessary to explore the causes and impact of

* Correspondence: joemer.maravilla@uqconnect.edu.au
[1]School of Public Health, The University of Queensland, Herston, QLD, Australia
[2]Institute for Social Science Research, The University of Queensland, Indooroopilly, QLD, Australia
Full list of author information is available at the end of the article

repeated pregnancy on maternal, child and neonatal health, not only in the Philippines, but also among other low- and middle-income countries.

Introduction

The adolescent pregnancy epidemic in the Philippines has been acknowledged as one of the worst in the Western Pacific Region [1] with a recent prevalence of 13.6% among 15–19 year olds. The Philippines is the only country in this region with no significant decline in adolescent fertility in the past decades [2] from 56 per 1000 in 1973 to 57 per 1000 in 2013 [2, 3]. In order to address this entrenched public health issue, preventive policies and programs have been implemented [4, 5], and epidemiological studies have been developed to provide evidence of the current sexual health and behaviour of Filipino adolescents [6]. However, these measures have put little emphasis on the more serious problem of repeated adolescent pregnancies.

Repeated adolescent pregnancy, which is defined as a subsequent pregnancy among adolescents aged 10–19 years [7] is known to affect around 18% of adolescent mothers in the USA [7], Europe [8], and Australia [9]. Despite the evident chance of repeated adolescent pregnancy especially within 2 years postpartum [10], current research is unable to clearly establish its magnitude in developing countries such as the Philippines, nor how the trends have changed across time [11–13]. Although a World Health Organization (WHO) multi-country report [14] discussed the relationship between age and parity among Filipino adolescents, this study did not assess the prevalence of multi parity as its primary measure.

As a marker for adolescent reproductive health, repeated pregnancy reflects health disparities particularly among the disadvantaged adolescent population. Repeated pregnancy also indicates poor distribution and unequal access to reproductive health services [15] and inadequate service capacity of individual localities. It relates to low educational attainment, limited employment opportunities and poverty among adolescent mothers [15, 16]. It has been shown that repeated adolescent pregnancy leads to an increase in national health and welfare expenditure as a consequence of the long-term dependency of adolescents and their families on government assistance [15, 17].

An increasing trend of adolescent sexual activity [3] ongoing poor compliance with modern contraceptives [2, 18] and inadequate use of family planning services all suggest that repeated adolescent pregnancy is highly prevalent in the Philippines [12]. Analysis of existing nationally representative data can be helpful in evaluating the extent of this public health problem. In this study, we aim to determine the prevalence of repeated pregnancies and births among adolescents and young adults from a series of national surveys conducted between 1993 and 2013. Moreover, we intend to analyze the trend of repeated pregnancies and births by age groupings and potential macro-level confounders across two decades, with resulting trends perhaps reflecting the effectiveness of existing policies and programs in addressing this under-recognized adolescent health problem.

Methods

Population and sample

This study used the Philippine Demographic and Health Survey (DHS) from 1993, 1998, 2003, 2008, and 2013 which are cross-sectional surveys conducted every 5 years. This nationally representative survey involved a multi-stage sampling design up to the household level with enumeration areas distributed by region and type of residence using the most recent national census as its sampling frame. All women in the selected households which includes adolescents aged 15–19 years and young adults aged 20–24 years were interviewed using the Individual Woman's Questionnaire. This survey therefore excludes adolescents aged below 15 years. As shown in Appendix, the majority of the survey sample belonged to these age brackets which we will refer to as adolescents for the succeeding parts of this paper.

Outcome and socio-geographic measures

Repeated adolescent pregnancy/birth

An adolescent aged 15–19 years was considered as having experienced repeated pregnancy (RP) if she had experienced at least two pregnancies, including current pregnancies, which either resulted in a live birth and/or pregnancy loss. A case of repeated birth (RB) was defined as an adolescent with at least two live births. These definitions were adapted from related review papers [8] and the Centers for Disease Control and Prevention [7].

Year

Survey year was considered as a continuous variable in the analysis to measure the trend because of equal intervals between survey years. Thus, each unit increase in year variable translates to an actual five-year increase.

Age

Respondents were categorized by age into three and five groups. The three age groups include "15–18" which considers the legal age of consent (18) in the Philippines, "19–21" as the transition period, and "22–24" as young adults [19]. In sensitivity analysis we further subdivided age into five groups (i.e. "15–16", "17–18", "19–20", "21–22", and "22–24") to analyze in detail the trends per age.

Socio-geographic variables

Region refers to the three main island groups: Luzon, Visayas, and Mindanao. We disaggregated and compared all estimates by region since each island group has unique geographical and cultural characteristics. Further disaggregation per administrative region was not pursued, as the number of administrative regions had increased during the 1998. Type of residence was either rural or urban area where the respondent resided at the time of the survey. Based on their household's wealth score, adolescents were grouped into the household wealth quintiles "richest", "richer", "middle", "poorer", and "poorest" class.

Analyses

We calculated the mean, standard deviation and prevalence rate of RP and RB per year per age group. RP prevalence was calculated by dividing the number of adolescents with RP and the number of adolescents who experienced at least one pregnancy (including those currently pregnant) multiplied by 100. RB prevalence on the other hand was calculated by dividing the number of adolescents with RB and the number of adolescents who experienced at least one livebirth multiplied by 100. Deformalized survey weights were applied while calculating the prevalence.

We used the *ptrendi* package in Stata13 to perform Cochran–Armitage tests to determine the prevalence trend per age group using the chi-square statistic and meeting the assumptions of an additive model. Cochran–Armitage test is a modified Pearson's chi-square test which assesses the association between binary (i.e. RP and RB) and ordinal (i.e. year and age) categories. Multivariate logistic regression analysis with interaction effects for age (i.e. age groups using both three and five categories) and year was conducted while using repeated pregnancy and birth as binary outcome variables (i.e. yes or no). We measured the trend between two consecutive survey years to identify which periods had significant changes in prevalence. In addition, we analyzed trends using year and socio-geographic (i.e. region, type of residence, and wealth index) interaction per age group. For the purpose of this analysis, we used the three category age group as this was the only categorization which allowed a sufficient number of cases.

Results

Among women aged 15–24 years with at least one pregnancy ($n = 7091$), a large proportion (53.3%) were found among the 22–24 year olds. Despite the small proportion of adolescents captured by the surveys, the proportion of 15–18 year olds reported in the survey has increased over time from 7.64% ($n = 107$) in 1993 to 15.55% ($n = 213$) in 2013 (*see* Table 1).

Trend analysis per age group

Cochran–Armitage tests showed an overall decrease in the trend of RP (Chi2 = 127.60; $p < 0.001$) across 20 years among the 15–24 years old from a weighted RP prevalence ($WtPrev_{RP}$) of 58.12% in 1993 to 40.58% in 2013. There was also a general RB (Chi2 = 100.90; $p < 0.001$) reduction from weighted RB prevalence ($WtPrev_{RB}$) of 51.25% to 35.66%. However, within age groupings this decline was not observed among 15–18 years olds. In Fig. 1, we only found a slight decrease in RP prevalence from 20.39% in 1993 to 18.06% in 2013. RB prevalence also presented a minimal change with 0.69 decline among 15–18 and 0.80 decline among 17–18 years olds in this 20-year period (*see* Fig. 2). Further observations among 17–18 years olds showed a similar RP trend from 22.26 to 18.52%.

Similar results were found in the regression analysis. The RP trend among 15–18 year olds remained virtually unchanged across all surveys from 1993 to 2013 [Odds ratio (OR) =0.93; 95% Confidence interval (CI) =0.81–1.07]. There was a similar pattern of RB trend in this age group (OR = 0.87; CI = 0.72–1.06) following an apparent increase in prevalence from 1993 to 1998 (OR = 3.29; CI = 1.25–8.62). On the other hand, the older age groups showed a significant decline both for RP and RB with unadjusted ORs ranging from 0.83 to 0.87 (*see* Table 2). Analyses using five age categories showed no significant difference in the trends previously described. Trends among 15–16 and 17–18 year old adolescents remained unchanged, whereas a decreasing trend was apparent for those aged 19–20, 21–22 and 23–24.

Adjustments for regions, types of residence and wealth quintile suggested that the trends were not confounded by these factors across all age groups. Interestingly, wealth index was strongly associated with RP and RB as adolescents from the poorest quintile had shown higher odds in reference to richest quintile ($OR_{RP} = 5.41$, CI = 4.31–6.78; $OR_{RB} = 5.36$, CI = 4.17–6.89). Calculation of weighted prevalence confirmed this association with a $WtPrev_{RP}$ of 59.60% and $WtPrev_{RB}$ of 52.50%.

Change of prevalence between two consecutive survey years was also analyzed using the three age categories. We found that there was a decrease in RP prevalence among 15–18 from 1998 to 2003 (OR = 0.52; CI = 0.28–0.99), and among 22–24 from 1993 to 1998 (OR = 0.77; CI = 0.61–0.97) and 2003–2008 (OR = 0.71; CI = 0.58–0.88). A drop in RB prevalence was also found among 15–18 from 1998 to 2003 (OR = 0.32; OR = 0.13–0.81); and among 22–24 from 1993 to 1998 (OR = 0.74; CI = 0.58–0.93).

Trend per socio-geographic variable per age group

The constant RP trend among 15–18 and the decreasing RP trend among 22–24 were found in all regions, types

Table 1 Characteristics of the respondents

Characteristics	1993		1998		2003		2008		2013		TOTAL
	n	%	n	%	n	%	n	%	n	%	
Age (in 3 groups)											
15–18	107	7.64	124	9.74	128	9.54	165	11.97	213	12.55	**737**
19–21	460	32.86	449	35.27	429	31.97	479	34.74	580	34.18	**2397**
22–24	833	59.50	700	54.99	785	58.49	735	53.30	904	53.27	**3957**
Age (in 5 groups)											
15–16	14	1.00	19	1.49	21	1.56	33	2.39	45	2.65	**132**
17–18	93	6.64	105	8.25	107	7.97	132	9.57	168	9.90	**605**
19–20	268	19.14	268	21.05	269	20.04	300	21.75	352	20.74	**1457**
21–22	429	30.64	387	30.40	385	28.69	402	29.15	502	29.58	**2105**
23–24	596	42.57	494	38.81	560	41.73	512	37.13	630	37.12	**2792**
Region											
Luzon	685	48.93	523	41.08	728	54.25	699	50.69	870	51.27	**3505**
Visayas	275	19.64	244	19.17	187	13.93	229	16.61	232	13.67	**1167**
Mindanao	440	31.43	506	39.75	427	31.82	451	32.70	595	35.06	**2419**
Type of residence											
Urban	604	43.14	481	37.78	672	50.07	554	40.00	761	44.84	**3072**
Rural	796	56.86	792	62.22	670	49.93	825	59.83	936	55.16	**4019**
Wealth quintile											
Poorest	420	30.00	425	33.39	372	27.72	377	27.00	416	24.51	**2010**
Poorer	342	24.43	355	27.89	325	24.22	344	25.00	414	24.40	**1780**
Middle	292	20.86	210	16.50	272	20.27	256	18.56	389	22.92	**1419**
Richer	214	15.00	173	14.00	203	15.00	233	17.00	305	17.97	**1128**
Richest	132	9.43	110	8.64	170	12.67	169	12.26	173	10.19	**754**
With at least 1 birth[a]	1260	90.00	1124	88.30	1181	88.00	1163	84.34	1471	86.68	**6199**
With repeated pregnancy	825	58.93	680	53.42	662	49.33	571	41.41	704	41.48	**3442**
With repeated birth[b]	660	25.04	532	20.18	495	18.78	420	15.93	529	20.07	**2636**
TOTAL[+]	**1400**	**100**	**1273**	**100**	**1342**	**100**	**1379**	**100**	**1697**	**100**	**7091**

Abbreviations: *n*-Number of respondents
[a]Birth pertains to livebirth; [b] Adolescents with at least 1 pregnancy
Data captured in bold are highly significant

of residence and wealth quintiles (*see* Table 3). On the other hand, the decline of RP decline among 19–21 was only consistent across regions and types of residence. Only the poorer households showed a 20-year reduction when compared to the other four quintiles.

A similar pattern was observed for RB trend among those aged between 15 and 18 and 22–24. Unlike RP, the trend for RB among 19–21 year olds was inconsistent across the three socio-geographic variables. The decreasing trend was only found in Visayas and Mindanao region, rural communities, and poor wealth quintiles (*see* Fig. 3).

In each age group, we also conducted adjusted Wald tests to measure the difference of trend estimates between the categories of each socio-geographic variable. No differences were observed for 15–18. For 19–21, differences were only found between the RP trend estimates of poorest and poorer quintiles, and between the RB trend estimates rural and urban communities. For 22–24, differences between the trend estimates of poorest and richest, and between poorer and richest were found both for RP and RB.

Discussions

Despite the declining trends of RP and RB in older age groups, the prevalence among adolescents younger than 18 years showed no decrease across 20 years of data, remaining stable across all regions, types of residence, and wealth quintiles. The prevalence was high with approximately one in every five adolescents aged 15–18 years with a history of pregnancy experiencing RP while one in every ten of those who had a livebirth experienced RB.

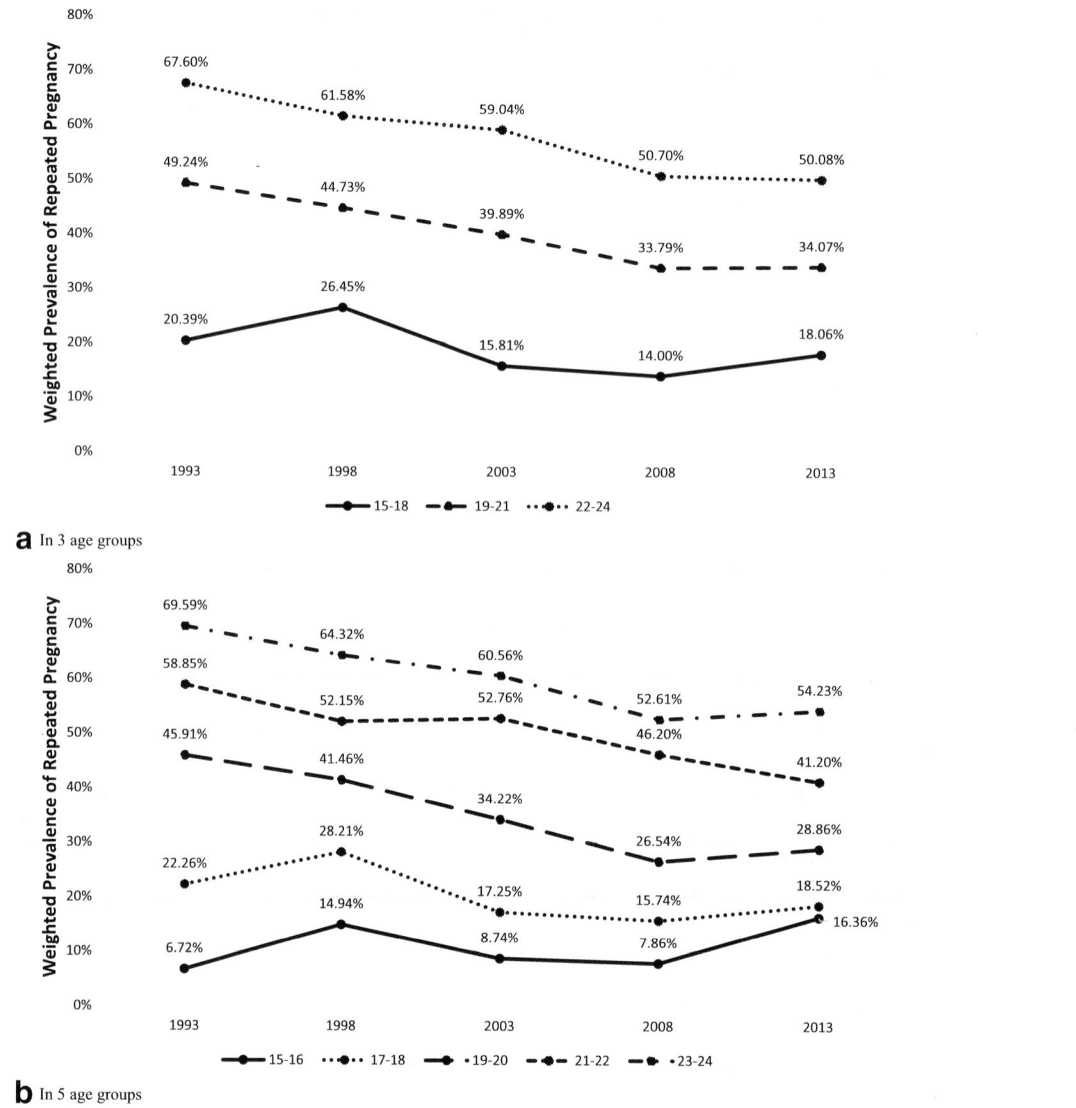

Fig. 1 Prevalence trends of adolescents with repeated pregnancy in the Philippines from 1993 to 2013 by age group. Caption: This figure presents the weighted prevalence of repeated pregnancy using age groups with (**a**) three and (**b**) five categories. Groups using the three categories include 15–18 years old, 19–21 years old and 22–24 years old while the five categories including 15–16 years old, 17–18 years old, 19–20 years old, 21–22 years old and 23–24 years old, as represented by each line on the graphs. The x-axis is the survey year arranged in chronological order while the y-axis the weighted prevalence

While the decreasing RP and RB trend among young adults can likely be attributed to their improved contraceptive use [20] and awareness of and participation in family planning (FP) strategies [3, 21]. The unchanged trend among adolescents may result from the unique socio-cultural characteristics and FP policies in the Philippines, wherein adolescents are prevented from accessing FP services, even after their first pregnancy. One of the possible explanations for this finding is that the strong influence of the Catholic church at the local level may have affected the health seeking behavior and the implementation of reproductive health programs among adolescents [22, 23].

Unclear and restricted health and health-related policies for adolescent mothers may also play a role. The initial adolescent health policy in the Philippines [24], which aimed to reduce unwanted pregnancies and provide adolescent-friendly health services, did not include strategies for dealing with the prevention of secondary pregnancies [25, 26]. This may have led to adolescents being discouraged to access essential health information and use birth control methods [23, 27].

Despite emphasizing the importance of health promotion and behavioral change, a recently introduced national law (Responsible Parenthood and Reproductive Health Act of 2012 or RH Law) and framework [4], did

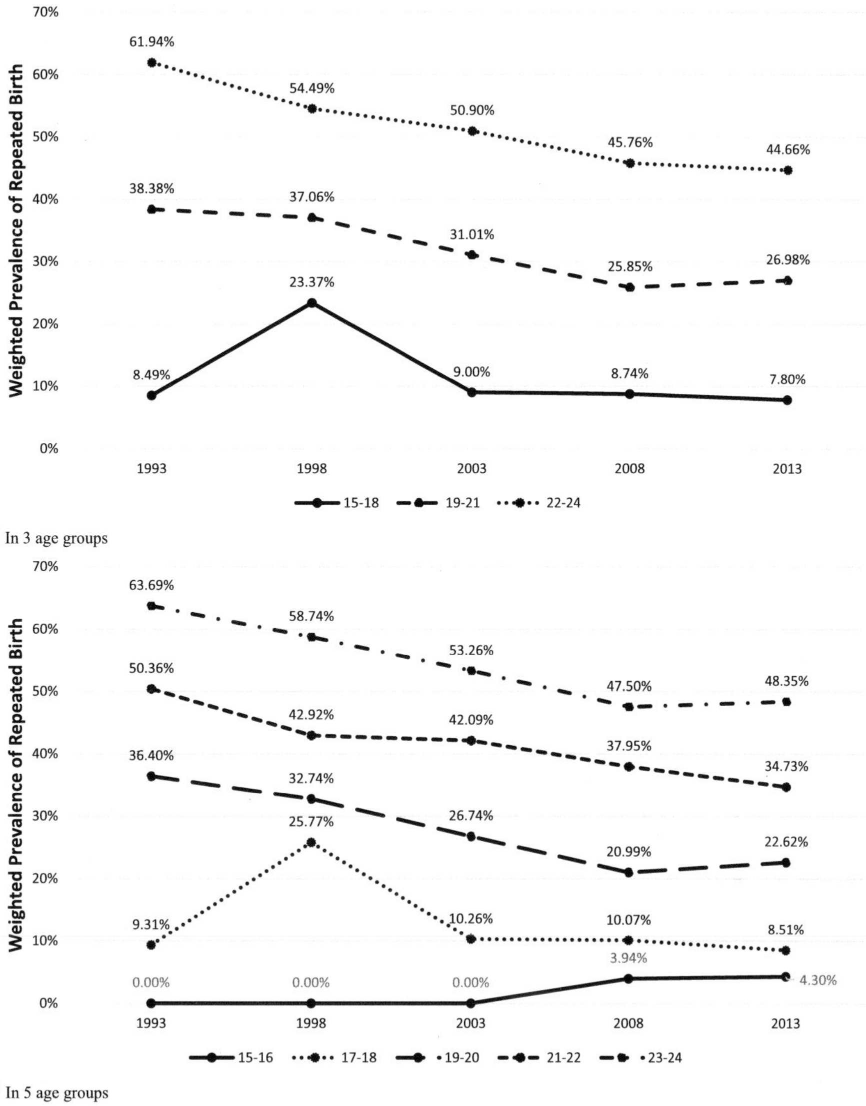

Fig. 2 Prevalence trends of adolescents with repeated birth in the Philippines from 1993 to 2013 by age group. Caption: This figure presents the weighted prevalence of repeated birth using age groups with (**a**) three and (**b**) five categories. Groups using the three categories include 15–18 years old, 19–21 years old and 22–24 years old while the five categories including 15–16 years old, 17–18 years old, 19–20 years old, 21–22 years old and 23–24 years old, as represented by each line on the graphs. The x-axis is the survey year arranged in chronological order while the y-axis the weighted prevalence

not embrace specific programmatic actions to address RP. The RH Law still prevents minors (i.e. below 18 years old) from accessing modern methods of contraception without parental consent and does not exempt adolescent mothers and adolescents who experienced miscarriage [28]. This policy restriction has already been found as a deterrent for adolescents to access contraceptives and counselling services in a review of evidence from 16 developing countries [29]. This study suggests that despite the availability of contraception, most of these developing countries retain barriers and restrictions towards the use of birth control methods, particularly among unmarried adolescents. In the context of this social and political environment, the RP/RB trends showed in this paper can be expected to continue for several years to come not only in the Philippines but also in other developing countries.

The role and reach of secondary prevention programs must be clarified due to the limited access to appropriate postnatal services (e.g. contraception, counselling, and educational support) for adolescent mothers. Health workers may also need to be trained to address the unique psychosocial characteristics and support the challenging developmental transition of very young mothers by enhancing adolescents' readiness and decision-making abilities to delay another pregnancy

Table 2 Trend analysis of repeated pregnancy and birth adolescents from 1993 to 2013 per age group

Year x Age Contrasts	Unadjusted Model			Adjusted Model [b]		
	OR	CI	*p*-value	AOR	CI	*p*-value
Repeated pregnancy						
Age (in 3 groups)						
15–18	0.93	0.81–1.07	0.330	0.96	0.82–1.11	0.566
19-21 [a]	0.85	0.80-0.90	< 0.001	0.86	0.81–0.92	< 0.001
22–24 [a]	0.83	0.79–0.87	< 0.001	0.84	0.80–0.88	< 0.001
Age (in 5 groups)						
15–16	1.24	0.79–1.96	0.351	1.35	0.82–2.23	0.234
17–18	0.91	0.79–1.06	0.229	0.93	0.80–1.09	0.382
19–20 [a]	0.82	0.76–0.89	< 0.001	0.82	0.76–0.90	< 0.001
21–22 [a]	0.84	0.79–0.89	< 0.001	0.85	0.80–0.91	< 0.001
23–24 [a]	0.84	0.80–0.89	< 0.001	0.85	0.80–0.90	< 0.001
Repeated birth						
Age (in 3 groups)						
15–18	0.87	0.72–1.06	0.181	0.90	0.73–1.10	0.311
19–21 [a]	0.87	0.81–0.93	< 0.001	0.88	0.83–0.95	< 0.001
22–24 [a]	0.84	0.80–0.88	< 0.001	0.85	0.82–0.89	< 0.001
Age (in 5 groups)						
15–16	2.15	0.54–8.57	0.275	2.47	0.54–11.46	0.245
17–18	0.87	0.72–1.07	0.186	0.90	0.73–1.11	0.316
19-20 [a]	0.83	0.76-0.89	< 0.001	0.85	0.77–0.93	0.001
21–22 [a]	0.86	0.80–0.92	< 0.001	0.87	0.82–0.94	< 0.001
23–24 [a]	0.85	0.80–0.90	< 0.001	0.86	0.81–0.91	< 0.001

Abbreviations: OR-Odds ratio; CI-95% Confidence Interval
[a]Significant during Cochran test at 0.001 level; [b] Adjusted for region, type of residence and wealth quintile

and/or use modern family planning methods. Given the high rate of unmet need for modern contraception among married adolescents [21], policy initiatives/reforms such as providing exemption on contraception to adolescent mothers may be needed to achieve a reduction in the trend seen in this paper.

Our findings also suggest that prevention programs aimed at those from the poorest quintile may be warranted due to the high RP/RB prevalence among this group. In the Philippines and other low- and middle-income countries (LMICs), attempts to reach out to households from the poorest sector have been undertaken through the Conditional Cash Transfer (CCT) Program [30, 31]. For example, the CCT program in Mexico has been found to indirectly reduce adolescent pregnancy and increase contraceptive use among adolescents and young adults [31]. The potential of cash incentive schemes can also be used as an opportunity to monitor and provide prevention programs to adolescent mothers, particularly within 24 months after their first pregnancy [10].

Our study uniquely explores the status of repeated pregnancy and birth in LMICs in the Asia-pacific Region. Most published reports on this topic are primarily from the USA, Europe, and Australia [32]. Of the few reports identified from LMICs, many used birth order (i.e. 2nd order or higher) and a different denominator (i.e. total number of adolescents) in the computation of prevalence. Despite the availability of possible data sources among LMICs [33], few studies have attempted to look specifically at the distribution of adolescents and young adults with RP/RB. Most of the reports available may include vital statistics which is limited to those only with livebirths and does not necessarily account for previous unsuccessful pregnancies.

By placing RP as an issue of crucial importance to the public health especially of LMICs, our paper makes a significant contribution to the literature calling for improvement of sexual and reproductive health of adolescents. The Global Strategy for Adolescent Health for 2030 recognized childbirth and pregnancy complications as one of the two leading causes of death among 15–19 year old girls [34]—addressing RP would help to reduce this. The absence of a reduction in RP trend over 20 years that we identified, signals the need for secondary prevention programs in line with WHO recommendations [35].

This study finds strength in our use of nationally-representative individual datasets instead of aggregate estimates. This prevents the risk of producing results affected by the ecological fallacy, particularly in the analysis of year-age interaction. Furthermore, we were able to perform more thorough analyses such as the adjustment of trend estimates for confounders (i.e. wealth quintile, region, and type of residence).

Limitations
Our study also has limitations. Recall bias and under-reporting are likely to produce bias in any surveys covering information of a sensitive nature. Insufficient record validation is common across the DHS surveys from all countries. However, the DHS' survey procedure enables cross-checking through repeated questions during the interview to reduce the effect of this validation issue. Additionally, our findings may not be comparable to longitudinal studies from developed countries that defined RP as an adolescent who became pregnant within 12–24 months of her first pregnancy/ delivery.

Future research
In addition to cross-sectional analyses that measure RP prevalence, epidemiological investigations are needed to explore the causes and outcomes of RP. Studies conducted in LMICs may identify different associations and dynamics due to the psychosocial and cultural

Table 3 Trend analysis of repeated pregnancy and birth among adolescents per socio-geographic variable in each age group

(Year x Characteristics Contrasts)	Repeated pregnancy									Repeated birth								
	15–18 years old			19–21 years old			22–24 years old			15–18 years old			19–21 years old			22–24 years old		
	OR	CI	p	OR	CI	p	OR	CI	p	OR	CI	p	OR	CI	p	OR	CI	p
Region																		
Luzon	0.82	0.66–1.02	0.08	0.88	0.81–0.96	**0.004**	0.80	0.75–0.86	**< 0.001**	0.86	0.65–1.14	0.291	0.92	0.84–1.02	0.118	0.84	0.79–0.90	**< 0.001**
Visayas	1.09	0.74–1.61	0.65	0.74	0.64–0.86	**< 0.001**	0.84	0.73–0.93	**0.001**	0.94	0.57–1.55	0.801	0.77	0.65–0.91	**0.002**	0.81	0.72–0.91	**< 0.001**
Mindanao	1.04	0.82–1.30	0.763	0.85	0.77–0.94	**0.001**	0.91	0.84–0.93	**0.017**	0.86	0.63–1.18	0.358	0.82	0.74–0.91	**< 0.001**	0.87	0.80–0.94	**0.001**
Type of residence																		
Urban	0.88	0.69–1.11	0.282	0.88	0.80–0.96	**0.006**	0.80	0.74–0.86	**< 0.001**	0.89	0.62–1.27	0.528	0.95	0.85–1.05	0.288	0.81	0.75–0.87	**< 0.001**
Rural	0.98	0.82–1.18	0.85	0.83	0.76–0.90	**< 0.001**	0.86	0.81–0.92	**< 0.001**	0.88	0.69–1.13	0.307	0.81	0.74–0.88	**< 0.001**	0.87	0.82–0.93	**< 0.011**
Wealth quintile																		
Poorest	0.95	0.75–1.20	0.677	0.9	0.81–1.00	0.056	0.90	0.81–0.99	**0.03**	0.82	0.59–1.14	0.239	0.88	0.79–0.98	**0.018**	0.90	0.82–1.00	**0.041**
Poorer	0.90	0.69–1.19	0.463	0.77	0.69–0.86	**< 0.001**	0.87	0.79–0.96	**0.005**	0.97	0.70–1.33	0.833	0.80	0.70–0.91	**0.001**	0.89	0.81–0.98	**0.018**
Middle	0.98	0.71–1.36	0.905	0.92	0.80–1.05	0.202	0.87	0.79–0.95	**0.003**	0.85	0.51–1.44	0.551	0.93	0.79–1.10	0.379	0.87	0.79–0.96	**0.004**
Richer	1.01	0.66–1.53	0.97	0.89	0.75–1.05	0.16	0.82	0.72–0.91	**< 0.001**	1.00	0.53–1.88	0.993	0.96	0.79–1.17	0.685	0.79	0.70–0.89	**< 0.001**
Richest	0.69	0.27–1.80	0.45	0.89	0.70–1.11	0.298	0.68	0.59–0.79	**< 0.001**	NC			0.99	0.76–1.29	0.927	0.73	0.62–0.86	**< 0.001**
Adjusted Wald Test	**F**	**p**		**F**	**p**		**F**	**p**		**F**	**p**		**F**	**p**		**F**	**p**	
Region																		
Luzon vs. Visayas	1.57	0.211		3.69	0.054		0.18	0.668		0.09	0.766		3.58	0.059		0.30	0.585	
Luzon vs. Mindanao	2.04	0.154		0.30	0.582		6.01	**0.014**		0.00	0.967		2.56	0.110		0.47	0.493	
Visayas vs. Mindanao	0.06	0.812		2.07	0.151		1.86	0.173		0.08	0.782		0.47	0.491		1.06	0.302	
Type of residence																		
Urban vs. Rural	0.54	0.462		0.94	0.33		2.62	0.106		0.00	0.951		5.21	**0.023**		2.34	0.127	
Wealth quintile																		
Poorest vs. Poorer	0.07	0.787		4.29	**0.039**		0.13	0.718		0.49	0.485		1.22	0.289		0.04	0.844	
Poorest vs. Middle	0.02	0.876		0.03	0.87		0.20	0.656		0.01	0.907		0.31	0.58		0.35	0.55	
Poorest vs. Richer	0.07	0.797		0.03	0.853		1.43	0.232		0.28	0.595		0.60	0.44		2.74	0.098	
Poorest vs. Richest	0.40	0.528		0.02	0.883		9.18	**0.003**		NA			0.65	0.419		5.00	**0.023**	
Poorer vs. Middle	0.15	0.70		3.64	0.057		0.01	0.933		0.16	0.689		1.90	0.169		0.14	0.705	
Poorer vs. Richer	0.18	0.668		1.87	0.172		0.83	0.363		0.01	0.93		2.27	0.133		2.37	0.124	
Poorer vs. Richest	0.28	0.599		1.14	0.285		7.86	**0.005**		NA			1.96	0.162		4.39	**0.036**	

Table 3 Trend analysis of repeated pregnancy and birth among adolescents per socio-geographic variable in each age group *(Continued)*

(Year x Characteristics Contrasts)	Repeated pregnancy									Repeated birth								
	15–18 years old			19–21 years old			22–24 years old			15–18 years old			19–21 years old			22–24 years old		
	OR	CI	p	OR	CI	p	OR	CI	p	OR	CI	p	OR	CI	p	OR	CI	p
Middle vs. Richer	0.01	0.915		0.09	0.763		0.75	0.387		0.14	0.709		0.06	0.801		1.47	0.226	
Middle vs. Richest	0.45	0.504		0.06	0.807		7.63	**0.006**		NA			0.15	0.70		3.25	0.072	
Richer vs. Richest	0.51	0.475		0.00	0.999		3.78	0.052		NA			0.03	0.866		0.65	0.42	

Abbreviations: OR-Odds ratio; CI-95% Confidence Interval; p-*p* value; F-F statistic; NC-No cases; NA-Not applicable; OR-Odds ratio
Data captured in bold are highly significant

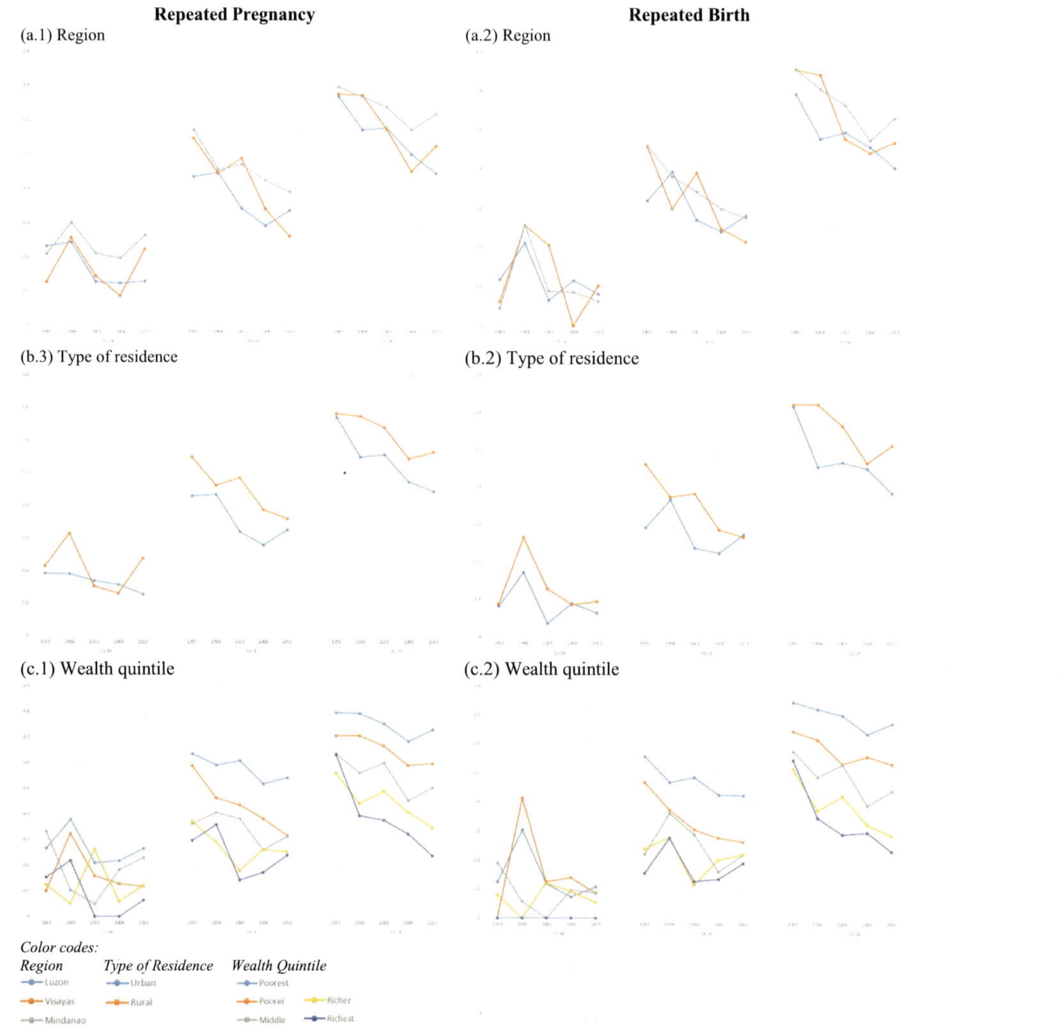

Fig. 3 Prevalence trend of repeated pregnancies and births among adolescents per socio-geographic variable in each age group. Caption: This figure presents the trend of the weighted prevalence of repeated pregnancies and births in each of the socio-graphic variable using the three age categories: 15–18 years old, 19–21 years old and 22–24 years old. The left column presents the weighted prevalence of repeated pregnancy while the right column presents repeated birth. In each graph, the x-axis is the survey year arranged in chronological order while the y-axis the weighted prevalence. The color of each line represents a category of each socio-geographic variable as shown at the bottom of the graph

Appendix

Table 4 Characteristics of National Demographic and Health Survey (NDHS) Philippines from 1993 to 2013

Characteristics	Year				
	2013	2008	2003	1998	1993
Sampling					
Frame	2010 Census	2000 Census	2000 Census	1995 Census	1990 Census
Design	Stratified Two-stage *First stage:* Systematic selection of 800 Enumeration Areas (EAs) distributed by region (17) and type of residence (rural, urban) *Second stage:* Systematic selection of 20 housing units per EA (maximum of 3 households per unit)	Stratified Three-stage *First stage:* Selection of PSUs *Second stage:* Selection of 794 EAs *Third stage:* Selection of 17 housing units per EA through systematic random sampling (maximum of 3 households per unit)	Stratified Three-stage Cluster *First stage:* Selection of 819 PSUs *Second Stage:* Selection of EAs per PSU *Third stage:* Systematic selection of 17 households per EA	Stratified Two-stage *First stage:* Selection of 752 EAs on 16 regions *Second Stage:* Systematic selection of households in urban while cluster sampling among rural areas	Stratified Two-stage *First stage:* Selection of 750 PSUs distributed among 14 regions Second stage: Selection of 20 households per PSU
Response Rates					
Households	99.2	99.3	99.1	98.7	99.2
Women (15–49 years old)	98.3	98.3	97.8	97.2	98
Sample Size					
Households	14,804	12,469	12,586	12,407	12,995
n of Women (15–19 years old) Weighted % distribution	3261 20%	2766 20.2%	2646 19.4%	2949 20.9%	3139 21%
n of Women (15–24 years old)	6070 37.3%	4909 36%	4860 35.6%	5190 37.3%	5741 38.6%

characteristics of and attitudes towards adolescent mothers in these countries. This type of study not only directs the development of specialized perinatal care, and psychosocial and welfare support but also places priority on those adolescents with RP.

A multi-country analysis would also be beneficial in obtaining a broader RP status especially in countries with similar characteristics. This would help international organizations to implement immediate action for RP in a global approach and prioritize countries with a high RP burden. Additionally, projection of RP prevalence at least until 2030 using country-level determinants such as contraceptive prevalence, poverty, literacy, and maternal-child mortality rates, may facilitate target setting for this potential adolescent reproductive health indicator.

Conclusion

There is a constant trend of one in every five adolescent mothers in the Philippines experiencing repeated pregnancy from 1993 to 2013 (across all regions, type of residence, and socio-economic status). These findings indicate the need for secondary prevention programs, particularly among the poorest households. Epidemiological investigations are also necessary to explore the causes and impacts of repeated pregnancy on maternal, child, and neonatal health in the Philippines and other low- and middle-income countries.

Abbreviations

CCT: Conditional Cash Transfer; CI: 95% Confidence Interval; DHS: Demographic and Health Survey; FP: Family planning; LMICs: Low- and middle-income countries; OR: Odds ratio; RB: Repeated birth; RP: Repeated Pregnancy; WHO: World Health Organization; WtPrevRB: Weighted RB prevalence; WtPrevRP: Weighted RP prevalence

Acknowledgements

We also acknowledge the Demographic and Health Surveys Program for allowing us to access the all Philippine DHS datasets. This study was presented at the 15th World Congress on Public Health, Australia, April 3–7, 2017.

Funding

This study was supported by the University of Queensland International Scholarship.

Authors' contributions

JM conceptualized the study design, prepared the datasets, conducted the analysis, and drafted and revised the manuscript. KB conceptualized the study design, conducted the analysis, and revised the manuscript. RA conceptualized the study design, supervised the data analysis, and revised the manuscript. All authors approved the final manuscript as submitted and agreed to be accountable for all aspects of the work.

Competing interests

The authors declare that they have no competing interests. The authors have no financial relationships relevant to this article to disclose.

Author details
[1]School of Public Health, The University of Queensland, Herston, QLD, Australia. [2]Institute for Social Science Research, The University of Queensland, Indooroopilly, QLD, Australia. [3]Centre for Youth Substance Abuse Research, The University of Queensland, Herston, QLD, Australia.

References

1. World Health Organization-Western Pacific Region. Fact Sheet on Adolescent Health. 2015; http://www.wpro.who.int/mediacentre/factsheets/docs/fs_201202_adolescent_health/en/. Accessed June 30, 2015, 2015.
2. UNFPA, UNESCO and WHO. Sexual and Reproductive Health of young people in Asia and the Pacific: A review of issues, policies and programmes. Bangkok: UNFPA; 2015.
3. Philippine Statistics Authority, and ICF International. Philippines National Demographic and Health Survey 2013. Manila, Philippines, and Rockville, Maryland, USA: Philippine Statistics Authority, and ICF International; 2014.
4. Department of Health-Philippines. In: Health Do, editor. National policy and strategic framework on adolescent health and Development. Philippines: Department of Health; 2013.
5. Department of Health-Philippines. Behavior change communication strategies for preventing preventing adolescent pregnancy. Philippines: Department of Health; 2012. https://www.doh.gov.ph/sites/default/files/publications/SourcebookBCCStrategiesPreventingAdolescentPregnancy.pdf. Accessed 19 Feb 2016.
6. Natividad J. Teenage pregnancy in the Philippines: trends, correlates and data sources. J ASEAN Fed Endocr Soc. 2013;28(1):30–7.
7. Gavin L, Warner L, O'Neil ME, et al. Vital signs: repeat births among teens - United States, 2007-2010. Mmwr-Morbid Mortal W. 2013;62(13):249–55.
8. Rowlands S. Social predictors of repeat adolescent pregnancy and focussed strategies. Best Pract Res Clin Obstet Gynaecol. 2010;24(5): 605–16.
9. Lewis LN, Doherty DA, Hickey M, Skinner SR. Predictors of sexual intercourse and rapid-repeat pregnancy among teenage mothers: an Australian prospective longitudinal study. Med J Aust. 2010;193(6):338–42.
10. Stevens-Simon C, Kelly L, Singer D, Nelligan D. Reasons for first teen pregnancies predict the rate of subsequent teen conceptions. Pediatrics. 1998;101(1):E8.
11. Capanzana MV, Aguila DV, Javier CA, Mendoza TS, Santos-Abalos VM. Adolescent pregnancy and the first 1000 days (the Philippine situation). Asia Pac J Clin Nutr. 2015;24(4):759–66.
12. Hussain R, Finer L. Unintended pregnancy and unsafe abortion in the Philippines: context and consequences. In Brief. 2013;3 https://www.guttmacher.org/sites/default/files/report_pdf/ib-unintended-pregnancy-philippines.pdf. Accessed 15 June 2018.
13. Salvador JT, Sauce BRJ, Alvarez MOC, Rosario AB. The phenomenon of teenage pregnancy in the Philippines. Eur Scientific J. 2016;12(32).
14. Ganchimeg T, Ota E, Morisaki N, et al. Pregnancy and childbirth outcomes among adolescent mothers: a World Health Organization multicountry study. BJOG Int J Obstet Gynaecol. 2014;121:40–8.
15. Association of Maternal & Child Health Programs. Life course indicator: Repeat teen Birth Life course indicator online tool 2014; http://www.amchp.org/programsandtopics/data-assessment/LifeCourseIndicatorDocuments/LC-54%20Teen%20Births_Final-9-10-2014.pdf. Accessed February 12, 2016.
16. Penman-Aguilar A, Carter, M., Snead, M. C., Kourtis, A. P. Socioeconomic disadvantage as a social determinant of teen childbearing in the U.S. Vol 1282013.
17. National Campaign to Prevent Teen and Unplanned Pregnancy. Counting it up: The public costs of teen childbearing. 2014; https://thenationalcampaign.org/resource/public-costs-teen-childbearing-united-states. Accessed August 22, 2014.
18. Guttmacher Institute. Sexual and reproductive health of young women in the Philippines: 2013 data Update 2015.
19. Knoll LJ, Magis-Weinberg L, Speekenbrink M, Blakemore S-J. Social influence on risk perception during adolescence. Psychol Sci. 2015;26(5):583–92.
20. Melgar JD, Melgar AR, Cabigon JV. Family Planning in the Philippines. In: Zaman W, Masnin H, Loftus J, editors. Family Planning in Asia & the Pacific: Addressing the Challenges. Malaysia: International Council on Management of Population Programmes; 2012. http://icomp.org.my/FP%20in%20Asia%20and%20the%20Pacific%20Jan%202012.pdf.
21. Demographic Research and Development Foundation, and University of the Philippines Population Institute. 2013 YAFS4 Key Findings. Quezon City, Philippines: Demographic Research and Development Foundation, and University of the Philippines Population Institute; 2014.
22. Ogena NA. Development concept of adolescence: the case of adolescents in the Philippines. Philipp Popul Rev. 2014;3(1).
23. Varga CA, Zosa-Feranil I. Adolescent reproductive health in the Philippines: status, policies, programs, and issues. Washington, DC: The Futures Group International, POLICY Project; 2003.
24. Department of Health-Philippines. Adolescent & Youth Health (AYH) policy. Manila: Department of Health; 2000.
25. Sedgh G, Finer LB, Bankole A, Eilers MA, Singh S. Adolescent pregnancy, birth, and abortion rates across countries: levels and recent trends. J Adolesc Health. 2015;56(2):223–30.
26. Corcoran J, Pillai VK. Effectiveness of secondary pregnancy prevention programs: a meta-analysis. Res Soc Work Pract. 2007;17(1):5–18.
27. Pogoy AM, Verzosa R. Coming NS, Agustino RG. Lived experiences of early pregnancy among teenagers: a phenomenological study. Eur Scientific J. 2014;10(2).
28. Government of the Philippines. Republic act no. 10354: An act providing for a national policy on responsible parenthood and reproductive healthy on responsible parenthood and reproductive health. In: Gazette-Philippines. 2012; Document number:10534. http://www.gov.ph/2012/12/21/republic-act-no-10354/.
29. Chandra-Mouli V, McCarraher DR, Phillips SJ, Williamson NE, Hainsworth G. Contraception for adolescents in low and middle income countries: needs, barriers, and access. Reprod Health 2014;11(1):1.
30. World Bank. Philippines conditional cash transfer program : impact evaluation 2012. Washington, DC: World Bank; 2013.
31. Darney BG, Weaver MR, Sosa-Rubi SG, et al. The Oportunidades conditional cash transfer program: effects on pregnancy and contraceptive use among young rural women in Mexico. Int Perspect Sex Reprod Health. 2013;39(4): 205–14.
32. Maravilla, JC, Betts, KS, Couto e Cruz, C, and Alati, R. Factors influencing repeated teenage pregnancy: a review and meta-analysis. Am J Obstet Gynecol. 2017; 217(5). https://doi.org/10.1016/j.ajog.2017.04.02.
33. Gray N, Azzopardi P, Kennedy E, Willersdorf E, Creati M. Improving adolescent reproductive health in Asia and the Pacific. Asia Pac J Public Health. 2013;25(2):134–44.
34. Every Woman Every Child Strategy and Coordination Group. Global Strategy for Women's, Children's and Adolescent's Health 2016-2030. Italy: United Nations; 2015.
35. Chandra-Mouli V, Camacho AV, Michaud P-A. WHO guidelines on preventing early pregnancy and poor reproductive outcomes among adolescents in developing countries. J Adolesc Health. 2013;52(5):517.

Permissions

All chapters in this book were first published in RH, by BioMed Central; hereby published with permission under the Creative Commons Attribution License or equivalent. Every chapter published in this book has been scrutinized by our experts. Their significance has been extensively debated. The topics covered herein carry significant findings which will fuel the growth of the discipline. They may even be implemented as practical applications or may be referred to as a beginning point for another development.

The contributors of this book come from diverse backgrounds, making this book a truly international effort. This book will bring forth new frontiers with its revolutionizing research information and detailed analysis of the nascent developments around the world.

We would like to thank all the contributing authors for lending their expertise to make the book truly unique. They have played a crucial role in the development of this book. Without their invaluable contributions this book wouldn't have been possible. They have made vital efforts to compile up to date information on the varied aspects of this subject to make this book a valuable addition to the collection of many professionals and students.

This book was conceptualized with the vision of imparting up-to-date information and advanced data in this field. To ensure the same, a matchless editorial board was set up. Every individual on the board went through rigorous rounds of assessment to prove their worth. After which they invested a large part of their time researching and compiling the most relevant data for our readers.

The editorial board has been involved in producing this book since its inception. They have spent rigorous hours researching and exploring the diverse topics which have resulted in the successful publishing of this book. They have passed on their knowledge of decades through this book. To expedite this challenging task, the publisher supported the team at every step. A small team of assistant editors was also appointed to further simplify the editing procedure and attain best results for the readers.

Apart from the editorial board, the designing team has also invested a significant amount of their time in understanding the subject and creating the most relevant covers. They scrutinized every image to scout for the most suitable representation of the subject and create an appropriate cover for the book.

The publishing team has been an ardent support to the editorial, designing and production team. Their endless efforts to recruit the best for this project, has resulted in the accomplishment of this book. They are a veteran in the field of academics and their pool of knowledge is as vast as their experience in printing. Their expertise and guidance has proved useful at every step. Their uncompromising quality standards have made this book an exceptional effort. Their encouragement from time to time has been an inspiration for everyone.

The publisher and the editorial board hope that this book will prove to be a valuable piece of knowledge for researchers, students, practitioners and scholars across the globe.

List of Contributors

Ruth Nimota Nukpezah
Department of Nursing, University for development studies, Tamale, Ghana

Samuel Victor Nuvor
School of Medical Sciences, University of Cape Coast, Cape Coast, Ghana

Jerry Ninnoni
School of Nursing and Midwifery, University of Cape Coast, Cape Coast, Ghana

Patience A. Afulani, Nadia Diamond-Smith and Beth Phillips
School of Medicine, Institute for Global Health Sciences, University of California, San Francisco, USA

Shreya Singhal
Community Empowerment Lab, Lucknow, India

May Sudhinaraset
Jonathan and Karin Fielding School of Public Health, University of California, Los Angeles, USA

Zhongchen Luo
Nursing Department, Guizhou Provincial People's Hospital, Guiyang, China

Lingling Gao and Juanjuan Zhao
School of Nursing, Sun Yat-sen University, 74, Zhongshan Road II, Guangzhou 510089, China

Ronald Anguzu
School of Public Health, Makerere University, Kampala city, Uganda

Mohamed M. Ali
UNDP-UNFPA-UNICEF-WHO-World Bank Special Programme of Research, Development and Research Training in Human Reproduction (HRP), World Health Organization, 20 Avenue Appia, 1211 Geneva, Switzerland

John Cleland
Department of Population Health, Faculty of Epidemiology and Population Health, London School of Hygiene and Tropical Medicine, Keppel Street, London WC1E 7HT, UK

Sarah Neal and Chloe Harvey
Department of Social Statistics and Demography, University of Southampton, Southampton, UK

Venkatraman Chandra-Mouli
Human Reproduction Programme/ Department of Reproductive Health and Research, World Health Organization, Geneva, Switzerland

Sonja Caffe
Pan American Health Organization, 525 23rd Street, NW, Washington DC, USA

Alma Virginia Camacho
SRH Team, Latin America and the Caribbean Regional Office, United Nations Population Fund, Panama City, Panama

Aline Labat, Michèle Dramaix, Wei-Hong Zhang and Sophie Alexander
Université Libre de Bruxelles, Ecole de Santé Publique, Research Center: Policies and Health Systems - International Health, 808, Route de Lennik, 1070 Brussels, Belgium

Marta Medina
Hera, Right to Health and Development, Reet, Belgium

Mohammed Elhassein, Afrina Karim and Kim E. Dickson
UNFPA, Freetown, Sierra Leone

Mohammad B. Jalloh
FOCUS 1000, NGO, Freetown, Sierra Leone

M. M. Dynes, E. Bernstein, D. Morof and F. Serbanescu
Centers for Disease Control and Prevention, Division of Reproductive Health, Atlanta, USA

L. Kelly and A. Ruiz
Centers for Disease Control and Prevention, Division of Reproductive Health (CDCF Contractor), Atlanta, USA

W. Mongo
Engender Health, Washington, DC, USA

P. Chaote
Regional Medical Officer, Kigoma, Kigoma Region, Tanzania

R. N. Bujari
AMCA Inter Consult, Dar es Salaam, Tanzania

Rebecca Kippen
School of Rural Health, Monash University, 26 Mercy St, Bendigo, VIC 3552, Australia

Edith Gray and Ann Evans
School of Demography, The Australian National University, Building 9, Acton, ACT 2601, Australia

Elizabeth Kemigisha
Mbarara University of Science and Technology, Mbarara, Uganda
International Centre for Reproductive Health, Faculty of Medicine and Health Sciences, Ghent University, Ghent, Belgium

Katharine Bruce, Viola N. Nyakato, Gad Ndaruhutse Ruzaaza and Wendo Mlahagwa
Mbarara University of Science and Technology, Mbarara, Uganda

Anna B. Ninsiima and Gily Coene
RHEA, Centre of Expertise on Gender, Diversity and Intersectionality, Vrije Universiteit Brussel, Brussels, Belgium

Kristien Michielsen and Els Leye
International Centre for Reproductive Health, Faculty of Medicine and Health Sciences, Ghent University, Ghent, Belgium

Boris Martinez
Wuqu' Kawoq | Maya Health Alliance, 2a. Calle 5-43 Zona 1, Santiago Sacatepéquez, Guatemala
Department of Medicine, Saint Peter's University Hospital, New Brunswick, NJ, USA

Enma Coyote Ixen and Michel Juarez
Wuqu' Kawoq | Maya Health Alliance, 2a. Calle 5-43 Zona 1, Santiago Sacatepéquez, Guatemala

Rachel Hall-Clifford
Departments of Sociology and Anthropology and Public Health, Agnes Scott College, Decatur, GA, USA

Ann C. Miller
Department of Global Health and Social Medicine, Harvard Medical School, Boston, MA, USA

Aaron Francis and Camilo E. Valderrama
Department of Biomedical Informatics, Emory University, Atlanta, GA, USA

Lisa Stroux
Institute of Biomedical Engineering, Department of Engineering Science, University of Oxford, Oxford, UK

Gari D. Clifford
Department of Biomedical Informatics, Emory University, Atlanta, GA, USA
Department of Biomedical Engineering, Georgia Institute of Technology and Emory University, Atlanta, GA, USA

Peter Rohloff
Wuqu' Kawoq | Maya Health Alliance, 2a. Calle 5-43 Zona 1, Santiago Sacatepéquez, Guatemala
Division of Global Health Equity, Brigham and Women's Hospital, Boston, MA, USA

Andrea Solnes Miltenburg and Johanne Sundby
Institute of Health and Society, Department of Community Medicine and Global Health, Faculty of Medicine, University of Oslo, Oslo, Norway

Richard Forget Kiritta
Department of Obstetrics and Gynaecology, Sekotoure Regional Referral Hospital, Mwanza, Mwanza Region, Tanzania

Tarek Meguid
Department of Obstetrics and Gynaecology, Mnazi Mmoja Hospital, Zanzibar, Tanzania

Roosbelinda Cárdenas
International Planned Parenthood/Western Hemisphere Region, New York, USA
Hampshire College, Amherst, USA

Ana Labandera, Fernanda Chiribao, Ivana Leus and Silvia Avondet
Iniciativas Sanitarias, Montevideo, Uruguay

Sarah E. Baum
Ibis Reproductive Health, Oakland, USA

Jennifer Friedman
International Planned Parenthood/Western Hemisphere Region, New York, USA

Bwalya C. Bwalya
Ministry of Education, Matero Girls Secondary School, Lusaka, Zambia

Doreen Sitali, Kumar Sridutt Baboo and Joseph M. Zulu
Departments of Public Health, School of Medicine, University of Zambia, Lusaka, Zambia

Geetanjali Katageri and Ashalata Mallapur
Department of Obstetrics and Gynaecology, S Nijalingappa Medical College, Bagalkot, Karnataka, India

Umesh Charantimath, Anjali Joshi, Chandrashekhar Karadiguddi, Geetanjali Mungarwadi, Avinash Kavi, Shivaprasad Goudar and Mrutyunjaya Bellad
KLE Academy of Higher Education and Research's J N Medical College, Belagavi, Karnataka, India

Marianne Vidler, Sumedha Sharma and Beth A. Payne
Department of Obstetrics and Gynaecology, University of British Columbia, Vancouver, BC, Canada

Umesh Ramadurg
Department of Community Medicine, S Nijalingappa Medical College, Bagalkot, Karnataka, India

Sheshidhar Bannale
Department of Pharmacology, S Nijalingappa Medical College, Bagalkot, Karnataka, India

Sangamesh Rakaraddi
Department of Anatomy, S Nijalingappa Medical College, Bagalkot, Karnataka, India

Diane Sawchuck
Department of Research, Vancouver Island Health Authority, British Columbia, Canada

Richard Derman
Global Affairs, Thomas Jefferson University, Philadelphia, USA

Laura A. Magee and Peter von Dadelszen
School of Life Course Sciences, Faculty of Life Sciences and Medicine, King's College London, London, UK

Rahat Qureshi
Division of Women and Child Health, Aga Khan University, Karachi, Sindh, Pakistan

Nianqing Wan, Li Cai, Ting Zhang and Yajun Chen
Department of Maternal and Child Health, School of Public Health, Sun Yat-sen University, Guangzhou 510000, China

Weiqing Tan and Jiewen Yang
Health Promotion Centre for Primary and Secondary Schools of Guangzhou Municipality, Guangzhou 510000, China

Cho Lee Wong
The Nethersole School of Nursing, Faculty of Medicine, The Chinese University of Hong Kong, Room 824, Esther Lee Building, Shatin, New Territories, Hong Kong

Miriam Clark and Rohanna Buchanan
Oregon Social Learning Center, 10 Shelton McMurphey Blvd, Eugene, OR 97401, USA

Rachel Kovensky and Leslie D. Leve
Prevention Science Institute, 6217 University of Oregon, Eugene, OR 97403, USA

Eman S. Mohammed, Amany E. Seedhom and Eman M. Mahfouz
Public Health and Preventive Medicine, Faculty of Medicine, Minia University, Minia 1666, Egypt

Paraskevi Stylianou-Riga and Thalia Papadouri
Neonatal Intensive Care Unit, "Archbishop Makarios III" Hospital, Nicosia, Cyprus

Panayiotis Kouis, Paraskevi Kinni and Panayiotis K. Yiallouros
Medical School, University of Cyprus Shakolas Educational Center of Clinical Medicine, Palaios Dromos Lefkosias Lemesou 215/6, 2029 Aglantzia, Nicosia, Cyprus

Mamas Theodorou
Faculty of Economics and Management, Open University of Cyprus, Nicosia, Cyprus

Aparna Jain and Elizabeth Tobey
Population Council, 4301 Connecticut Avenue NW, Suite 280, Washington DC 20008, USA

Hussein Ismail and Annabel Erulkar
Population Council, Heritage Plaza, 4th floor, Bole Medhaneialem Road, Addis Ababa, Ethiopia

Michael O N Kunnuji and Idongesit Eshiet
Department of Sociology, University of Lagos, Lagos, Nigeria

Chinyere C P Nnorom
Department of Sociology/Psychology/Criminology and Security Studies, Faculty of Management and Social Sciences, Alex Ekwueme Federal University Ndufu-Alike Ikwo (AE-FUNAI), Abakaliki, Ebonyi State, Nigeria

Stefanie Theuring and Gundel Harms
Institute of Tropical Medicine and International Health, Charité- Universitätsmedizin, Augustenburger Platz 1, 13353 Berlin, Germany

Alimamy Philip Koroma
Department of Obstetrics and Gynecology, Princess Christian Maternity Hospital, Freetown, Sierra Leone

Joemer C. Maravilla and Kim S. Betts
School of Public Health, The University of Queensland, Herston, QLD, Australia
Institute for Social Science Research, The University of Queensland, Indooroopilly, QLD, Australia

Rosa Alati
School of Public Health, The University of Queensland, Herston, QLD, Australia
Institute for Social Science Research, The University of Queensland, Indooroopilly, QLD, Australia
Centre for Youth Substance Abuse Research, The University of Queensland, Herston, QLD, Australia

Index